THIRD EDITION

COMPREHENSIVE
RADIOGRAPHIC
PATHOLOGY

THIRD EDITION

COMPREHENSIVE RADIOGRAPHIC PATHOLOGY

Ronald L. Eisenberg, MD, JD, FACR

Chairman of Imaging, Department of Radiology
Highland General Hospital
Oakland, California
Clinical Professor of Radiology
University of California at San Francisco and Davis

Nancy M. Johnson, BA, RT (R) (CV) (CT) (QM)

Faculty, Medical Radiography Program
GateWay Community College
Phoenix, Arizona

An Affiliate of Elsevier

An Affiliate of Elsevier

11830 Westline Industrial Drive
St. Louis, Missouri 63146

Publishing Director: Andrew Allen
Acquisitions Editor: Jeanne Wilke
Senior Developmental Editor: Linda Woodard
Publishing Services Manager: John Rogers
Senior Project Manager: Beth Hayes
Senior Designer: Kathi Gosche
Cover Design: Jenny Hobein, Studio Montage

TG/MVY

Printed in the United States of America

Last digit is the print number: 9 8 7 6 5 4

Acknowledgments

I would like to acknowledge and thank the
following technologists:

Kathleen Murphy, MBA, RDMS;
Norma Mesa, RT (R) (CT);
Cyndi Smith, RT (R);
Bartram Pierce, RT (R) (MR);
Jeanne Dial, CNMT;
and Daniel Bandy, MS, CNMT.

Nancy Johnson

The unnumbered figures in Chapters 2 through 10
were borrowed from Thibodeau GA, Patton KT:
Anatomy and physiology, ed 2, St. Louis, 1993, Mosby.

Reviewers

RACHEL BAILEY, BS, RT (R)
Program Director, School of Radiologic Technology
Columbia–St. Mary's Hospitals
Milwaukee, Wisconsin

KELLI WELCH HAYNES, MSRS, RT (R)
Assistant Professor & Clinical Coordinator
Northwestern State University
Shreveport, Louisiana

JEANNIE KILGORE, MED, BS, RT (R)
Program Director/Instructor Radiologic Technology
Clovis Community College
Clovis, New Mexico

JENNIFER S. THOMAS, MS, RT (R)(MR)
Program Director
Southeast Arkansas College
Pine Bluff, Arkansas

Preface

Understanding the basic principles of pathology is an essential part of the radiologic technologist's training. Knowing how disease processes work and recognizing the radiographic appearance of specific diseases can aid the technologist in selecting proper modalities and determining the need for repeat radiographs in different situations. This kind of knowledge enables the radiologic technologist to become a more competent professional and a contributing member of the diagnostic team.

■ Content and Organization

Fully illustrated and well organized, *Comprehensive Radiographic Pathology* meets the needs of today's student and practicing radiographers. The book opens with a preliminary chapter on pathology that introduces the pathologic terms used throughout the text. This chapter also describes the advantages and limitations of six widely used modalities: ultrasound, CT, MRI, nuclear medicine, single-photon emission computed tomography (SPECT), and positron-emission tomography (PET).

Each of the remaining chapters is a systematic approach to the diseases involving a specific organ system. These chapters begin with an overview of physiology. For each of the most common pathologic conditions associated with the system, there is a brief description of the disease and its clinical manifestations, followed by imaging findings and treatment. Summary tables follow each major discussion, reiterating the location, radiographic appearance, and treatment of the diseases just presented.

"Radiographer Notes" offer helpful suggestions for producing optimal radiographs of the organ system featured in each chapter. Information especially relevant to radiologic technologists is included, such as technique adjustments for patients with specific conditions and special patient handling requirements. If multiple imaging modalities can be used, the most appropriate initial procedure is indicated, as well as the sequence in which various imaging studies should be performed.

Other chapter features include a listing of prerequisite knowledge and goals and objectives. Finally, each chapter ends with a series of review questions to help readers assess their comprehension of the material. An answer key is found at the back of the book, along with several appendixes, an extensive glossary, and a list of major prefixes, roots, and suffixes to help readers determine the meaning of unfamiliar words.

■ New Content and Features

This edition features discussions of three new modalities—nuclear medicine, SPECT, and PET—and updated discussions of common modalities that were previously included: ultrasound, computed tomography, and magnetic resonance imaging. Hundreds of new images using these modalities, as well as plain-film radiography, have been added to update existing content and to illustrate new discussions.

New content also includes a discussion of respiratory syncytial virus and an expanded section on pulmonary mycosis.

Navigating the chapters is easier than ever with a new standardized heading scheme for the systems chapters. Another tool for finding information quickly is the summary table that follows each major discussion of common pathologies. The tables list the diseases just presented and their location in the body, and summarize the radiographic appearance and treatment of each disease.

■ Electronic Ancillaries

An electronic image collection on CD-ROM that includes the images from the book is available for those teaching a course with the text, providing an easy-to-use and cost-effective alternative to traditional pathology slide sets.

Contents

THIRD EDITION

COMPREHENSIVE RADIOGRAPHIC PATHOLOGY

Introduction to Pathology

■ **Prerequisite Knowledge**

The student should have a basic knowledge of the normal anatomy and physiology of the human body. A good foundation in medical terminology, including word roots, prefixes, and suffixes (see Appendix A) will be most helpful for assimilating the somewhat difficult information presented in this and future chapters. In addition, proper learning and understanding of the material will be facilitated if the student has some clinical experience in all areas of radiography of the human body and film evaluation, including a concept of the changes in technique required to compensate for density differences produced by underlying pathologic conditions.

■ **Goals**

To acquaint the student radiographer with basic medical terminology used to describe various pathologic conditions occurring in the human body (including hereditary diseases, immune reactions, and acquired immunodeficiency syndrome) and to introduce the student to some specialized imaging techniques

■ **Objectives**

1. To be able to classify the more common diseases in terms of their attenuation of x-rays
2. To be familiar with the changes in technical factors required for obtaining optimal quality radiographs in patients with various underlying pathologic conditions
3. To understand and be able to define or describe all bold-faced terms in this chapter
4. To be able to describe inflammation, edema, infarction, hemorrhage, and neoplasia
5. To be able to describe the various alterations of cell growth
6. To be able to describe the various immune reactions of the body

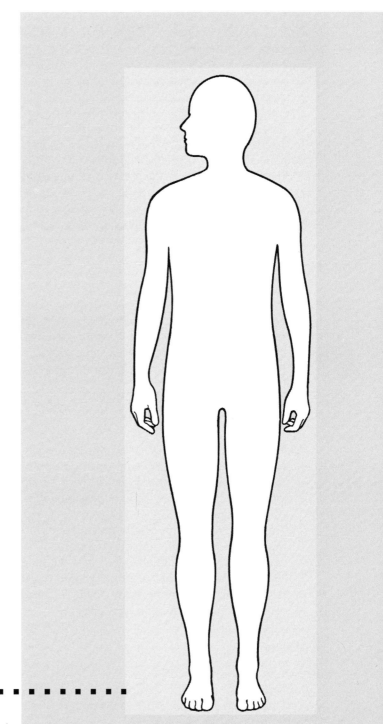

CHAPTER 1

■ ■ ■ ■ ■ ■ ■ Radiographer Notes

Radiography of patients with underlying pathologic conditions can present problems for even the most experienced radiographers. Adjustments in patient position may be necessary to prevent excessive pain caused by the body's response to trauma or certain disease processes. A change in routine projections may be indicated to visualize subtle alterations in the normal radiographic appearance. Many disease processes also alter the density of the structures being radiographed and therefore require changes in technique. For example, extensive edema may require an increased technique, whereas severe atrophy may require a decreased technique. Unless the radiographer has access to previous films with recorded exposure factors, a standard technique chart should be used to determine the initial exposures. Any necessary adjustments can then be made on subsequent films.

The box on p. 3 lists the relative attenuations of x-rays that can be expected in advanced stages of various disease processes. In chest radiography, 110 to 125 kilovolts (kV) is optimal; therefore adjust milliampere-second (mAs) factors to control density. In skeletal radiography, when bone *quality* changes are expected, the best exposure factor to change is the kilovolt level (beam quality change for structural change). When bone *quantity* changes, the milliampere-seconds value is the exposure factor to change to control density (beam quantity increases to ensure that enough radiation reaches the film without changing the contrast). For example, in os-

teoporosis there is a decrease in bone quantity and quality; however, a decrease in kilovolts produces a higher-quality image. The normal kilovolt level easily penetrates the diseased bone, producing a low-contrast image with loss of visibility of detail.

Certain diseases suppress the normal immune response. Immunocompromised patients (such as those with advanced leukemia) may require special care to prevent their acquiring a disease from the radiographer. Personal protective equipment (PPE) aids in preventing the spread of microorganisms to the patient as well as to the healthcare worker. The patient may have to be placed in protective isolation (or "reverse" isolation), and the radiographer may be required to wear mask, gown, and gloves before approaching the patient.

Diseases such as AIDS and hepatitis require that the radiographer wear rubber or latex gloves to be protected against exposure to blood and body fluids, which could contaminate any area near the patient. When examining a patient with AIDS who has a productive cough, the radiographer must wear a mask and possibly protective eye goggles if there is a need to be very close to a patient's face. It is important to remember that many patients having radiographic procedures have not been diagnosed and thus all patients should be treated as though they may have a communicable disease. Therefore whenever exposure to any type of body secretion or blood may occur, the healthcare worker should wear appropriate personal protective equipment.

7. To be able to describe AIDS and the precautions necessary when taking a radiograph of patients with AIDS or any patient with whom contact with any body fluid is possible (Standard Precautions)
8. To be able to describe briefly the theory of image production with ultrasound, computed tomography (CT), magnetic resonance imaging (MRI), nuclear medicine, single-photon emission computed tomography (SPECT), and positron-emission tomography (PET)

■ **Disease**

Pathology is the study of diseases that can cause abnormalities in the structure or function of various organ systems. In essence, a disease is the pattern of the

body's response to some form of injury. Diseases may be hereditary or may result from a broad spectrum of traumatic, infectious, vascular, or metabolic processes. They may reflect alterations of cell growth, as in **neoplasia** (tumors), or they may even be caused by physicians and their treatment **(iatrogenic).** In some cases the underlying cause is unknown, and the disease is termed **idiopathic.**

This chapter discusses several basic reactions of the body that characterize the underlying mechanisms for the radiographic manifestations of most pathologic conditions. These processes include **inflammation, edema, ischemia** and **infarction, hemorrhage,** and alterations of cell growth leading to the development of **neoplasms** (tumors). In addition, this chapter deals with **hereditary** diseases, as well as immune reactions and the **acquired immunodeficiency syndrome** (AIDS).

. . . .

Relative Attenuation of X-rays in Advanced Stages of Diseases

SKELETAL SYSTEM
Additive (increased attenuation)
  Acromegaly
  Acute kyphosis
  Callus
  Charcot's joint
  Chronic osteomyelitis (healed)
  Exostosis
  Hydrocephalus
  Marble bone
  Metastasis (osteosclerotic)
  Osteochondroma
  Osteoma
  Paget's disease
  Proliferative arthritis
  Sclerosis
Destructive (decreased attenuation)
  Active osteomyelitis
  Active tuberculosis
  Aseptic necrosis
  Atrophy (disease or disuse)
  Blastomycosis
  Carcinoma
  Coccidioidomycosis
  Degenerative arthritis
  Ewing's tumor (in children)
  Fibrosarcoma
  Giant cell tumor
  Gout
  Hemangioma
  Hodgkin's disease
  Hyperparathyroidism
  Leprosy
  Metastasis (osteolytic)
  Multiple myeloma
  Neuroblastoma
  New bone (fibrosis)
  Osteitis fibrosa cystica
  Osteoporosis/osteomalacia
  Radiation necrosis
  Solitary myeloma

RESPIRATORY SYSTEM
Additive (increased attenuation)
  Actinomycosis
  Arrested tuberculosis (calcification)
  Atelectasis
  Bronchiectasis
  Edema
  Empyema
  Encapsulated abscess
  Hydropneumothorax
  Malignancy
  Miliary tuberculosis
  Pleural effusion
  Pneumoconiosis
    Anthracosis
    Asbestosis
    Calcinosis
    Siderosis
    Silicosis
  Pneumonia
  Syphilis
  Thoracoplasty
Destructive (decreased attenuation)
  Early lung abscess
  Emphysema
  Pneumothorax

CIRCULATORY SYSTEM
Additive (increased attenuation)
  Aortic aneurysm
  Ascites
  Cirrhosis of the liver
  Enlarged heart

SOFT TISSUE
Additive (increased attenuation)
  Edema
Destructive (decreased attenuation)
  Emaciation

. . . .

From Thompson TT: *Cahoon's formulating x-ray techniques*, ed 9, Durham, NC, 1979, Duke University Press.

Inflammation

Acute inflammation is the initial response of body tissues to local injury. The various types of injury include those caused by blunt or penetrating trauma, infectious organisms, and irritating chemical substances. Regardless of the underlying cause, the inflammatory response consists of four overlapping events that occur sequentially:

1. Alterations in blood flow and vascular permeability
2. Migration of circulating white blood cells to the interstitium of the injured tissue
3. Phagocytosis and enzymatic digestion of dead cells and tissue elements
4. Repair of injury by regeneration of normal parenchymal cells or proliferation of granulation tissue and eventual scar formation

The earliest bodily response to local injury is dilation of arterioles, capillaries, and venules, leading to a dramatic increase in blood flow in and around the injury site. This **hyperemia** produces the heat and redness associated with inflammation. As hyperemia develops, the venules and capillaries become abnormally **permeable,** allowing passage of protein-rich plasma across vessel walls into the interstitium. This inflammatory **exudate** in the tissues results in the swelling associated with inflammation, which produces pressure on sensitive nerve endings and causes pain. The protein-rich exudate of inflammation must be differentiated from a **transudate,** a low-protein fluid such as that seen in the pulmonary edema that develops in congestive heart failure.

Very early in the inflammatory response, leukocytes (white blood cells, especially neutrophils and macrophages) of the circulating blood migrate to the area of injury. These white blood cells cross the capillary walls into the injured tissues, where they engulf and enzymatically digest infecting organisms and cellular debris, a process called **phagocytosis.**

The removal of necrotic debris and any injurious agents such as bacteria makes possible the repair of the injury that triggered the inflammatory response. In many tissues, such as the lung after pneumococcal pneumonia, regeneration of parenchymal cells permits reconstitution of normal anatomic structure and function. However, some tissues, such as the heart after myocardial infarction, cannot heal by regeneration. A fibrous **scar** replaces the area of destroyed tissue with **granulation tissue.** Granulation tissue refers to a combination of young developing capillaries and actively proliferating fibroblasts, which produce connective tissue fibers (collagen) that replace the dead tissue. Eventually, the strong connective tissue contracts to produce a fibrous scar. In the abdomen, such

fibrous adhesions can narrow loops of intestine and result in an obstruction. The accumulation of excessive amounts of collagen (more common in African Americans) may produce a protruding, tumorlike scar known as a **keloid.** Unfortunately, surgery to remove a keloid is usually ineffective because the subsequent incision tends to heal in the same way.

Many injuries heal by a combination of regeneration and scar tissue formation. An example is the response of the liver to repeated and persistent alcoholic injury; the result is cirrhosis, in which irregular lobules of regenerated liver cells are crisscrossed and surrounded by bands of scar tissue.

The five clinical signs of acute inflammation are **rubor** (redness), **calor** (heat), **tumor** (swelling), **dolor** (pain), and **loss of function.** The localized heat and redness result from increased blood flow in the microcirculation at the site of injury. The swelling occurs because the exudate increases the amount of interstitial fluid, resulting in pressure on nerve endings and thus pain.

Acute inflammation can also lead to systemic manifestations. Fever is especially common in inflammatory conditions associated with the spread of organisms into the bloodstream. The number of circulating white blood cells also increases (leukocytosis).

Some bacterial organisms (such as staphylococci and streptococci) produce **toxins** that damage the tissues and incite an inflammatory response. The presence of **pyogenic** bacteria leads to the production of a thick, yellow fluid called **pus,** which contains dead white blood cells, inflammatory exudate, and bacteria. A **suppurative** inflammation is one that is associated with pus formation. When a pyogenic infection occurs beneath the skin or in a solid organ, it produces an **abscess,** a localized, usually encapsulated, collection of pus. All pyogens, wherever they become implanted, have the ability to invade blood vessels to produce **bacteremia,** with the potential involvement of other organs and tissues in the body.

A **granulomatous** inflammation manifests as a distinct pattern seen in relatively few diseases, including tuberculosis, syphilis, and sarcoidosis. A **granuloma** is a localized area of chronic inflammation, often with central necrosis. It is characterized by the accumulation of macrophages, some of which fuse to form multinucleated giant cells.

Edema

Edema is the accumulation of abnormal amounts of fluid in the intercellular tissue spaces or body cavities. Localized edema results from an inflammatory reaction, whereas generalized edema occurs with pronounced swelling of subcutaneous tissues throughout the body **(anasarca).** Localized edema may result from inflammation, with the escape of protein-rich intravascular fluid into the extravascular tissue. It may also result from a local obstruction to lymphatic drainage; for example, in **filariasis,** a parasitic worm causes lymphatic obstruction, and the resulting localized edema is termed **elephantiasis.** Generalized edema occurs most frequently in patients with congestive heart failure, cirrhosis of the liver, and certain forms of renal disease. Because of the effect of gravity, generalized edema is usually most prominent in dependent portions of the body. Thus ambulatory patients tend to accumulate fluid in tissues around the ankles and lower legs, whereas in hospitalized patients who are nonambulatory or sedentary, the edema fluid collects most prominently in the lower back and sacral areas and in the lung.

Extravascular fluid can also accumulate in serous cavities to produce pleural and pericardial effusions and peritoneal ascites. Edema may produce minimal clinical symptoms or be potentially fatal. If localized to the subcutaneous tissues, large amounts of edema may cause minimal functional impairment. In contrast, pulmonary edema, pericardial effusion, or edematous swelling of the brain may have dire consequences.

Ischemia and infarction

Ischemia refers to an interference with the blood supply to an organ or part of an organ, depriving the organ's cells and tissues of oxygen and nutrients. Ischemia may be caused by a narrowing of arterial structures, as in atherosclerosis, or by thrombotic or embolic occlusion. Depending on several factors, occlusion of an artery or vein may have little or no effect on the involved tissue, or it may cause death of the tissue and even of the individual. A major determinant is the availability of an alternative or newly acquired route of blood supply (collateral vessels). Other factors include the rate of development of the occlusion, the vulnerability of the tissue to hypoxia, and the oxygen-carrying capacity of the blood. Slowly developing occlusions are less likely to cause tissue death (necrosis) because they provide an opportunity for the development of alternative pathways of flow. Ganglion cells of the nervous system and myocardial muscle cells undergo irreversible damage if deprived of their blood supply for 3 to 5 minutes. Anemic or cyanotic patients tolerate arterial insufficiency less well than normal individuals do, and thus occlusion of even a small vessel in such an individual may lead to death of tissue.

An **infarct** is a localized area of ischemic necrosis within a tissue or organ produced by occlusion of either its arterial supply or its venous drainage. The two most common clinical forms of infarction are myocardial and pulmonary. Almost all infarcts result from thrombotic or embolic occlusion. Infrequent causes include twisting of an organ (volvulus), compression of the blood supply of a loop of bowel in a hernia sac, or trapping of a viscus under a peritoneal adhesion.

Severe arterial disease of the lower extremities may result in necrosis of several toes or a large segment of the foot, a condition called **gangrene.** A frequent presenting symptom in diabetic patients is ischemia of the foot that may progress to infarction and result in gangrene.

Infarctions tend to be especially severe because they occur more often in the patients least able to withstand them. Thus infarcts tend to occur in elderly individuals with advanced atherosclerosis or impaired cardiac function. The periods after surgery and delivery also have increased occurrence of infarctions.

Hemorrhage

The term **hemorrhage** implies rupture of a blood vessel. Rupture of a large artery or vein is almost always caused by some form of injury, such as trauma, atherosclerosis, or inflammatory or neoplastic erosion of the vessel wall. Hemorrhage may be external, or the blood may be trapped within body tissues, resulting in an accumulation termed a **hematoma.** The accumulation of blood in a body cavity results in hemothorax, hemopericardium, hemoperitoneum, or hemarthrosis (blood in a joint). Minimal hemorrhages into the skin, mucous membranes, or serosal surfaces are called **petechiae;** slightly larger hemorrhages are termed **purpura.** A large (greater than 1 to 2 cm) subcutaneous hematoma, or bruise, is called an **ecchymosis.**

The significance of hemorrhage depends on the volume of blood loss, the rate of loss, and the site of the hemorrhage. Sudden losses of up to 20% of the blood volume or slow losses of even larger amounts may have little clinical significance. The site of the hemorrhage is critical. For example, an amount of bleeding that would have little clinical significance in the subcutaneous tissues may cause death when located in a vital portion of the brain. Large amounts of external bleeding lead to the chronic loss of iron from the body and anemia. In contrast, internal hemorrhages into body cavities, joints, or tissues permit the iron to be recaptured for the synthesis of hemoglobin and the development of normal red blood cells.

Alterations of cell growth

Changes in the number and size of cells, their differentiation, and their arrangement may develop in response to physiologic stimuli. **Atrophy** refers to a reduction in the size or number of cells in an organ or tissue, with a corresponding decrease in function. It must be distinguished from **hypoplasia** and **aplasia,** in which failure of normal development accounts for small size.

An example is the **disuse atrophy** that occurs with immobilization of a limb by a plaster cast. The muscle mass of the encased limb reduces dramatically. Because the cast also removes the stress and strain from the enclosed bone that normally stimulates new bone formation, normal bone resorption continues unchecked and the loss of calcified bone can be detected on radiographs. In this situation, there is rapid recovery from the atrophic appearance when the cast is removed and normal function is resumed.

Pathologic, irreversible atrophy may be caused by loss of innervation or hormonal stimulation or by decreased blood supply. For example, stenosis of a renal artery may cause atrophy of the kidney with shrinkage of individual nephrons and loss of interstitial tissue.

Hypertrophy refers to an increase in the size of the cells of a tissue or organ in response to a demand for increased function. This must be distinguished from **hyperplasia,** an increase in the *number* of cells in a tissue or organ. Hypertrophy occurs most often in cells that cannot multiply, especially those in myocardial and peripheral striated muscle. Myocardial hypertrophy is necessary to maintain cardiac output despite increased peripheral resistance in patients with arterial hypertension or aortic valve disease. After the loss of a normal kidney, hypertrophy of the kidney on the opposite side occurs in an attempt to continue adequate renal function.

Examples of hyperplasia include (1) proliferation of granulation tissue in the repair of injury and (2) the increased cellularity of bone marrow in patients with hemolytic anemia or after hemorrhage. Hyperplasia of the adrenal cortex is a response to increased adrenocorticotropic hormone (ACTH) secretion; hyperplasia of the thyroid gland occurs with increased thyrotropic hormone secretion by the pituitary gland.

Dysplasia is a loss in the uniformity of individual cells and their architectural orientation; it is typically associated with prolonged chronic irritation or inflammation. Removal of the irritant may result in a return to normal, but often the tissue change persists, and it may evolve into a totally abnormal growth pattern. Thus dysplasia is generally considered at least potentially premalignant—a borderline lesion that may heal or progress to cancer.

Neoplasia

Neoplasia, from the Latin word for "new growth," refers to an abnormal proliferation of cells that are no longer controlled by the factors that govern the growth of normal cells. Neoplastic cells act as parasites, competing with normal cells and tissues for their metabolic needs. Thus tumor cells may flourish and the patient becomes weak and emaciated, a condition termed **cachexia.**

Neoplasms are commonly referred to as tumors; indeed, the study of neoplasms is called **oncology,** derived from the Greek word *oncos,* meaning "tumor." Although the word *tumor* originally referred to any swelling, which could also be produced by edema or hemorrhage in tissue, the word now refers almost exclusively to a neoplasm.

Neoplasms are divided into benign and malignant categories on the basis of their potential clinical behavior. **Benign** tumors closely resemble their cells of origin in structure and function. They remain localized, without spreading to other sites, and thus can usually be surgically removed with resultant survival of the patient.

Nevertheless, some benign tumors can have severe consequences because of their position or hormonal secretion. For example, a benign pituitary tumor can cause pressure atrophy and destruction of the surrounding gland, and a benign tumor of the islets of Langerhans in the pancreas can produce excessive amounts of insulin resulting in possibly fatal low levels of blood glucose. Other potentially dangerous benign tumors include those arising in the brain or spinal cord, which may influence central nervous system function. Tumors of the trachea or esophagus may occlude the air supply or make it impossible to swallow.

Malignant neoplasms invade and destroy adjacent structures and spread to distant sites (metastasize), causing death. Malignancies tend to be poorly differentiated so that it may be impossible to determine the organ from which they originate. Malignant tumors are collectively referred to as **cancers.** This term is derived from the Latin word for "crab," possibly because the fingerlike projections that extend into underlying tissue resemble crablike claws.

All tumors, both benign and malignant, have two basic components: (1) the parenchyma, made up of proliferating neoplastic cells, and (2) the supporting stroma, made up of connective tissue, blood vessels, and possibly lymphatic vessels. The parenchyma of the neoplasm largely determines its biological behavior and is the component that determines how the tumor is named.

Most benign tumors consist of parenchymal cells that closely resemble the tissue of origin. Their names come from adding the suffix *-oma* to the cell type from which the tumor arose. For example, benign tumors of fibrous tissue are termed **fibromas,** whereas benign cartilaginous tumors are **chondromas.** The term **adenoma** is applied to benign epithelial neoplasms that grow in glandlike patterns. Benign tumors that form large cystic masses are called **cystadenomas. Lipomas** consist of soft fatty tissue, **myomas** are tumors of muscle, and **angiomas** are tumors composed of blood vessels. An epithelial tumor that grows as a projecting mass on the skin or from an inner mucous membrane (such as the gastrointestinal tract) is termed a **papilloma** or a **polyp.**

Malignant neoplasms of epithelial cell origin are called **carcinomas,** from the Greek word *karkinos,* meaning "crab." Carcinomas affect epithelial tissues, skin, and mucous membranes lining body cavities. **Adenocarcinoma** refers to malignancies of glandular tissues such as the breast, liver, and pancreas, and of the cells lining the gastrointestinal tract. **Squamous cell carcinoma** denotes a cancer in which the tumor cells resemble stratified squamous epithelium, as in the lung and head and neck regions. At times, the tumor grows in such a bizarre pattern that it is termed **undifferentiated** or **anaplastic** (without form).

Sarcomas are highly malignant tumors arising from connective tissues such as bone, muscle, and cartilage. Although they are less common than carcinomas, sarcomas tend to spread more rapidly.

Substantial evidence exists indicating that most tumors arise from a single cell (monoclonal origin). The rate of growth generally correlates inversely with the level of parenchymal differentiation. Thus well-differentiated tumors tend to grow slowly, whereas bizarre, undifferentiated neoplasms have a rapid growth rate.

Although the cause of cancer is still unknown, many possible causative factors (carcinogens) have been implicated. Chemical carcinogens may cause structural alteration of the DNA molecule (mutation), which may lead to the development of a neoplasm. Examples of chemical carcinogens include air and water pollution, cigarette smoke, asbestos, and a variety of other substances used in industry, food, cosmetics, and plastics. The development of specific types of cancer in certain families suggests a possible genetic predisposition. Excessive exposure to ultraviolet radiation (sunshine) may lead to the development of skin cancer. Survivors of the atom bomb who received huge doses of radiation have demonstrated a high incidence of leukemia. A greater-than-expected rate of leukemia was also seen in persons working with x-radiation before the need for proper protection was appreciated.

The study of experimental animal tumors has offered convincing evidence that DNA and RNA viruses can induce neoplastic transformation. Viruses that invade normal cells may alter their genetic material, leading to the abnormal cell divisions and rapid growth observed in malignant tumors.

The clinical symptoms of cancer vary with the site of malignancy. A blood-tinged stool, a change in bowel activity (e.g., intermittent constipation and diarrhea), or intestinal obstruction is suggestive of gastrointestinal malignancy. Difficulty in swallowing **(dysphagia)** or loss of appetite **(anorexia),** especially if accompanied by rapid weight loss, suggests a neoplasm in the esophagus or stomach. Hematuria may indicate kidney or bladder cancer, whereas difficulties in urination (e.g., urgency, a burning sensation, an inability to start the stream of urine) in an elderly man may be a sign of prostate tumor. Hemoptysis (coughing up blood), a persistent cough, or hoarseness may suggest a neoplasm in the respiratory tract. Severe anemia may develop from internal bleeding or from malfunction of the bone marrow caused by growth of a malignant lesion in the skeleton.

It should be stressed that these clinical symptoms may also be caused by benign disease. Nevertheless, because they may signal an underlying malignancy, they should be carefully investigated to exclude the presence of cancer.

Pain is frequently not an early sign of cancer. Unfortunately, pain may be appreciated only when the malignancy has spread too extensively to be curable. Secondary infections are common and an increasing cause of death. Most cancer patients are immunologically compromised, either because of their original disease or as a result of radiation or chemotherapy. In addition to having typical bacterial and viral infections, immunocompromised patients with malignancy are especially susceptible to unusual **opportunistic** infections such as *Pneumocystis carinii* pneumonia and **cytomegalovirus.**

Some cancers that are still at a curable stage can be detected by screening procedures. Routine mammography may identify nonpalpable breast cancer; a Papanicolaou (Pap) smear may show otherwise unsuspected cancer of the cervix. Surgical removal of these small tumors without metastatic spread offers an excellent prognosis.

Malignant neoplasms disseminate to distant sites by one of three pathways: (1) seeding within body cavities, (2) lymphatic spread, and (3) hematogenous spread.

Seeding (diffuse spread) of cancers occurs when neoplasms invade a natural body cavity. For example, a tumor of the gastrointestinal tract may penetrate the wall of the gut (visceral peritoneum), permitting metastases to enter the peritoneal cavity and implant at distant sites. A similar sequence may occur with lung cancers in the pleural cavity. Neoplasms of the central nervous system (medulloblastoma, ependymoma) may spread from the cerebral ventricles by means of the cerebrospinal fluid to reimplant on the meningeal surfaces within the brain or in the spinal cord.

Lymphatic spread is the major metastatic route of carcinomas, especially those of the lung and breast. The pattern of lymph node involvement depends on the site of the primary neoplasm and the natural lymphatic pathways of drainage of that region. Carcinomas of the lung metastasize first to the regional bronchial lymph nodes and then to the tracheobronchial and hilar nodes. Carcinoma of the breast usually arises in the upper outer quadrant and first spreads to the axillary nodes. Medial breast lesions may drain through the chest wall to nodes along the internal mammary artery.

The **hematogenous spread** of cancer is a complex process involving several steps. Tumor cells invade and penetrate blood vessels, traveling as neoplastic emboli in the circulation. These emboli of tumor cells are trapped in small vascular channels of distant organs, where they invade the wall of the arresting vessel and infiltrate and multiply in the adjacent tissue. The localization of hematogenous metastases tends to be determined by the vascular connections and anatomic relationships between the primary neoplasm and the metastatic sites. For example, carcinomas arising in abdominal organs such as the gastrointestinal tract tend to metastasize to the liver because of the flow of portal vein blood to that organ. Cancers arising in midline organs close to the vertebral column (e.g., prostate, thyroid) tend to embolize through the paravertebral venous plexus to seed the vertebral column. Neoplasms in organs drained by the inferior and superior vena cava, such as the kidney, tend to metastasize to the lung. However, several well-defined patterns of metastatic spread cannot be easily explained by vascular-anatomic relationships. Some examples include the tendency for carcinoma of the lung to involve the adrenal glands, simultaneous metastatic deposits in the brain and adrenal glands, and pituitary metastases occurring from breast carcinomas.

The **grading** of a malignant tumor assesses aggressiveness, or degree of malignancy. The grade of a tumor usually indicates its biological behavior and may allow prediction of its responsiveness to certain therapeutic agents. **Staging** refers to the extensiveness of a tumor at its primary site and the presence or absence of metastases to lymph nodes and distant organs such as the liver, lungs, and skeleton. The staging of a tumor aids in determining the most appropriate therapy. Well-localized tumors without evidence of metastases may be surgically removed. Fast-growing, undifferentiated tumors such as those found in patients with Hodgkin's disease may respond best to **radiation therapy.** Cancer of the prostate responds to **hormonal therapy,** either by the removal of the sources of male gonadal hormones that stimulate tumor growth or by the administration of female gonadal hormone (estrogen) that inhibits it. **Chemotherapy** uses one or a combination of cytotoxic substances that kill neoplastic cells, but these drugs may injure many normal cells and result in significant complications.

■ Hereditary Diseases

Hereditary diseases pass from one generation to the next through the genetic information contained in the nucleus of each cell. They reflect an abnormality in the DNA (deoxyribonucleic acid), which provides the blueprint for protein synthesis in the cell. In many hereditary diseases, an error in a single protein molecule leads to enzyme defects; membrane receptor and transport system defects; alterations in the structure, function, or quantity of nonenzyme proteins; and unusual drug reactions.

The most common hereditary abnormality is an enzyme deficiency. This leads to a metabolic block that results in a decreased amount of a substance needed for normal function, or in an accumulation of a metabolic intermediate that may cause injury. An example of the first mechanism is albinism, the absence of pigmentation resulting from an enzymatic deficiency that prevents the synthesis of the pigment melanin. An example of the second mechanism is phenylketonuria, in which the absence of an enzyme leads to the accumulation of toxic levels of the amino acid phenylalanine.

A defect in the structure of the globin molecule leads to the development of the hemoglobinopathies such as sickle cell disease and thalassemia. An example of a genetically determined adverse reaction to drugs is glucose 6-phosphate dehydrogenase deficiency, in which an insufficient amount of the enzyme results in a severe hemolytic anemia in patients receiving a common antimalarial drug.

Despite our extensive knowledge of the biochemical basis of many genetic disorders, there are a large number of conditions for which the underlying mechanism is still unknown. This list includes cystic fibrosis (Chapter 2), neurofibromatosis, retinoblastoma, familial colonic polyposis (Chapter 4), and Huntington's disease (Chapter 7).

Each human cell contains 46 chromosomes divided into 23 pairs. The chromosomes, in turn, contain thousands of genes, each of which is responsible for the synthesis of a single protein. Forty-four of the chromosomes are called **autosomes;** the other two are the X and Y chromosomes, which determine the sex of the person. A combination of XY chromosomes results in a male, whereas an XX configuration results in a female.

Each person inherits half of his or her chromosomes from each parent. If the genes inherited from each parent are the same for a particular trait, the person is **homozygous** for that trait. If the genes differ (e.g., one for brown eyes and one for blue eyes), the person is **heterozygous** for that trait. **Dominant** genes always produce an effect regardless of whether the person is homozygous or heterozygous; **recessive** genes manifest themselves only when the person is homozygous for the trait. In determining eye color, brown is dominant, whereas blue is recessive. It must be remembered that although a recessive trait must have been contributed by both parents, the possibility exits that neither parent demonstrates that trait. For example, two parents, each with one gene for brown eyes and one gene for blue eyes, would show the dominant brown coloration, although they could each contribute a blue-eye gene to their offspring, who would manifest the recessive blue-eye trait.

For some traits, the genes are **codominant,** so that both are expressed. An example is the AB blood type, in which the gene for factor A is inherited from one parent and that for factor B is inherited from the other.

Mutations are alterations in the DNA structure that may become permanent hereditary changes if they affect the gonadal cells. Mutations may result from radiation, chemicals, or viruses. They may have minimal effect and be virtually undetectable or be so serious that they are incompatible with life, causing the death of a fetus and spontaneous abortion.

Autosomal dominant disorders are transmitted from one generation to the next. These disorders affect females and males, and both can transmit the condition. When an affected person marries an unaffected person, half the children (on the average) will have the disease. The clinical manifestations of autosomal dominant disorders can be modified by reduced penetrance and variable expressivity. **Reduced penetrance** means that not everyone who has the gene will demonstrate the trait; **variable expressivity** refers to the fact that a dominant gene may manifest somewhat differently in different individuals (e.g., polydactyly may be expressed in the toes or in the fingers as one or more extra digits). Examples of autosomal dominant disorders include achondroplasia (Chapter 3), neurofibromatosis, Marfan's syndrome (Chapter 11), and familial hypercholesterolemia.

Autosomal recessive disorders result only when a person is homozygous for the defective gene. The trait does not usually affect the parents, although siblings may show the disease. On average, siblings have a one-in-four chance of being affected; two out of four will be carriers of the gene, and one will be normal. Recessive genes appear more frequently in a family, and close intermarriage (as between first cousins) increases the risk of the particular disease. Unlike autosomal dominant diseases, the expression of the defect tends to be uniform in autosomal recessive diseases and the age of onset is frequently early in life. Examples of autosomal recessive disorders include phenylketonuria (Chapter 11), cystic fibrosis (Chapter 2), galactosemia, glycogen and lipid storage diseases (Chapter 11), Tay-Sachs disease, and sickle cell anemia (Chapter 8).

Sex-linked disorders generally result from defective genes on the X chromosome, because the Y chromosome is small and carries very few genes. Most of these conditions are transmitted by heterozygous female carriers virtually only to sons, who have only the single, affected X chromosome. Sons of a heterozygous woman have a one-in-two chance of receiving the mutant gene. An affected man does not transmit the disorder to sons, but all his daughters carry the genetic trait. In rare cases a female may have the sex-linked disease if she is homozygous for the recessive gene. Virtually all sex-linked disorders are recessive. The most common example of a sex-linked disorder is color blindness. Other conditions include glucose 6-phosphate dehydrogenase deficiency, and some types of hemophilia (Chapter 8) and muscular dystrophy (Chapter 11).

Disorders of immunity

The immune reaction of the body provides a powerful defense against invading organisms by allowing it to recognize foreign substances **(antigens),** such as bacteria, viruses, fungi, and toxins, and to produce **antibodies** to counteract them. The antibody binds together with the antigen to make the antigen harmless. Once antibodies have been produced, a person becomes **immune** to the antigen.

Antibodies, or **immunoglobulins,** form in lymphoid tissue, primarily in the lymph nodes, thymus gland, and spleen. Although an infant has some immunity at birth, most immunity is acquired either naturally by exposure to a disease or artificially by immunization. There are two types of artificial immunity, active and passive. In **active immunity,** a person forms antibodies to counteract an antigen in the form of a vaccine or a toxoid. A **vaccine** consists of a low dose of dead or deactivated bacteria or viruses. Although these organisms cannot cause disease, they are foreign proteins containing antigens that stimulate the body to produce antibodies against them. A **toxoid** is a chemically altered **toxin,** the poisonous material produced by a pathogenic organism. As with a vaccine, the toxin cannot cause disease but does trigger the development of antibodies. Examples of active immunity are the vaccines given to prevent smallpox, polio, measles, tetanus, and diphtheria. Active immunity persists for a long time, although a relatively long time is required to build up immunity, and a booster shot frequently gives a stronger effect.

Passive immunity refers to the administration of a dose of preformed antibodies from the immune serum of an animal, usually a horse. This type of immunity acts immediately but lasts for a relatively short time. It is used in situations when a person is exposed to a serious disease (hepatitis, rabies, tetanus) but has no immunity against it and thus requires an immediate supply of antibodies to prevent a possibly fatal infection.

Several fundamental mechanisms of immunologic responses to antigens exist. The first type is a rapidly occurring reaction in which antigens are attacked by antibodies previously bound to the surface of mast cells. The mast cells release **histamine,** which causes a local increase in vascular permeability and smooth muscle contraction. Disorders resulting from localized reactions of this type (which probably have a genetically determined predisposition) include hay fever, asthma, and gastrointestinal allergies. Generalized, or systemic, **anaphylactic** reactions are characterized by hypotension and vascular collapse (shock) with urticaria (hives), bronchiolar spasm, and laryngeal edema. This reaction causes acute death in patients who are hypersensitive ("allergic") to the sting of bees, wasps, and other insects and to medications such as penicillin and the iodinated contrast materials used in radiology.

In the second type of immune reaction, called a cytotoxic reaction, either the antigen is a component of a cell or it attaches to the wall of red blood cells, white blood cells, platelets, or vascular endothelial cells. The reaction with an antibody leads to cell destruction by lysis or phagocytosis. Examples of a cytotoxic immune reaction include the transfusion reaction occurring after the administration of ABO-incompatible blood, and erythroblastosis fetalis, the hemolytic anemia of the Rh-positive newborn whose Rh-negative mother has produced anti-Rh antibodies.

The third type of immune reaction, a delayed reaction, occurs in an individual previously sensitized to an antigen. As an example, the first time a person touches poison ivy no reaction occurs. However, on the next exposure to poison ivy, antibodies are present to attack the antigen, and the patient develops the typical rash and irritation. A similar process produces a reaction to tuberculosis, leprosy, many fungal diseases, and other infections. This process also represents the principal component of rejection in organ transplants.

Acquired immunodeficiency syndrome

AIDS, which most commonly affects young homosexual men and intravenous drug abusers, is characterized by a profound and sustained impairment of cellular immunity that results in recurrent or sequential opportunistic infections and a particularly aggressive form of Kaposi's sarcoma. AIDS has also

been reported in a substantial number of hemophiliacs, in recipients of transfusions, and increasingly in heterosexual partners of affected individuals. AIDS is attributable to infection with retroviruses known as human immunodeficiency viruses (HIV). This immune deficiency predominantly involves the lungs, gastrointestinal tract, and central nervous system. Pulmonary infections are extremely common in patients with AIDS and are frequently caused by organisms that only rarely produce disease in individuals with normal immune systems. About 60% of AIDS victims develop one or more attacks of *Pneumocystis carinii* pneumonia, which is characterized by a sudden onset, a rapid progression to diffuse lung involvement, and a considerable delay in resolution. *Pneumocystis carinii* cannot be cultured, and the disease usually is fatal if untreated. An open-lung biopsy is often necessary to make the diagnosis if a sputum examination reveals no organisms in a patient suspected of having this disease.

Gastrointestinal manifestations of AIDS include a variety of sexually transmitted diseases involving the rectum and colon, infectious processes (such as shigellosis, amebiasis, candidiasis, and giardiasis), and alimentary tract dissemination (spread) of Kaposi's sarcoma. Kaposi's sarcoma, a systemic disease, characteristically affects the skin and causes an ulcerated hemorrhagic dermatitis. Metastases to the small bowel, which are relatively common, consist of multiple reddish or bluish red nodules that intrude into the lumen of the bowel (Figure 1-1). Similar lesions can develop throughout the gastrointestinal tract. Central ulceration of the metastases causes gastrointestinal bleeding and a characteristic radiographic appearance of multiple "bull's-eye" lesions simulating metastatic melanoma.

About 40% of all AIDS victims have neurologic symptoms, most commonly progressive dementia. Patients who develop mass lesions of the brain commonly have focal neurologic symptoms and signs.

Radiographic appearance

The typical early radiographic finding of *P. carinii* pneumonia is a hazy, perihilar, granular infiltrate that spreads to the periphery and appears predominantly interstitial. In later stages the pattern progresses to patchy areas of air-space consolidation with air bronchograms, indicating the alveolar nature of the process (Figure 1-2). The radiographic appearance may closely resemble pulmonary edema or bacterial pneumonia.

MRI best demonstrates the multiple manifestations of AIDS in the central nervous system, where areas of increased signal intensity can be seen on T2-weighted images. Atypical brain abscesses and

Figure 1-1 Kaposi's sarcoma. Small bowel study shows multiple intramural nodules (predominantly involving the jejunum) that distort the mucosal pattern and produce contour defects and intraluminal lucencies. (From Bryk D, et al: Kaposi's sarcoma of the intestinal tract: roentgen manifestations, *Gastrointest Radiol* 3:425, 1978.)

Figure 1-2 *Pneumocystis carinii* pneumonia. Diffuse bilateral air-space consolidation is suggestive of severe bacterial pneumonia or pulmonary edema.

meningeal infection often occur, most commonly related to toxoplasmosis, cryptococcosis, cytomegalovirus, and herpesvirus (Figure 1-3). Increasing evidence indicates that cerebral infections may manifest from the human immunodeficiency virus itself. Patients with AIDS also have a high incidence of lymphoma involving the central nervous system.

Treatment

Although much research has been initiated, no cure for AIDS has been found. Currently, treatment assists in maintaining quality of life and management of symptoms as they manifest. Antiviral drugs assist in suppressing the HIV infection. A healthy lifestyle free of stress, alcohol, and illegal drugs is recommended. HIV carriers should avoid infections if possible because they may accelerate the HIV process.

■ Specialized Imaging Techniques

Ultrasound

Ultrasound is a widely accepted cross-sectional imaging technique because of its low cost, availability, and ability to differentiate cystic (gallbladder), solid (liver), and complex (liver tumor) tissue. Ultrasound (Figure 1-4) is a noninvasive imaging modality that utilizes high-frequency sound waves produced by electrical stimulation of a specialized crystal. When the high-frequency sound waves pass through the body, their intensity is reduced by different amounts, depending on the acoustic properties of the tissues through which they travel. The crystal mounted in a transducer sends the signal and also acts as a receiver to record echoes reflected back from the body whenever the sound wave strikes an interface between two tissues that have different acoustic properties. The transducer records the tiny changes of the signal's pitch and direction. A water–tissue interface can produce strong reflections **(echoes),** whereas a solid tissue mass that contains small differences in composition can cause weak reflections. The display of the ultrasound image on a television monitor shows both the intensity level of the echoes and the position in the body from which they were scanned. Ultrasound images may be displayed as static gray-scale images or as multiple (video) images that permit movement to be viewed in real time. Depending on the equipment used, the interactions of the tissue with the sound wave determine how the tissue or organ is visualized and described.

In general, fluid-filled structures have intense echoes at their borders, no internal echoes, and good transmission of the sound waves. **Anechoic** tissue or structures (which are echo free, or lacking a signal) transmit sound waves easily and appear as the dark region on the image; examples are the gallbladder and

Figure 1-3   Neurologic manifestations of acquired immunodeficiency syndrome. **A,** Computed tomographic scan shows multiple ring-enhancing lesions caused by cryptococcal brain abscesses. **B,** Magnetic resonance image, after intravenous administration of contrast medium, demonstrates multiple enhancing abscesses caused by toxoplasmosis.

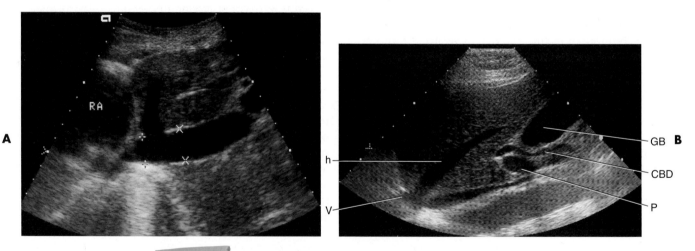

Figure 1-4   Ultrasound images of normal abdomens. **A,** Right atrium of the heart *(RA)*, the inferior vena cava (marked for measurement), and the hepatic vein joining the inferior vena cava. **B,** Gallbladder *(GB)*, common bile duct *(CBD)*, portal vein *(P)*, hepatic vein *(h)*, and inferior vena cava *(V)*.

Sonogram of the abdomen of a woman with a multiple pregnancy. Cranial architecture is normal in fetus *A* and abnormal in fetus *B,* which documented fetal demise ×2, of fetuses B and C.

Figure 1-5   Ultrasound images of the abdomen. **A,** Transverse right kidney demonstrates a hyperechoic area *(white)* within the mass caused by renal cell carcinoma. **B,** Gallbladder *(GB)* and aorta *(AO)* are hypoechoic compared to the pancreas. Focal masses *(arrows)* within the pancreas are all isoechoic (i.e., similar in density).

a distended urinary bladder. Solid structures (e.g., a gallbladder with gallstones) produce internal echoes of variable intensity. Because the solid structure tends to attenuate the sound waves, the posterior margin appears less sharply defined than the anterior margin, and only a portion of the beam is transmitted. The terms **hyperechoic** and **echogenic** indicate that the tissue structure exhibits a relatively strong reflection, a bright intensity appearing light gray to white on the image (e.g., stones and bone). **Hypoechoic** tissue exhibits relatively weak reflections that appear dark gray to gray on the image (e.g., the gastrointestinal tract). The term **isoechoic** is used to describe two structures that have the same echogenicity even though the tissue may not be the same; for example, liver tissue is isoechoic to renal cortex. Complex tissue types have both anechoic and echogenic areas (Figure 1-5).

The major advantage of ultrasound is its safety. There has been no evidence of any adverse effect on human tissues at the intensity level currently used for diagnostic procedures. Therefore ultrasound is the modality of choice for examinations of children and pregnant women, in whom a potential danger exists from the radiation exposure of other imaging studies. Ultrasound is by far the best technique for evaluating fetal age and placenta placement, congenital anomalies, and complications of pregnancy (Figure 1-6). Abdominal ultrasound is used extensively to evaluate the intraperitoneal and retroperitoneal structures, to detect abdominal and pelvic abscesses, and to diagnose obstruction of the biliary and urinary tracts. Pelvic ultrasound images the prostate gland, detecting and accurately staging neoplasms. Pelvic imaging is performed by a transabdominal (organs), transvaginal (uterus), or transrectal (prostate gland) approach.

Vascular or color-flow Doppler studies assess the patency of major blood vessels, demonstrating obstructions (stenoses), blood clots, plaques, and emboli. The color-flow duplex system, in which conventional real-time imaging is integrated with Doppler imaging (to produce quantitative data) and with color, depicts motion and the direction and velocity of blood flow. The color and intensity represent the direction of flow and the velocity, respectively (e.g., in the carotid artery).

Other uses of ultrasound include breast imaging (to differentiate solid from cystic masses) (Figure 1-7),

Figure 1-7   Ultrasound image of a breast. The sonogram shows an anechoic mass *(C)* with a well-defined back wall and distal enhancement *(arrows)*.

Figure 1-8   Ultrasound image of a wrist demonstrating the musculoskeletal architecture. A cystic structure (15 mm × 5 mm) can be seen near the dorsal aspect of base of the fourth and fifth metacarpals.

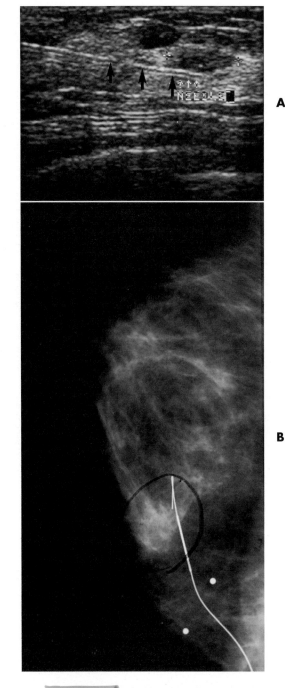

Figure 1-9   Ultrasound-guided localization. **A,** Ultrasound needle localization for surgical biopsy of the breast. **B,** Mammography image verifying needle localization.

musculoskeletal imaging (to detect problems with tendons, muscles, and joints, and soft-tissue fluid collections or masses) (Figure 1-8), and as an imaging guide for invasive procedures (biopsies, aspirations, and drain placement) (Figure 1-9).

Ultrasound is a quick, inexpensive procedure for evaluating postoperative complications, although it may be difficult to perform in some patients because of overlying dressings, retention sutures, drains, and open wounds, which may prevent the transducer from being in direct contact with the skin. In children with open fontanelles, ultrasound can image the intracranial structures. High-resolution, real-time ultrasound systems can assist surgeons during operative procedures.

Figure 1-10   Normal computed tomographic scan of lower abdomen. *a*, Aorta; *G*, gallbladder; *L*, Liver; *S*, spine.

This technique has been applied to the neurosurgical localization of brain and spine neoplasms, to the evaluation of intraventricular shunt tube placement, to the localization of renal calculi, and to surgical procedures involving the hepatobiliary system and pancreas.

The role of ultrasound imaging has expanded as a result of the availability of multifrequency transducers (2 megahertz to 15 megahertz) and advances in software (signal-processing) technology. The resultant higher-resolution images are used in musculoskeletal, breast, and small-parts imaging. The latest technologies include harmonic imaging (which involves a broad band of low frequencies and can suppress reflection from surrounding tissue) to reduce image noise and artifact, sonoCT real-time compound imaging (a combination of multiple lines of sight that increases image clarity and provides more diagnostic information), and contrast agents (microbubble echo-enhancing agents) that increase vasculature definition. Harmonic imaging produces diminished noise images, increasing the resolution in a hypersthenic patient so that patient size does not prevent obtaining diagnostic images. SonoCT real-time compound imaging provides a wider field of view in real time, which allows visualization of an entire fetus in a single pass. Contrast agents, injectable stabilized gas bubbles (less than 5 μm), and perfluorochemicals (inert dense fluids) increase the differentiation of tissues and enhance visibility of detail in tumors, vessel stenosis, heart studies, and ultrasound hysterosalpingography.

The major limitation of ultrasound is the presence of acoustic barriers, such as air, bone, and barium. For example, air reflects essentially the entire ultrasound beam, so that structures beneath cannot be imaged. This special problem interferes with imaging of the solid abdominal organs (e.g., the pancreas) in a patient with adynamic ileus, and it is the major factor precluding the ultrasound examination of the thorax. For an ultrasound examination of the pelvis, the patient usually drinks a large amount of fluid to fill the bladder, thus displacing the air-filled bowel from the region of interest.*

Computed tomography

CT produces cross-sectional tomographic images by first scanning a slice of tissue from multiple angles with a narrow x-ray beam, then calculating a relative linear attenuation coefficient (representing the amount of radiation absorbed in tissue for the various tissue elements in the section), and finally displaying the computed reconstruction as a gray-scale image on a television monitor. Unlike other imaging modalities (except for the more recent MRI), CT permits the radiographic differentiation of a variety of soft tissues from each other (Figure 1-10). CT is extremely sensitive to slight (1%) differences in tissue densities; for comparison, detection by conventional screen-film

*For more information on ultrasound imaging, refer to the following Internet sites: www.aium.org, www.sdms.org, and www.ardms.org.

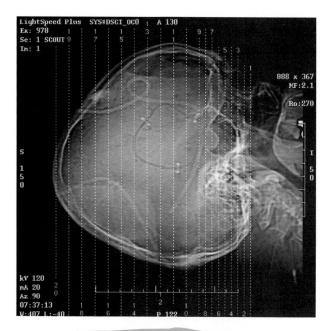

Figure 1-11   Computed tomographic scout image with overlying grid representing scan slices.

radiography requires differences in tissue density of at least 5%. Thus, in the head, CT can differentiate between blood clots, white matter and gray matter, cerebrospinal fluid, cerebral edema, and neoplastic processes.

The CT number reflects the attenuation of a specific tissue relative to that of water, which is arbitrarily assigned a CT number of 0 and appears gray on the image. The highest CT number (1000) represents bone, which appears white, and the lowest CT number (−1000) denotes air, which appears black. Fat has a CT number less than 0, whereas soft tissues have CT numbers higher than 0. Technical improvements in CT instrumentation and tube heat unit capacity have greatly reduced the time required to produce a single slice (1 to 2 seconds), and this permits the CT evaluation of virtually any portion of the body. In most instances, some type of preliminary film is obtained (either a radiograph or a CT-generated image) for localization, the detection of potentially interfering high-density material (metallic clips, barium, electrodes), and correlation with the CT images. An overlying grid with numeric markers permits close correlation between the subsequent CT scans and the initial scout film (Figure 1-11).

The intravenous injection of iodinated contrast material has become an integral part of many CT examinations. Scanning during or immediately after the administration of contrast material permits the differentiation of vascular from nonvascular solid structures.

Differences in the degree and the time course of contrast enhancement may permit the detection of neoplastic or infectious processes within normal parenchymal structures. Because of its relatively low CT number, fat can serve as a natural contrast material and can outline parenchymal organs. In patients with malignant lesions, the loss of adjacent fat planes strongly suggests tumor extension. For abdominal studies, especially those of the pancreas and retroperitoneum, dilute oral contrast material is frequently given to demonstrate the lumen of the gastrointestinal tract, and it permits the distinction between loops of bowel and solid abdominal structures.

In high-resolution CT, thin sections (1.5- to 2.0-mm slices) are used to produce a very detailed display of lung anatomy. High-resolution CT is far more sensitive and specific than plain chest radiographs (or conventional CT) for the diagnosis of parenchymal lung disease (Figure 1-12).

A fairly new CT technology is spiral (helical) scanning. In this technique, continual CT scanning is performed as the patient moves through the gantry (unlike the multiple single scans in conventional CT). This permits much faster scanning without respiratory motion and provides data that can be easily reformatted in coronal and sagittal planes as well as in the standard axial plane. The newest scanners with subsecond scanning abilities produce images of the chest (taking 30 to 40 seconds to complete the scan protocol) that demonstrate the pulmonary arteries without motion and can detect pulmonary emboli. CT imaging protocols for some procedures (e.g., obtaining images of the kidneys and liver) may require three-phase scanning (an arterial phase, a venous phase, and an excretory phase) to demonstrate all anatomic (tissue) structures (Figure 1-13). The single-scan protocol changed with subsecond scanning because the intravenous bolus injection appears very dense on the image and may obscure the pathologic features. Subsecond scanning requires delayed scanning, second and third phases to demonstrate a higher sensitivity than single-slice scanning. Subsecond scanning also produces abdominal studies with much less peristaltic motion, which results in a higher-quality examination. Spiral CT allows reconstruction of images in three dimensions and can demonstrate vascular lesions without the need for arteriography (Figure 1-14). With the thin slices of spiral scanning and the addition of three-dimensional software, the reconstruction can produce virtual colonoscopy and bronchoscopy images. The next-generation scanner performs multiple slices (multidetectors producing four to eight slices) per rotation, offers pitch variability (table movement) and variable rotation speed of

Figure 1-12 High-resolution computed tomographic scan of the lung. **A,** A pneumothorax can be seen in the right side of the lung of an emphysematous patient, and blebs (high-density areas) in the left lung. **B,** Visualization of catheter placement in the treatment for the pneumothorax.

Figure 1-13 Three-phase computed tomography scanning protocol for an abdomen. **A,** Arterial phase demonstrating the abdominal aorta and kidney.

Figure 1-14 Computed tomographic angiography. **A,** Special software is used to demonstrate the abdominal aorta, the renal arteries, the superior mesenteric artery, and the iliac arteries. **B,** Three-dimensional software in a femoral arterial run-off is used to demonstrate the popliteal arteries.

the tube, and contains software programming for instantaneous three-dimensional images (Figure 1-15).

Magnetic resonance imaging

MRI, once called nuclear magnetic resonance (NMR), has in a few short years become an important clinical tool for a variety of conditions (Figure 1-16). It has become the modality of choice for imaging the central nervous system and spine. It is also the first line of imaging for most conditions of the musculoskeletal system, and it is a problem solver in the abdomen and pelvis.

Although the physics of MRI is beyond the scope of this book, the basic technique consists of inducing hydrogen atoms (protons) to alternate between a high-energy state and a low-energy state by absorbing and then releasing, or transferring, energy. This absorption of energy is accomplished by placing the anatomic part to be imaged in a strong static magnetic field and directing a radiofrequency (RF) pulse of a specific frequency at the area. As protons absorb energy, they move into a high-energy state. After a predetermined time, the RF pulse is turned off and the protons begin to release, or transfer, their absorbed energy as they move back to a low-energy state. This process is called relaxation and it occurs over time. Two types of relaxation, T1 and T2, occur simultaneously. A listening device called a receiver coil, placed near the anatomic site, is able to detect and calculate the time it takes for both T1 and T2 relaxation types. A complex computer program named Fourier transform translates the information from the receiving coil into a computer-generated gray-scale image.

To generate an MR image, the radiographer selects a group of scanning parameters referred to as a pulse sequence. This pulse sequence contains a set of RF pulses and their timing, which is usually represented by a specific echo time (TE) and a repetition time (TR). The TE is the time between the end of the last RF pulse and the point when the receiving coil "listens" for the MR signal (known as an echo). The TR is the time it takes to play out the entire set of RF pulses before repeating. The most commonly used pulse sequences are termed spin-echo (SE) and fast, or turbo, spin-echo (FSE). By varying the TE and TR, the radiographer is able to produce an image that is weighted, demonstrating T1 relaxation or T2 relaxation, proton density, or a combination of all three, which allows a superb display of the differences between normal and abnormal tissues. In general, a pulse sequence using a short TR (500 to 700 msec) and a short TE (20 to 30 msec) provides a T1-weighted image. A pulse sequence using a long TR (2000 to 2500 msec) and a long TE (60 to 80 msec) provides a T2-weighted image. A pulse sequence using a short TE (15 to 30 msec) and an intermediate TR (2000 msec) provides a proton-density, or spin-density, image.

Although the degree of signal intensity of various substances on MR scans is complex and depends on multiple factors, some generalizations can be made. On T1-weighted images, substances causing high signal intensity (i.e., appearing bright) include fat, subacute hemorrhage, highly proteinaceous material (e.g., mucus), slow flowing blood, and intravenous contrast material (e.g., gadolinium). Water, as in cerebrospinal fluid or simple cysts, has a relatively low

Figure 1-15 Three-dimensional computed tomographic images. **A,** Skull of 3-year-old girl with closed sutures (craniosynostosis) and shape deformity. **B,** Three-dimensional cut-away illustrating the base of a normal skull. The mandible has been removed from the image.

Figure 1-16 MR image of normal upper abdomen. Transverse scan shows liver *(L)* and branches of portal veins *(white arrows)*. Gallbladder *(GB)* has high intensity in this fasting person. Pancreas *(black arrow)* and stomach *(S)* are easily seen. Inferior vena cava *(I)*, aorta *(A)*, and main portal vein *(P)* are seen with signal void because they contain flowing blood.

Figure 1-17 MR image of normal brain. **A,** T1-weighted spin-echo image (TE = 9 msec, TR = 466 msec). The ventricles and cerebral spinal fluid areas appear dark, and the white and gray matter are shades of gray. **B,** T2-weighted fast spin-echo image (TE = 101 msec, TR = 4500 msec). The cerebrospinal fluid produces a high signal intensity (white area) on the image. **C,** Sagittal T2-weighted fast spin-echo image (TE = 104 msec, TR = 4000 msec) demonstrates cerebral cortex, ventricles, pons, and cerebellum. (Courtesy Bartram J. Pierce, RT, (R) (MR), Good Samaritan Medical Center, Corvallis, Ore.)

signal intensity and appears dark. Soft tissue has an intermediate level of signal intensity (Figure 1-17, *A*).

On T2-weighted images, water has a high signal intensity (it appears bright), whereas muscle and other soft tissues (including fat) tend to have lower signal intensity and appear intermediate to dark. Cortical bone, calcium, air, and fast-flowing blood appear very dark on most imaging sequences (see Figure 1-17, *B* and *C*).

MRI has many of the advantages offered by other imaging modalities, without the associated disadvantages, and it is complementary to other modalities. Like ultrasound, MRI produces images in multiple planes without the use of ionizing radiation. Unlike ultrasound, MRI depends less on the operator's skill and the habitus of the patient and can penetrate bone without significant decrease in intensity (i.e., without attenuation), so that the underlying tissue can be clearly imaged. The ability to image directly in any plane allows the best visualization of normal and abnormal anatomy.

Unlike other imaging modalities that depend on information from one parameter (such as CT, which depends on electron density), MRI derives information from multiple biological parameters, such as proton density (Figure 1-18, *A*) and T1 and T2 relaxation times. MRI provides excellent spatial resolution, equal to that of CT, and far better contrast resolution of soft tissue. The intravenous injection of contrast material is unnecessary with MRI because flowing blood produces a signal void that contrasts sharply with adjacent structures.

Although MRI demonstrates improved sensitivity for detection of abnormal tissue, up to now it has not shown significantly improved specificity. In the head, for example, infarction, edema, tumor, infection, and

Figure 1-18 MR image of sagittal lumbar spine with small disk protrusion at L4-L5 and slightly dessicated disk spaces. **A,** Proton density fast spin echo demonstrating disk protrusion. **B,** Fat suppressed image. Spinal fluid has high intensity and spinal nerves have a lower intensity signal. (Courtesy Bartram J. Pierce, RT (R) (MR), Good Samaritan Medical Center, Corvallis, Ore.)

demyelinating disease all produce identically high signal intensity on T2-weighted images. The introduction of intravenous contrast materials and different types of pulse sequences are helping increase specificity.

Disadvantages of MRI include a longer scanning time, leading to image degradation resulting from patient and physiologic motion. Patient claustrophobia is a possibility, and monitoring a patient in a somewhat closed environment may be difficult. Furthermore, imaging patients with pacemakers (which may not operate properly) or ferromagnetic intracranial aneurysm clips (which may slip and result in hemorrhage) is contraindicated.

MR angiography permits high-quality images of the arterial and venous systems without the need for contrast material (Figure 1-19, *A*). Recent advances using rapidly infused intravenous contrast (e.g., gadolinium chelates) coupled with subsecond scanning result in superb diagnostic images of the arterial and venous systems without the need for invasive catheter angiography (Figure 1-19, *B* and *C*). This modality and CT angiography have substantially supplanted contrast angiography for the diagnosis of vascular disease.

Spectroscopic examinations using high magnetic fields to assess various chemical elements permit the sophisticated biochemical analysis of tissues in vivo. Two major clinical applications include staging carcinoma of the prostate and follow-up of brain tumors after treatment. Improved hardware and software and the development of specific magnetic contrast agents should improve the specificity of this modality to make MRI the imaging procedure of choice for a broad spectrum of clinical applications.

New and faster sequencing pulses and stronger gradients produce diffusion and perfusion images that have expanded the clinical applications of MRI. Diffusion imaging relies on the movement of molecules and random thermal motion. (In this instance, random movement of water is known as diffusion.) This application of diffusion gradients requires the use of pulses to cancel normal tissue random motion, recording a high signal in tissue with reduced diffusion because of edema. Utilizing ultrafast echo-planar imaging techniques, this altered diffusion can be imaged within minutes from the onset of symptoms. MR perfusion imaging illustrates microcirculation (demonstrating blood volume) with an increased signal intensity by using an enhancement agent (e.g., rapidly infused gadolinium) or motion-sensitive gradients (e.g., diffusion imaging uses RF inversion of saturation pulses). These images of the brain, visceral organs (e.g., the liver), and myocardium demonstrate circulation in viable tissue, which helps to distinguish old from new infarctions or ischemic regions. Minor tissue characteristics show morphologic changes: for example, diffusion-weighted images show how much tissue has been affected by altered blood flow (e.g., as after an infarction), whereas perfusion images demonstrate the region of tissue that continues to be at risk. In brain or liver tissue, malignancies have increased tissue metabolism or perfusion and demonstrate an increased signal (i.e., a bright image). In cerebral blood volume, an area of stroke demonstrates a low perfusion and appears dark. Currently, diffusion and perfusion imaging assist in demonstrating stroke lesions early, increasing the possibility of revascularization with immediate treatment. Myocardial images acquired at rest or after exercise may demonstrate a decreased signal, indicating ischemic or infarcted tissue.

Figure 1-19   MR angiography. **A,** Collapsed view of the cerebrum showing a normal circle of Willis. **B,** Gadolinium enhancement of the abdomen demonstrates renal and mesentery arteries. **C,** The venous phase demonstrates the portal circulation in the same patient. (Courtesy of Bartram J. Pierce, RT (R) (MR), Good Samaritan Medical Center, Corvallis, Ore.)

One of the unique advantages of MRI is its ability to acquire images with selective tissue suppression. The tissue most often suppressed in routine imaging is fat. Fat-suppressed images require heavy weighting (i.e., saturation or full magnetization) on the T1 sequence to ensure a large contrast difference between fat and water. Fat saturation techniques produce images in which fat gives off little or no signal (see Figure 1-18, *B*). This technique effectively demonstrates small lesions when there are only sub-

tle differences with increasing lesion conspicuity in a normal T1-weighted image. Fat-suppression images are employed when imaging the skull base and the soft tissues of the neck, the abdomen, and the pelvis. When bone marrow is being imaged, fat suppression accentuates marrow edema, such as is found in stress fractures and bone bruises.

Functional MR (fMR) allows the localization of specific regions of the brain that correspond to various functions, such as the motor, sensory, memory, vision, and language functions. The technique used to create fMR images applies an ultrafast gradient to generate a functional map that is laid over a high-resolution anatomic image. The image maps brain activity because the increased blood flow to the activated cerebral cortex produces a signal change. The combined images allow the diagnostician to precisely plan interventions that will spare specific functional areas. Future uses of fMR will be in the evaluation of stroke, epilepsy, pain, and behavioral problems.

Nuclear medicine

In radiography, ionizing radiation interacts with tissue to produce an image. In nuclear medicine, however, the patient ingests, or is injected with, a radiopharmaceutical that emits radiation, and an image is created from the signals radiating from the patient (Figure 1-20). The dose of radiopharmaceutical is calculated on the basis of the specific half-life and decay rate of its attached radionuclide. The amount of ionizing radiation to the patient in a nuclear medicine study is similar to that in a plain radiographic examination. The injected radionuclide does not produce the pharmacologic side effects or complications seen with radiographic iodinated contrast agents, making the study safer for all patients with an iodine allergy.

A gamma camera with a sodium iodide crystal detects the ionizing radiation emitted from the patient. Interaction of the gamma rays with the crystal produces light scintillation, which is converted to a digital signal on a computer monitor. The scintigraphic image, which defines the distribution of the radioactive nuclide, represents the physiologic map of the organ or system being imaged.

The physiologic map produced by some nuclear medicine procedures allows changes to be detected earlier than plain radiographic images because the functional perspective makes it more sensitive, which may lead to an earlier diagnosis and thus a better prognosis. Abnormal radionuclide images demonstrate hot spots (produced by an increase in uptake that is directly proportional to the emission of gamma radiation) or cold spots (which reflect a decreased uptake).

The images obtained using nuclear medicine techniques are excellent for documenting organ physiology, but they can be lacking in anatomic information. Plain radiographic images can therefore be useful for correlative purposes.

New technology has expanded the role of nuclear medicine to include tumor imaging. These studies help determine tumor size, location, and recurrence. Because radiopharmaceuticals differ in their ability to demonstrate various tumors, a choice is made on the basis of the suspected diagnosis (Figure 1-21). The scintigraphic images can be used to document diagnoses and for treatment management.

Single-photon emission computed tomography

Single-photon emission computed tomography (SPECT) represents another aspect of nuclear medicine imaging (Figure 1-22). The radiopharmaceuticals used in SPECT are the same as those used in planar nuclear medicine. The SPECT camera is a gamma camera with the ability to rotate independently around the patient. With the aid of a computer, it can create three-dimensional slices at any level in the body. The three-dimensional images are created by initially acquiring projections 180 to 360 degrees around the patient. The software then performs a reconstruction of the raw data to produce a three-dimensional image that is "sliced" up into transverse, sagittal, and coronal sections, very much like CT or MRI. To gather the tomographic information, a detector array rotates around the patient 360 degrees. This is similar to a CT scanner, but in SPECT, instead of the source (the x-ray tube) and the detector array moving simultaneously, the source (the patient) emits the signal while the detector array rotates. The signal, which the computer reconstruction algorithm analyzes, determines the position and strength of the data to create an image. Because the position and attenuation coefficients are unknown, the information must be inferred by the signal detector system, resulting in decreased resolution and sensitivity.

The gamma camera, which detects the gamma rays used in SPECT, has a collimator containing multiple parallel channels to allow the rays to pass. By placing the collimator in front of the camera and moving the camera, attenuation prevents many of the gamma rays from reaching the camera, decreasing the amount of data collected. Attenuation also occurs when gamma rays interact with the body. Compton scattering and photoelectric effect take place and lead to a loss of image contrast. To compensate for this loss, the computer reconstruction software must correct for attenuation.

Today, a disadvantage of SPECT is the gamma camera, which allows imaging of a region of interest that is only the size of the camera. As technology improves, the resolution and sensitivity of this modality will increase. Currently, the advantage of SPECT is that it costs half the price of PET imaging. SPECT imaging provides useful information in evaluating patients with many disease states: coronary artery disease, ventricular function disorders, ventricular wall

A   **B**

Figure 1-20 Nuclear medicine bone scan (technetium 99m–labeled bone scintigraphy). This normal scan demonstrates the anterior **(A)** and posterior **(B)** perspectives in a patient with hypercalcemia.

Figure 1-21　This 24-hour indium-111 octreotide scan illustrates multiple hepatic carcinoma metastases.

Figure 1-22　SPECT images of the brain reconstructed into three planes of view: transverse **(A)**, sagittal **(B)**, and coronal **(C)**.

motion abnormalities (Figure 1-23), infection, tumors (evaluation and staging), strokes, focal seizures, and traumatic brain injuries.

Positron-emission tomography

In positron-emission tomography (PET), as in nuclear medicine procedures, a radionuclide tracer is used to produce images (Figure 1-24). However, here the radiopharmaceutical is different because it decays by positron emission. A positron emitted from the radionuclide tracer interacts with an electron. This "annihilation" interaction produces two high-energy photons (gamma rays) in opposite directions (separated by 180 degrees). If both gamma rays are detected simultaneously within the field, the computer can localize the interaction and add these signals to the image distribution. Detection of only one interaction will not be counted in the distribution since the computer must receive two signals simultaneously to satisfy the program. These simultaneous signals produce multiple lines of response, which determine the location of the signal and produce an image. The tracer in the radionuclide represents a naturally occurring substance in the body, such as carbon, oxygen, nitrogen, or glucose. The imaging distribution of these molecules creates a finely detailed metabolic representation of the area of interest. The body or organ metabolism illustrates the biochemistry of the tissue, distinguishing diseased or dead tissue from healthy or normal tissue, and demonstrating tissue viability. Thus PET images the

Figure 1-23   Single photon emission computed tomography images of the normal heart in three planes of view, completed at rest *(Rst)* and stress *(St)* levels, with image reconstruction. **A,** Short axis *(SA)* shows the coronal heart plane. **B,** Horizontal long axis *(HLA)* shows the oblique trans-axial plane. **C,** Vertical long axis *(VLA)* shows the oblique sagittal plane.

Figure 1-24   Normal positron-emission tomographic scan with multiplanar body imaging. **A,** Coronal plane. **B,** Projection plane. **C,** Sagittal plane. Bladder *(curved arrow)*, heart *(open arrows)*, and kidney *(solid arrows)*.

distribution of the gamma rays in the specific organs of interest and provides diagnosticians with a biological map.

With PET imaging, multiple detectors (sometimes in excess of 8000) receive the signal, and computerized software converts the raw data to a three-dimensional image in three planes: axial, coronal, and sagittal. In PET imaging, attenuation correction is resolved by performing a transmission scan on each patient. The computer reconstruction software then corrects for each patient's individual body contour and attenuation factor. This attenuation correction to the image

resolution and sensitivity of PET images produces higher-quality images compared to SPECT. Radiation exposure rates to the patient for PET imaging are similar to those in nuclear medicine studies; however, the technologist receives higher doses because of the energy level of the radionuclide.

PET is especially useful in three medical specialties: oncology, cardiology, and neurology. For oncology patients, this imaging modality can accurately image the whole body with one pass, permitting the detection of metastases in multiple organs as well as aiding in tumor staging. Because PET produces a metabolic im-

Figure 1-25 Positron-emission tomography used to assess effectiveness of chemotherapy. **A,** Image prior to therapy. **B,** After chemotherapy, the image demonstrates decreased uptake of ^{18}F-fluorodeoxyglucose (FDG).

Figure 1-26 Normal positron-emission tomography images of the heart. Cardiology procedure demonstrating: **A,** short axis; **B,** long vertical axis (LVA) using ^{18}F-fluorodeoxyglucose (FDG); and **C,** horizontal long axis (HLA) with normal perfusion.

age, follow-up scans can be used to demonstrate the effectiveness of radiation or chemotherapy treatment by documenting any changes (Figure 1-25). In cardiology patients, PET assists in screening for coronary artery disease by demonstrating myocardial perfusion (flow rates, flow reserves, and viable myocardium) (Figures 1-26 and 1-27).

In neurologic patients, PET can be used to evaluate for stroke and to identify epileptic foci for surgical intervention (Figure 1-28). The scanning environment (i.e., sound and light) may influence the scan results because these stimuli can affect the metabolism of the temporal and occipital regions of the brain; therefore the environment needs to be strictly controlled. Brain disorders that can be demonstrated by PET imaging include Parkinson's disease, schizophrenia, Huntington's disease, and Alzheimer's disease. Oxygen, carbon monoxide, and glucose (used most often) are tracers that are used in brain imaging to demonstrate different aspects of cerebral function. Unlike the anatomic map produced by CT and MRI, the physiological map provided by PET may permit earlier demonstration of abnormalities and lead to prompt treatment interventions and a better prognosis.

Figure 1-27 Positron-emission tomography images demonstrating myocardial viability. Cardiac resting and artificial stress (adenosine) perfusion images of the short axis using $^{13}NH_3^-$ ammonia. **A,** At rest, perfusion is normal. **B,** After artificial stress, uptake in the inferolateral wall is decreased. **C,** Viability scan with ^{18}F-fluorodeoxyglucose (FDG) suggests ischemia of the right coronary artery and the left circumflex coronary artery. Perfusion of the region indicates that the myocardium remains viable.

Figure 1-28 Positron-emission tomography image of the brain. Normal ^{18}F-fluorodeoxyglucose (FDG) uptake in the brain is indicated by the symmetric and consistent blood flow and metabolism in three planes. **A,** Axial or transverse. **B,** Coronal. **C,** Sagittal.

QUESTIONS

1. The accumulation of abnormal amounts of fluid in the spaces between cells or in body cavities is termed _____.

2. _____ is the process by which white blood cells surround and digest infectious organisms.

3. A tumorlike scar is referred to as a(n) _____.

4. Inflammation with pus formation is termed _____.

5. An interruption in the blood supply to an organ or body part is referred to as _____.

6. A localized area of ischemic necrosis in an organ or tissue is termed a(n) _____.

7. A swelling caused by bleeding into an enclosed area is termed _____.

8. A decrease in function of an organ or tissue because of a reduction in the size or number of cells is termed _____.

9. The term _____ means new growth.

10. The term for benign epithelial neoplasms that have a glandlike pattern is _____.

Match the definitions with the following terms.

11. _____ Soft fatty tumors

12. _____ Tumors composed of blood vessels

13. _____ Malignant neoplasms of epithelial cell origin

14. _____ Tumors of muscle

15. _____ Large, cystic, benign tumor masses

16. _____ Malignant tumors from connective tissues such as bone, muscle, and cartilage

17. _____ Without form

18. _____ Loss of appetite

19. _____ Difficulty in swallowing

20. _____ Coughing up blood

21. _____ Major metastatic route of carcinomas

22. _____ Assessing the aggressiveness of a malignant tumor

23. _____ Refers to extensiveness of a tumor and whether or not it has metastasized

24. _____ Use of cytotoxic substances that kill neoplastic cells and may cause injury to normal cells

25. _____ Foreign substances produced by invading organisms

26. _____ Consists of a low dose of dead or deactivated bacteria or viruses

27. _____ Critical reaction that can cause death

28. _____ Tumor cells grow well; patient becomes weak and emaciated

29. _____ Opportunistic infection

30. _____ Epithelial tumor that grows as a projecting mass arising on the skin or on a mucous membrane

A. Cachexia
B. Myomas
C. Dysphagia
D. Lymphatic
E. Staging
F. Lipomas
G. Hemoptysis
H. Cystadenomas
I. Angiomas
J. Grading
K. Vaccine
L. Antigen
M. Polyp
N. Chemotherapy
O. Sarcomas
P. Anorexia
Q. Carcinomas
R. *Pneumocystis carinii* pneumonia
S. Anaphylactic
T. Anaplastic

BIBLIOGRAPHY
General radiology

Eisenberg RL: *Diagnostic imaging in internal medicine,* New York, 1985, McGraw-Hill.

Eisenberg RL: *Diagnostic imaging in surgery,* New York, 1986, McGraw-Hill.

Juhl JH, Crummy AB: *Essentials of radiologic imaging,* Philadelphia, 1987, Lippincott.

Putman CE, Ravin CE: *Textbook of diagnostic imaging,* Philadelphia, 1988, Saunders.

Ultrasound

Hagen-Ansert SL: *Text of diagnostic ultrasonography,* St Louis, 2001, Mosby.

Mittelstaedt CA: *Abdominal ultrasound,* New York, 1987, Churchill Livingstone.

Sarti DA: *Diagnostic ultrasound: text and cases,* St Louis, 1987, Mosby.

Computed tomography

Greenberg M, Greenberg BM: *Essentials of body computed tomography,* Philadelphia, 1983, Saunders.

Lee JKT, Sagel SS, Stanley RJ: *Computed body tomography with MRI correlation,* New York, 1989, Raven Press.

Moss AA, Gamsu G, Genant HK: *Computed tomography of the body,* Philadelphia, 1992, Saunders.

Seeram E: *Computed tomography: physical principles, clinical applications and quality control,* Philadelphia, 2001, Saunders.

Magnetic resonance imaging

Edelman RR, Hesselink JR: *Clinical magnetic resonance imaging,* Philadelphia, 1990, Saunders.

Stark DD, Bradley WG: *Magnetic resonance imaging,* St Louis, 1993, Mosby.

Westbrook C, Kaut C: *MRI in practice,* Malden, Mass, 1998, Blackwell Science.

Nuclear medicine, SPECT, and PET

Hood KH: *Single-photon computed tomography (SPECT),* http://cfii.lbl.gov/-budinger/medIechdocs/SPECT.html.

Scarfone C: *SPECT image acquisition and processing,* Duke University Medical Center, 1995, www.bae.ncsu.edu/bae/courses/bae590f/1995/scarfone/gen.html.

SPECT of the brain, http://jura.stir.ac.uk/teaching/spect/tomographic.html.

TRIUMF (Canada's national laboratory for particle and nuclear physics): *Positron emission tomography (PET),* 1998, www.triumf.ca/welcome/petscan.html.

CHAPTER 2

Respiratory System

■ **Prerequisite Knowledge**

The student should have a basic knowledge of the anatomy and physiology of the respiratory system. In addition, proper learning and understanding of the material will be facilitated if the student has some clinical experience in chest radiography and film evaluation, including a concept of the changes in technique required to compensate for density differences produced by the underlying pathologic conditions.

■ **Goals**

To acquaint the student radiographer with the pathophysiology and radiographic manifestations of all of the common and some of the unusual disorders of the respiratory system

■ **Objectives**

1. To be able to classify the more common diseases in terms of their attenuation of x-rays
2. To be familiar with the changes in technical factors required to obtain optimal-quality radiographs for patients with various underlying pathologic conditions
3. To understand and be able to define or describe all bold-faced terms in this chapter
4. To be able to describe the physiology of the respiratory system
5. To be able to identify anatomic structures on both diagrams and radiographs of the respiratory system
6. To be able to describe the more common pathologic conditions affecting the respiratory system, as well as their radiographic manifestations

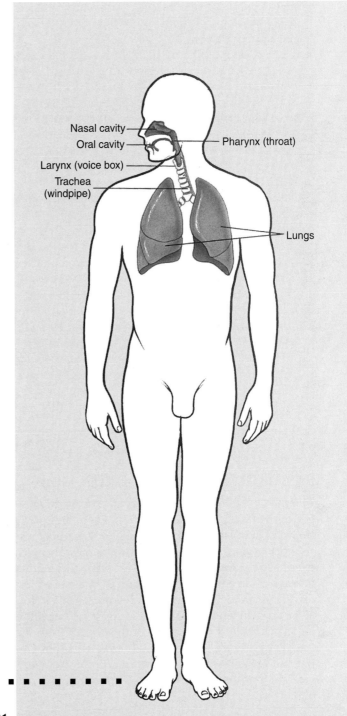

▪ ▪ ▪ ▪ ▪ ▪ Radiographer Notes

Proper positioning and the correct exposure factors are especially important in radiography of the respiratory system, because to make a precise diagnosis, radiologists must be able to detect subtle changes in pulmonary and vascular structures. Ideally, follow-up studies should be performed with the same exposure factors used when making the initial radiographs. By maintaining exposure factors, any density changes can be attributed to true pathologic findings rather than to mere technical differences.

All chest radiography should be performed with the patient in full inspiration (inhalation), except when expiration films are used for those few pathologic conditions requiring expiration films. In an ideal film the upper 10 posterior ribs should be visualized above the diaphragm. Poor expansion of the lungs may cause a normal-size heart to appear enlarged and makes it difficult to evaluate the lung bases. To obtain a full-inspiration radiograph, the patient should be instructed to take a deep breath, exhale, and inhale again (thus accomplishing maximal inspiration), at which time the exposure should be made. This technique avoids the *Valsalva effect*, which is a forced expiration against the closed glottis that increases the intrapulmonary pressure. The Valsalva effect results in compression and a large decrease in the size of the heart and adjacent blood vessels, and thus it is difficult to evaluate heart size and pulmonary vascularity accurately.

The patient must be precisely positioned for chest radiography to ensure symmetry of the lung fields and a true appearance of the heart and pulmonary vasculature. Whenever possible, all chest radiographs should be taken with the patient in the erect position. The only exception is for the patient with a suspected pathologic condition that requires a lateral decubitus position. Although recumbent radiographs may be necessary in immobile or seriously ill patients, they are less than satisfactory because in this position the abdominal contents tend to prevent the diaphragm from descending low enough to permit visualization of well-expanded lung bases or fluid levels. A 72-inch source-image receptor distance should be used when possible to minimize magnification of the heart and mediastinal structures. Correct positioning with absence of rotation in the frontal projection can be demonstrated by symmetry of the sternoclavicular joints. The shoulders must be rolled forward (anteriorly) to prevent the scapulas from overlying the lungs. In large-breasted women, it is often necessary to elevate and separate the breasts to allow good visualization of the lung bases. Nipple shadows of both men and women occasionally appear as soft-tissue masses. If the nature of these soft-tissue masses is unclear, it may be necessary to repeat the examination using small lead markers placed on the nipples. Collimation of the radiograph is required to reduce scattered radiation, although it is essential that both costophrenic angles be visualized. However the radiographer obtains a diagnostic image, it is necessary to label the image appropriately.

Radiographs exhibiting a long scale of contrast are necessary to visualize the entire spectrum of densities within the thoracic cavity (including those of the mediastinum, heart, lung markings,

▪ Physiology of the Respiratory System

The major role of the respiratory system is the oxygenation of blood and the removal of the body's waste products in the form of carbon dioxide. The upper respiratory system, which consists of the nasopharynx, oropharynx, and larynx, provides structure for the passage of air into the lower respiratory system. The lower respiratory system, which consists of the trachea, bronchi, and bronchioles, is composed of tubular structures responsible for conducting air from the upper respiratory structures. With the use of the upper and lower respiratory structures, the air from outside the body enters the lungs. The single trachea branches out into two bronchi (one to each lung), which in turn branch out into progressively smaller bronchioles to produce a structure termed the bronchial tree because its appearance resembles an inverted tree. The tracheobronchial tree is lined with a mucous membrane (the respiratory epithelium) containing numerous hairlike projections called cilia. During inspiration, the air is moistened and warmed as it enters the lungs. The cilia act as miniature sweepers to prevent dust and foreign particles from reaching the lungs. When the ciliary blanket works correctly, the particles are moved away from the lungs to be coughed up or swallowed. Any damage to the res-

and pulmonary vasculature) and the surrounding bony thorax. Most authorities agree that a minimum of 120 kilovolts-peak (kVp) should be used with an appropriate ratio grid for all adult chest radiography. If it is necessary to decrease the overall density, this should be accomplished by reduction of the milliampere-seconds (mAs) rather than of the kVp. Decreasing the kVp tends to enhance the bony thorax, which may obscure vascular details and cause underpenetration of the mediastinal structures. In general the density and contrast should be such that the thoracic vertebrae and intervertebral disk spaces are faintly visible through the shadow of the mediastinum without obscuring the lung markings and pulmonary vascularity. When producing radiographs for line placement, make sure to use the appropriate technical factors to demonstrate the line and possible chest pathology (pneumothorax or hemothorax) that may result from line placement.

Short exposure times (10 msec or less) must be used in chest radiography because longer times may not eliminate the involuntary motion of the heart. Automatic exposure devices are generally recommended, and they help to ensure that follow-up studies will have a similar film density. An exception is the expiration (exhalation) chest radiograph, which should be exposed with a manual technique because the preset density of an automatic exposure device may cause excessive blackening of the lungs and thus obscure a small pneumothorax.

Compensatory filters are sometimes needed to overcome the broad range of different tissue densities within the chest. They are especially important to allow good visualization of the mediastinum without overexposing the lungs. The use of compensatory filters generally requires that the radiographic exposure be twice that used in the absence of additional filtration.

To demonstrate fluid levels, the patient should be in an erect position, and a horizontal x-ray beam must be used. Any angulation of the beam prevents a parallel entrance to the air–fluid interface and obscures the fluid level. In some clinical situations (e.g., when there is a small pneumothorax, or pleural thickening as opposed to free pleural fluid), it is necessary to use a horizontal beam with the patient placed in the lateral decubitus position.

Certain pathologic conditions of the respiratory system require that the radiographer alter the routine technical factors. Some disorders produce increased density, which attenuates more of the x-ray beam, whereas others decrease the density of the lungs so there is less attenuation by the pulmonary tissue. It is important to remember that these changes may vary for a single disease, because the chest structures attenuate more or less of the x-ray beam depending on the stage of the disease process. Unless the radiographer has access to previous films with recorded techniques, the initial exposures should be made using a standard technique chart. Adjustments and technical factors can then be made, if necessary, on subsequent films. See the Box in Chapter 1 labeled Relative Attenuation of X-rays in Advanced Stages of Diseases for a list of the changes in attenuation factors expected in advanced stages of various disease processes.

piratory epithelium and its cilia permits particles (entering with the inspired or inhaled air) to proliferate and produce a disease process.

The vital gas exchange within the lung (called external respiration) takes place within the alveoli, extremely thin-walled sacs surrounded by blood capillaries, which represent the true parenchyma of the lung. Oxygen in the inhaled air diffuses from the alveoli into the blood capillaries, where it attaches to hemoglobin molecules in red blood cells and circulates to the various tissues of the body (called internal respiration). Carbon dioxide, a waste product of cellular metabolism, diffuses in the opposite direction, passing from the blood capillaries into the alveoli and then exiting the body during expiration (or exhalation). Because individual alveoli are extremely small, chest radiographs can demonstrate only a cluster of alveoli and their tiny terminal bronchioles, which are the basic anatomic units of the lung; a cluster of alveoli is termed the acinus.

Respiration is controlled by a center in the medulla at the base of the brain. The level of carbon dioxide in the blood regulates the respiratory center. Even a slight increase in the amount of carbon dioxide in the blood increases the rate and depth of breathing, as when an individual exercises. The accumulation of waste gases that must be removed from the body (as well as the body's need for additional oxygen) causes the respiratory center to stimulate the muscles of respiration—the diaphragm and the intercostal muscles between the ribs. Contraction of the muscles of respiration causes the volume of the chest cavity to increase. This decreases the pressure within the lungs and forces air to move into the lungs through the tracheobronchial tree. As the respiratory muscles relax, the volume of the chest cavity decreases, and air is forced out of the lungs. Special muscles of expiration (abdominal and internal intercostal muscles) may be needed for difficult breathing or in patients with decreased gas exchange as occurs in emphysema.

Unlike most other organs, the lung has two different blood supplies. The pulmonary circulation is a low-pressure, low-resistance system through which oxygen enters and carbon dioxide exits the circulatory system. The bronchial circulation, which is a part of the high-pressure systemic circulation, supplies oxygenated blood to nourish (or support) the lung tissue itself.

A double-walled membrane consisting of two layers of pleura encases the lungs. The visceral pleura is the inner layer that adheres to the lung, whereas the parietal pleura lines the inner chest wall (the thoracic cavity). Between the two layers of pleura is a potential space, which normally contains only a small amount of fluid to lubricate the surfaces to prevent friction as the lungs expand and contract. The airtight space between the lungs and the chest wall has a pressure a bit less than that in the lungs. This difference in pressure acts like a vacuum to prevent the lungs from collapsing. An inflammatory or neoplastic process that involves the pleura may produce fluid within the potential space (a pleural effusion).

■ Congenital/Hereditary Diseases

Cystic fibrosis

Cystic fibrosis (mucoviscidosis) is a hereditary disease characterized by the secretion of excessively viscous mucus by all the exocrine glands; it is caused by a defective gene in the middle of chromosome 7. Cystic fibrosis is the most common clinically important genetic disorder among white children. Ninety percent of the morbidity and mortality related to cystic fibrosis occurs as a result of respiratory involvement.

In the lungs, thick mucus secreted by mucosa in the trachea and bronchi blocks the air passages. These mucous plugs lead to focal areas of lung collapse. Recurrent pulmonary infections are common, because bacteria that are normally carried away by mucosal secretions adhere to the sticky mucus produced in this condition. In the pancreas, blockage of the ducts by mucous plugs prevents pancreatic enzymes from entering the duodenum. This impairs the digestion of fat, resulting in failure of the child to gain weight and

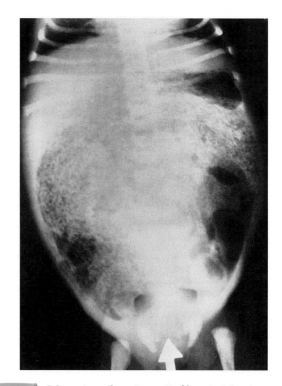

Figure 2-1 Meconium ileus in cystic fibrosis. Massive small bowel distention with profound soap-bubble effect of gas mixed with meconium. (From Swischuk LE: *Radiology of the newborn and young infant,* Baltimore, 1980, Williams & Wilkins.)

the production of large, bulky, foul-smelling stools. In about 10% of newborns with cystic fibrosis, the thick mucus causes obstruction of the small bowel (meconium ileus) (Figure 2-1). Bowel perforation with subsequent fatal peritonitis may occur.

Involvement of the sweat glands in cystic fibrosis causes the child to perspire excessively. This leads to a loss of large amounts of salt (sodium, potassium, and chloride), two to three times the normal amount. This makes the patients extremely susceptible to heat exhaustion in hot weather. The presence of excessive chloride on the skin is the basis for the "sweat test," a simple and reliable test for cystic fibrosis.

Radiographic appearance

Radiographically, cystic fibrosis causes generalized irregular thickening of linear markings throughout the lungs that, when combined with the almost invariable hyperinflation, produces an appearance similar to that of severe chronic lung disease in adults (Figure 2-2).

Treatment

Patient well-being depends on the use of prophylactic antibiotics, chest physiotherapy, and improved airflow. Prophylactic antibiotics reduce the risk of lung infections that may cause permanent lung damage

Figure 2-2 Cystic fibrosis. Multiple small cysts superimposed on diffuse, coarse, reticular pattern.

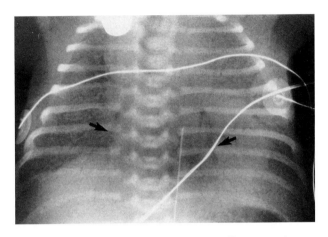

Figure 2-3 Hyaline membrane disease. Diffuse granular pattern of pulmonary parenchyma associated with air bronchograms *(arrows)*.

or bronchiectasis. Chest physiotherapy prevents lungs from filling with viscous mucus by keeping the mucus moving. Improved airflow depends on the use of bronchiodilators. A new drug to help control pulmonary infections is deoxyribonuclease (DNase), an enzyme that digests the DNA of bacterial and inflammatory cells in the lungs.

Hyaline membrane disease

Hyaline membrane disease, also known as idiopathic respiratory distress syndrome (IRDS), is one of the most common causes of respiratory distress in the newborn. It primarily occurs in premature infants, especially those who have diabetic mothers or who have been delivered by cesarean section. Hypoxia and increasing respiratory distress may not be immediately evident at birth but almost always appear within 6 hours of delivery.

The progressive underaeration of the lungs in hyaline membrane disease results from a lack of **surfactant.** Surfactant consists of a mixture of lipids, proteins, and carbohydrates that creates a high surface tension. Normally the alveolar cell walls produce lipoprotein, which maintains the surface tension within the alveoli. This permits the alveoli to remain inflated so that atelectasis does not occur. This disease process results from surfactant deficiency resulting from cell immaturity or birth trauma.

Radiographic appearance

In addition to pronounced underaeration, the radiographic hallmark of hyaline membrane disease is a finely granular appearance of the pulmonary parenchyma (Figure 2-3). A peripherally extending air bronchogram develops because the small airways dilate and stand out clearly against the atelectasis in the surrounding lung.

Treatment

New treatment advances for this disease include the use of an artificial surfactant, which offers the best therapy to reduce morbidity and mortality from this disease process.

The treatment of hyaline membrane disease includes the use of positive-pressure ventilators that pump air (often with high concentrations of oxygen) into the lungs through an endotracheal tube. The positive-pressure ventilator ensures satisfactory levels of tissue oxygenation. The high ventilator pressure may cause leakage of air from overinflated alveoli or small terminal bronchioles, leading to interstitial emphysema, pneumothorax, and pneumopericardium, all of which further decrease the expansion of the lungs.

■ Inflammatory Disorders of the Upper Respiratory System

Croup

Croup is primarily a viral infection of young children that produces inflammatory obstructive swelling localized to the subglottic portion of the trachea. The edema causes inspiratory stridor or a barking cough, depending on the degree of laryngeal obstruction.

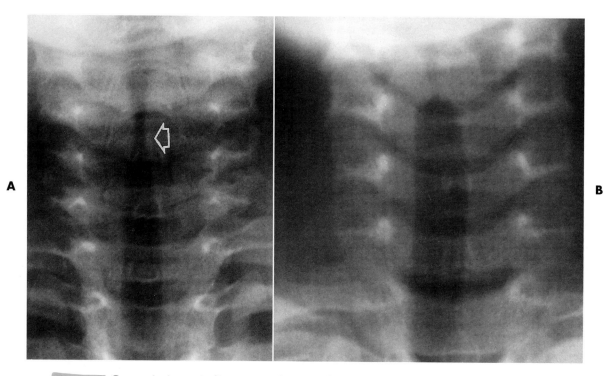

Figure 2-4 Croup. **A,** Arrow indicates smooth, tapered narrowing of subglottic portion of trachea (the Gothic arch sign). **B,** Normal trachea with broad shouldering in subglottic region.

Summary of Findings for Congenital and Hereditary Disorders

DISORDER	LOCATION	RADIOGRAPHIC APPEARANCE	TREATMENT
Cystic fibrosis	Bronchi	Irregular thickening of linear markings throughout lung Hyperinflation	Prophylactic antibiotics Chest physiotherapy Bronchodilators
Hyaline membrane disease	Alveoli	Minute granular densities in parenchyma Air bronchogram	Artificial surfactant Positive pressure ventilation

Radiographic appearance

Frontal radiographs of the lower neck show a characteristic smooth, fusiform, tapered narrowing of the subglottic airway caused by the edema (Figure 2-4, *A*), which is unlike the broad shouldering normally seen (Figure 2-4, *B*).

Treatment

A cool mist helps alleviate the breathing difficulty in patients with croup. At home, many use the steam from a hot shower for 15- to 20-minute intervals. When breathing continues to be difficult, medical attention should be sought. Corticosteroid treatment is used in severe cases to help reduce swelling.

Epiglottitis

Acute infections of the epiglottis, most commonly caused by *Haemophilus influenzae* in children, causes thickening of epiglottic tissue and the surrounding pharyngeal structures. The incidence of epiglottitis has decreased dramatically since the inception of the *Haemophilus influenzae* group B (HiB) vaccine as a routine childhood immunization.

Radiographic appearance

On lateral projections of the neck using soft-tissue techniques, a rounded thickening of the epiglottic shadow gives it the configuration and approximate size of an adult's thumb (Figure 2-5), in contrast to the

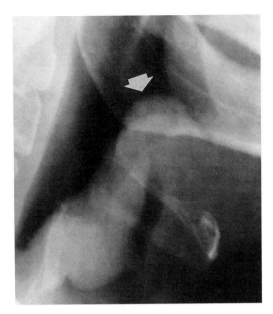

Figure 2-5   Epiglottitis. Lateral radiograph of neck demonstrates wide, rounded configuration of inflamed epiglottis *(arrow)*. (From Podgore JK, Bass JW: *J Pediatr* 88:154-155, 1976.)

Summary of Findings for Inflammatory Disorders of the Upper Respiratory System

DISORDER	LOCATION	RADIOGRAPHIC APPEARANCE	TREATMENT
Croup	Subglottic trachea Larynx	Smooth, tapered narrowing	Steam, mist tent, O_2
Epiglottitis	Supraglottic area or supraglottis	Fat epiglottic shadow	ER—intubation Antibiotics for infection

normal, narrow epiglottic shadow resembling an adult's little finger.

Treatment

Prompt recognition of acute epiglottitis is imperative because the condition may result in sudden complete airway obstruction. Because of its severity, epiglottitis requires hospitalization so that the patient may be monitored. Intubation may become necessary to restore normal respiration. Also, antibiotics may have to be administered to treat the infection, and corticosteroids to reduce the swelling.

■ Inflammatory Disorders of the Lower Respiratory System

Pneumonia

Acute pneumonia is an inflammation of the lung that can be caused by a variety of organisms, most commonly bacteria and viruses. Regardless of the cause, pneumonias tend to produce one of three basic radiographic patterns.

ALVEOLAR PNEUMONIA

Alveolar, or **air-space, pneumonia,** exemplified by pneumococcal pneumonia, is produced by an organism that causes an inflammatory exudate that replaces air in the alveoli so that the affected part of the lung is no longer air containing but rather appears solid, or radiopaque (Figure 2-6). The inflammation spreads from one alveolus to the next by way of communicating channels, and it may involve pulmonary segments or an entire lobe (lobar pneumonia).

Radiographic appearance

Consolidation of the lung parenchyma with little or no involvement of the airways produces the characteristic air-bronchogram sign (Figure 2-7). The sharp contrast between air within the bronchial tree and the surrounding airless lung parenchyma permits the normally invisible bronchial air column to be seen radiographically. The appearance of an air bronchogram requires the presence of air within the bronchial tree, which suggests that the bronchus is not completely occluded at its origin. An air bronchogram excludes

Figure 2-6 Alveolar pneumonia (pneumococcal). Homogeneous consolidation of right upper lobe and medial and posterior segments of right lower lobe. Note associated air bronchograms *(arrows)*.

Figure 2-8 Bronchopneumonia (staphylococcal). Ill-defined consolidation at right base.

Figure 2-7 Air-bronchogram sign in pneumonia. Frontal chest radiograph demonstrates air within intrapulmonary bronchi in patient with diffuse alveolar pneumonia of left lung.

the diagnosis of a pleural or mediastinal lesion, because there are no bronchi in these regions. Because air in the alveoli is replaced by an equal or almost equal quantity of inflammatory exudate, and because the airways leading to the affected portions of the

lung remain open, there is no evidence of volume loss in alveolar pneumonia.

BRONCHOPNEUMONIA

Bronchopneumonia, typified by staphylococcal infection, is primarily an inflammation that originates in the bronchi or the bronchiolar mucosa and spreads to adjacent alveoli. Because alveolar spread of the infection in the peripheral air spaces is minimal, the inflammation tends to produce small patches of consolidation. Bronchial inflammation causing airway obstruction leads to atelectasis with loss of lung volume.

Radiographic appearance

The small patches of consolidation may be seen radiographically as opacifications that are scattered throughout the lungs but are separated by an abundance of air-containing lung tissue (Figure 2-8); air bronchograms are absent. If consolidation causes obstructed airways, atelectasis is evident.

INTERSTITIAL PNEUMONIA

Interstitial pneumonia is most commonly produced by viral and mycoplasmal infections. In this type of pneumonia the inflammatory process involves predominantly the walls and lining of the alveoli and the interstitial supporting structures of the lung, the alveoli septa.

Radiographic appearance

The interstitial dispersal of the infection produces a linear or reticular pattern (Figure 2-9). When seen on end, the thickened interstitium may appear as multiple small nodular densities. Left untreated, interstitial

Figure 2-9 Interstitial pneumonia (viral). Diffuse peribronchial infiltrate with associated air-space consolidation obscures heart border (shaggy heart sign). Patchy alveolar infiltrate is present in right upper lung. (From Eisenberg R: *Atlas of signs in radiology*, Philadelphia, 1984, Lippincott.)

Figure 2-10 Pneumonia. CT scan demonstrates single lobe infiltrate by increased density of lung tissue on the left side.

pneumonia may cause "honeycomb lung," which is demonstrated by computed tomography (CT) as cystlike spaces and dense fibrotic walls (Figure 2-10).

Treatment

Extensive inflammation of the lung can cause a mixed pattern of alveolar, bronchial, and interstitial pneumonias, and this pattern appears as opacifications representing pulmonary consolidation. Treatment for these types of pneumonias usually includes regimented doses of an antibiotic to eradicate the cause. Rest, hydration, and deep-breathing techniques (supportive therapy) help in treating the infectious process.

ASPIRATION PNEUMONIA

The aspiration of esophageal or gastric contents into the lung can lead to the development of pneumonia. Aspiration of esophageal material can occur in patients with esophageal obstruction (e.g., tumor, stricture, achalasia), diverticula (Zenker's), or neuromuscular swallowing disturbances. Aspiration of liquid gastric contents is most often related to general anesthesia, tracheostomy, coma, or trauma.

Radiographic appearance

Both types of aspiration cause multiple alveolar densities, which may be distributed widely and diffusely throughout both lungs (Figure 2-11). Because the ana-

Figure 2-11 Aspiration pneumonia. Bilateral, nonsegmental air-space consolidation.

tomic distribution of pulmonary changes is affected by gravity, the posterior segments of the upper and lower lobes are most commonly affected, especially in debilitated or bedridden patients.

Treatment

For effective treatment, early diagnosis of aspiration pneumonia and the prompt institution of corticosteroid and antibiotic therapy are essential to improve the otherwise grave prognosis.

Lung abscess

A lung abscess is a necrotic area of pulmonary parenchyma containing purulent (puslike) material. A lung abscess may be a complication of bacterial pneumonia, bronchial obstruction, aspiration, a foreign body, or the hematogenous spread of organisms to the lungs either in a patient with diffuse bacteremia or as a result of septic emboli. Aspiration, which is the most common cause of lung abscesses, frequently occurs in the right lung because the right main bronchus is more vertical than the left. The necrotic parenchyma becomes encapsulated by a fibrous wall, which encases the necrotic material. Unlike abscesses involving other organs, lung abscesses create an opening into the airway that can expand the extent of the infection.

Clinically, a patient with a lung abscess has a fever and cough and produces copious amounts of foul-smelling sputum. An important complication of lung abscess is the development of a brain abscess, which is produced by infected material carried by the blood from the lung to the left side of the heart and then on to the brain.

Radiographic appearance

The earliest radiographic finding of lung abscess is a spherical density that characteristically has a dense center with a hazy, poorly defined periphery. If there is communication with the bronchial tree, the fluid contents of the cavity are partly replaced by air, producing a typical air–fluid level within the abscess (Figure 2-12). A cavitary lung abscess usually has a thickened wall with a shaggy, irregular inner margin. CT can assist in the diagnostic process to demonstrate an ill-defined outer wall and rule out empyema (Figure 2-13).

Treatment

The treatment for lung abscesses varies according to the cause. Specific therapy to control and eradicate the underlying organism is utilized as well as supplemental treatment to alleviate possible complications. The patient also receives supportive therapy to help the lung mobilize the purulent material and to ensure pulmonary volume.

Tuberculosis

Tuberculosis is caused by *Mycobacterium tuberculosis*, a rod-shaped bacterium with a protective waxy coat that permits it to live outside the body for a long time. Tuberculosis spreads mainly by droplets in the air, which are produced in huge numbers by the cough-

Figure 2-12 Lung abscess (bacterial pneumonia). Large, thick-walled left upper lobe abscess with air-fluid level *(arrow)* and associated infiltrate.

Figure 2-13 Lung abscess. CT scan demonstrates multiloculated capsule with air–fluid level.

ing of an infected patient. Therefore it is essential that respiratory precautions be followed when radiographing patients with active disease. The organisms may be inhaled from sputum that has dried and turned into dust. They are rapidly killed by direct sunlight but may survive a long time in the dark. Tuberculosis also may be acquired by drinking the milk of infected cows. However, routine pasteurization of milk has virtually eliminated this route of infection.

Unlike most bacteria, mycobacteria do not stain reliably by Gram's method. However, once stain is

- -

Summary of Findings for Inflammatory Disorders of the Lower Respiratory System

DISORDER	LOCATION	RADIOGRAPHIC APPEARANCE	TREATMENT
Pneumococcal pneumonia	Lobar/segment	Lobe/segment opacification	Antibiotic
Staphylococcal pneumonia	Bronchial airway/ alveoli	Patchy opacification with air bronchogram	Antibiotic
Viral or mycoplasmic pneumonia	Alveolar/interstitial	Linear or reticular pattern	Antibiotic
Aspiration pneumonia	Alveolar (lobe/ segment)	Patchy opacification	Corticosteroid and antibiotic
Lung abscess	Most common in right lung	Encapsulated opaque mass with air-fluid level	Appropriate antibiotic for specific organism, aid in expectoration of purulent material

- -

taken up, it is difficult to decolorize mycobacteria by either acid or alcohol, and thus the organisms are often called acid-fast bacilli.

Tuberculosis is primarily a disease of the lungs, although it can spread to involve the gastrointestinal, genitourinary, and skeletal systems. In the initial tuberculous infection (the primary lesion), a collection of inflammatory cells collects around a clump of tuberculosis bacilli to form a small mass (tubercle) that is visible to the naked eye. The outcome of this initial infection depends on the number of bacilli and the resistance of the infected tissue. If the resistance is good and the dose is small, the proliferation of fibrous tissue around the tumor limits the spread of infection and produces a mass of scar tissue. In the lung, tuberculous scars are commonly found in the posterior apical segments. They often contain calcium, which is deposited as healing occurs.

A larger dose of bacilli or lower patient resistance tends to permit the disease to progress slowly. Within the center of the tubercle, the bacilli kill inflammatory cells, so that the core becomes a necrotic, Swiss cheese–like mass (caseation). The caseous material may eventually become liquefied to form a cavity. Coalescence of several small cavities can result in the formation of a large cavity, which may contain an air–fluid level. Rupture of blood vessels crossing a cavity causes bleeding and the coughing up of blood (hemoptysis). An overwhelming infection with low resistance causes diffuse destruction throughout the lung, with the formation of huge cavities and often a fatal outcome.

The tuberculin skin test can detect previous tuberculous infection. The purified protein derivative (PPD) of the tuberculosis bacillus is injected into the skin and the injection site examined 2 to 3 days later. A visible and palpable swelling 10 mm in diameter or larger indicates that the individual has developed antibodies to a previous exposure to the bacilli. If there is no such reaction, the individual has either not been exposed to the tuberculosis bacilli or is anergic (i.e., immunologically nonreacting). The tuberculin test is not positive during an acute infection or for several weeks thereafter. One must consider the 3- to 6-week incubation period and the fact that the tuberculin skin test does not become positive until 2 to 10 weeks after infection.

PRIMARY TUBERCULOSIS

Primary pulmonary tuberculosis has traditionally been considered a disease of children and young adults. However, with the dramatic decrease in the prevalence of tuberculosis (especially in children and young adults), primary pulmonary disease can develop at any age.

Radiographic appearance

There are four basic radiographic patterns of primary pulmonary tuberculosis. (1) The infiltrate may be seen as a lobar or segmental air-space consolidation that is usually homogeneous, dense, and well defined (Figure 2-14). The apical lordotic projection best demonstrates the apices without superimposition of bony structures (Figure 2-15). (2) Associated enlargement of hilar or mediastinal lymph nodes is very common (Figure 2-16). (3) Indeed, the combination of a focal parenchymal lesion and enlarged hilar or mediastinal lymph nodes produces the classic primary complex (the Ghon lesion), an appearance strongly suggestive of primary tuberculosis. (4) Pleural effusion is common, especially in adults

Figure 2-14   Primary tuberculosis. Consolidation of right upper lobe.

Figure 2-16   Primary tuberculosis. Enlargement of right hilar lymph nodes without discrete parenchymal infiltrate.

Figure 2-15   Apical lordotic projection. Lung apices can be seen without bony superimposition.

Figure 2-17   Primary tuberculosis. Unilateral right tuberculous pleural effusion without parenchymal or lymph node involvement.

(Figure 2-17). Most primary tuberculous effusions are unilateral and clear rapidly with treatment.

Miliary tuberculosis refers to dissemination of the disease by way of the bloodstream. Radiographically, this produces innumerable fine discrete nodules (granulomas) distributed uniformly throughout both lungs (Figure 2-18).

Tuberculous pneumonia may resolve completely and leave a normal lung. However, if necrosis and caseation develop, some fibrous scarring occurs.

Calcification may develop within both the parenchymal and the nodal lesions, and this may be the only residue of primary tuberculous infection on subsequent films. If the disease responds poorly to therapy and continues to progress (especially in patients with immunodeficiency or diabetes and in those receiving steroid therapy), the pneumonia may break down into multiple necrotic cavities or a single large abscess filled with caseous material (Figure 2-19).

Figure 2-18   Miliary tuberculosis.

Figure 2-20   Secondary tuberculosis. Bilateral fibrocalcific changes at apices. Notice upward retraction of hila.

Figure 2-19   Tuberculosis. Multiple large cavities with air-fluid levels in both upper lobes. Notice chronic fibrotic changes and upward retraction of hila.

SECONDARY (REACTIVATION) TUBERCULOSIS

Reactivation of organisms from previously dormant tubercles is termed a secondary lesion or re-infection tuberculosis. At times, the tuberculosis bacillus may remain inactive for many years before a secondary lesion develops, often because of a decrease in the body's immune defense. The diffuse, poorly defined lesion develops areas of caseous necrosis. Necrosis and liquefaction commonly lead to the development of tuberculous cavities, which typically have thick walls with ill-defined inner margins. Secondary pulmonary tuberculosis heals slowly with extensive fibrosis. Contraction of the fibrous scars causes loss of volume of the involved segment or lobe and a decrease in the size of the hemithorax. The trachea and other mediastinal structures are retracted to the involved side; in upper lobe disease the hilum is elevated.

Radiographic appearance

Secondary tuberculosis most commonly affects the upper lobes, especially the apical and posterior segments (Figure 2-20). It is initially seen as a nonspecific, hazy, poorly marginated alveolar infiltrate that often radiates outward from the hilum.

Because of the difficulty of radiographically determining the activity of secondary tuberculosis, comparison with previous films is essential. An unchanged appearance of fibrosis and calcification on serial films usually indicates evidence of "healing" of the tuberculous process. Nevertheless, even densely calcified lesions can contain central areas of necrosis in which viable organisms can still be found even after long periods of apparent inactivity. Of course, new cavitation or an increasing amount of pulmonary infiltrate indicates active disease.

TUBERCULOMA

A tuberculoma is a sharply circumscribed parenchymal nodule, often containing viable tuberculosis bacilli that can develop in either primary or secondary disease. Although the residual localized caseation may remain unchanged for a long period or permanently, a tuberculoma

Figure 2-21 Calcified tuberculoma. Large soft-tissue mass in left lung *(arrows)* that contains dense central calcification.

is potentially dangerous because it may break down at any time and lead to dissemination of the disease.

Radiographic appearance

Radiographically, tuberculomas appear as single or multiple pulmonary nodules, usually 1 to 3 cm in diameter. They can occur in any part of the lung but are most common in the periphery and in the upper lobes. A central nidus of calcification (which may be detectable only on tomograms) is strongly suggestive of the lesion representing a tuberculoma (Figure 2-21). However, the lack of calcification is of no diagnostic value.

Treatment

Tuberculosis treatment begins with a two-drug regimen to help prevent drug resistance through mutation. The most common drugs used today are isoniazid, rifampin, and pyrasinamide. The effectiveness of the treatment is evaluated regularly to be sure the patient's strain of *M. tuberculosis* has not become resistant to the drugs of choice.

Pulmonary mycosis

The term *pulmonary mycosis* means fungal infection of the lung. The two most common systemic fungal infections found in North America are histoplasmosis (endemic in the Mississippi and Ohio River valleys), and coccidioidomycosis (seen in the southwestern United States).

Histoplasmosis

Histoplasmosis, caused by the fungus *Histoplasma capsulatum,* is a common disease that often produces a radiographic appearance simulating that of tuberculosis. The primary form of histoplasmosis is usually relatively benign and often passes unnoticed.

Histoplasmosis can incite progressive fibrosis in the mediastinum. This can cause obstruction of the superior vena cava, pulmonary arteries, and pulmonary veins, as well as severe narrowing of the esophagus.

Diffuse calcification in the liver, spleen, and lymph nodes is virtually diagnostic of histoplasmosis, especially in areas in which the disease is endemic (e.g., the Mississippi and Ohio River valleys). These calcifications tend to be small, multiple, dense, and discrete, although occasionally they appear as moderately large, solidly calcified granulomas.

Coccidioidomycosis

Coccidioidomycosis is caused by a fungus, *Coccidioides immitis,* which is found in the desert soil of the southwestern United States. Coccidioidomycosis can develop from an acute infection to chronic or disseminated forms. The infection is transmitted through fungal spores in the air. Immunosuppressed patients are more susceptible, and the disease may progress rapidly in those with a compromised immune system.

Acute coccidioidomycosis has few or no symptoms in most cases. The symptoms emulate influenza. As in histoplasmosis, those who are infected often remain undiagnosed and the immune system builds antibodies to fight the infection. In chronic disease, the infection results in lung abscesses, which may rupture and infect the mediastinum and pleural cavity. The disease processes of chronic and disseminated coccidioidomycosis are similar to and may be indistinguishable from those of chronic histoplasmosis.

Radiographic appearance

Chest radiographs may demonstrate single or multiple areas of pulmonary infiltration; these most often appear in the lower lung and are frequently associ-

■ ■

Summary of Findings for Tuberculosis

DISORDER	LOCATION	RADIOGRAPHIC APPEARANCE	TREATMENT
Primary tuberculosis	Lobar or segmental	Consolidation is homogeneous, dense, and well defined	For all cases of tuberculosis, treatment is a two-drug regimen for 2 months or longer (isoniazid, rifampin, and pyrasinamide)
	Hilar and mediastinal lymph nodes	Hilar enlargement without parenchymal involvement	
	Parenchymal, hilar, and mediastinal nodes	Demonstrates Ghon lesion	
	Pleural cavity	Pleural effusion	
Miliary tuberculosis	Throughout lungs, and possible spread to other organs	Innumerable fine discrete nodules uniformly throughout lungs	
Tuberculous pneumonia	Parenchymal and nodal	Necrotic cavities or large abscess	
Secondary tuberculosis	Upper lobes and posterior segments	Extensive fibrotic changes with possible calcification	
Tuberculoma	Any part of lung, commonly in periphery and upper lobes	Single or multiple nodules, 1-3 cm	

■ ■

ated with hilar lymph node enlargement in primary histoplasmosis. Although this pattern simulates the primary complex of tuberculosis, pleural effusion rarely occurs with histoplasmosis. In children, striking hilar adenopathy, which may cause bronchial compression, may develop without radiographic evidence of parenchymal disease. Hilar lymph node calcification commonly occurs in adults and produces a "popcorn" radiographic appearance. Pulmonary histoplasmosis frequently manifests as a solitary, sharply circumscribed, granulomatous nodule (histoplasmoma), which is usually less than 3 cm in diameter and found most often in a lower lobe. Central, rounded calcification within the mass (the target lesion) is virtually pathognomonic of this disease (Figure 2-22). Multiple soft-tissue nodules scattered throughout both lungs may simulate miliary tuberculosis. These shadows may clear completely or may fibrose and persist, often appearing on subsequent chest radiographs as widespread punctate calcifications (Figure 2-23).

Coccidioidomycosis typically produces small pulmonary consolidations in the periphery of the parenchyma resembling extensive pneumonia (Figure 2-24).

Chronic histoplasmosis and advanced chronic coccidioidomycosis closely simulate the radiographic appearance of re-infection tuberculosis, as they both commonly exhibit cavitation and are found in an upper lobe.

Treatment

Fewer than 1% of patients with primary or chronic histoplasmosis or with coccidioidomycosis require any drug treatment. Restricted activity and bed rest is encouraged. When drug treatment is required, the drug of choice is amphotericin B.

Respiratory syncytial virus

Respiratory syncytial virus (RSV) affects approximately 50% of infants, of whom about 90,000, reported in 2002, are hospitalized for treatment. Of all bronchiolitis cases, 80% occur as a result of an RSV infection. RSV attacks the lower respiratory tract and causes necrosis of the respiratory epithelium of the bronchi and bronchioles, which leads to bronchiolitis. The necrotic material and edema from the infection cause bronchial obstruction. Bronchiolitis produces bronchial spasm, and interstitial pneumonia occurs as a result of the obstruction. The patient presents with only cold or flulike symp-

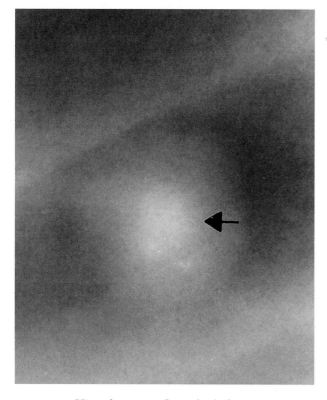

Figure 2-22   Histoplasmoma. Central calcification *(arrow)* in solitary pulmonary nodule.

Figure 2-23   Histoplasmosis. Diffuse calcifications in lungs produce snowball pattern.

Figure 2-24   Coccidioidomycosis. Posteroanterior and lateral views demonstrate consolidation caused by fungus in the left lung.

Figure 2-25 Respiratory syncytial virus. Bilateral fluffy pulmonary infiltrates, associated with hyperinflation, the features being consistent with respiratory syncytial virus pneumonia. (Courtesy Karen Brown, R.T. (R) (M), St. Joseph's Hospital and Medical Center, Phoenix, AZ.)

Summary of Findings for Pulmonary Mycosis

DISORDER	LOCATION	RADIOGRAPHIC APPEARANCE	TREATMENT
Primary histoplasmosis	Lower lung Hilar lymph nodes	Pulmonary infiltration Granulomatous nodule Hilar lymph node enlargement and/or calcification	<1% require treatment; amphotericin B Fluconazole for AIDS patients
Chronic histoplasmosis	Upper lobe	Zones of parenchymal consolidation Cavitation Calcified granulomas	<1% require treatment; amphotericin B Fluconazole for AIDS patients
Acute coccidioidomycosis	Peripheral parenchyma	Pneumonia appearance Coccidioidoma (granuloma)	None needed unless grave; amphotericin B
Chronic coccidioidomycosis	Peripheral parenchyma	Lung abscesses	None needed unless grave; amphotericin B

toms and therefore is not managed with the appropriate infection control procedures. Therefore, the virus has caused a high rate of nosocomial infection. Fomites carry the virus through droplets from the nose or throat, and the virus has the ability to persist for many hours on surfaces. Healthcare workers must use appropriate protective personal devices and dispose of them properly to protect themselves and others.

Radiographic appearance

The necrosis of the respiratory epithelium, if severe, appears radiographically as an interstitial pneumonia (Figure 2-25).

Treatment

Many children do not need drug therapy and recover simply through their immune response. Those children who require hospitalization receive antibiotics for infectious complications, and they may also be given the antiviral drug ribavirin. Most infected adults recover without treatment.

■ Diffuse Lung Disease

Chronic obstructive pulmonary disease

Chronic obstructive pulmonary disease (COPD) includes several conditions in which chronic obstruction of the airways leads to an ineffective exchange of respiratory gases and makes breathing difficult. In many cases, two disease processes coexist to cause the obstructive process. **Chronic bronchitis** is characterized by excessive tracheobronchial mucus production leading to the obstruction of small airways. **Emphysema** refers to the distention of distal air spaces as a result of the destruction of alveolar walls and the obstruction of small airways. **Asthma** occurs when

Summary of Findings for Respiratory Syncytial Virus

DISORDER	LOCATION	RADIOGRAPHIC APPEARANCE	TREATMENT
Respiratory syncytial virus	Bronchial epithelium	Interstitial pneumonia	No treatment needed in most cases Antibiotic and antiviral drugs (ribavirin)

the bronchioles go into spasm, causing decreased airflow and sometimes obstruction of the airway. Chronic dilatation of the bronchi or bronchioles indicates **bronchiectasis.** Factors that predispose to COPD include cigarette smoking, infection, air pollution, and occupational exposure to harmful substances such as asbestos.

CHRONIC BRONCHITIS

Chronic inflammation of the bronchi leads to severe coughing with the production of sputum. Bronchitis may be a complication of respiratory infection or the result of long-term exposure to air pollution or cigarette smoking. Of all chronic bronchitis cases, 90% are associated with cigarette smoking. The severity of the disease and how quickly the symptoms can be relieved is directly related to the number of cigarettes smoked.

The walls of the bronchi and bronchioles thicken and produce viscous mucus. Over an extended period, the mucous glands become hyperplastic.

Radiographic appearance

About half the patients with chronic bronchial disease demonstrate no changes on chest radiographs. The most common radiographic abnormality in chronic bronchitis is a generalized increase in bronchovascular markings ("dirty chest"), especially in the lower lungs (Figure 2-26). Thickening of bronchial walls and peribronchial inflammation can cause parallel or slightly tapered tubular line shadows ("tram lines") or may appear as thickening of bronchial shadows when viewed end on.

Eventually, excessive production of mucus and swelling of the bronchial mucosa may lead to narrowing of the airways and overinflation of the lungs (emphysema). Chest radiographs demonstrate hyperinflated lungs and a depressed diaphragm.

Treatment

In general, the treatment for chronic bronchitis is designed to improve symptoms, decrease any reversible

Figure 2-26   Chronic bronchitis. Coned view of right lower lung demonstrates an increase in coarseness in interstitial markings. Arrows point to characteristic parallel line shadows ("tram lines") outside the boundary of the pulmonary hilum. (From Eisenberg R: *Atlas of signs in radiology,* Philadelphia, 1984, Lippincott.)

processes, and prevent progression of the disease. Prophylactic antibiotic therapy reduces infections. Bronchial dilators reduce spasm and open airways. Expectorants assist in keeping the lungs clear. Although currently no cure exits, appropriate therapy can be expected to reduce severe flare-ups and minimize progression of the disease.

EMPHYSEMA

Emphysema is a crippling and debilitating condition in which obstructive and destructive changes in small airways (the acini or terminal bronchioles) lead to a dramatic increase in the volume of air in the lungs. In many patients, the development of emphysema is closely associated with heavy cigarette smoking.

Figure 2-27 Emphysema. Frontal **(A)** and lateral **(B)** projections of the chest demonstrate severe overinflation of lungs along with flattening and even a superiorly concave configuration of the hemidiaphragms. Also, the size and lucency of the retrosternal air space is increased, the AP diameter of the chest is increased, and the number and caliber of peripheral pulmonary arteries are reduced.

Other predisposing factors are chronic bronchitis, air pollution, and long-term exposure to irritants of the respiratory tract.

Irritating smoke, fumes, and pollutants injure the fine hairs (cilia) of the respiratory mucosa, which can no longer sweep away foreign particles. This causes mucosal inflammation and the secretion of excess mucus that plugs up the air passages and leads to an increase in airway resistance. Collateral air drift permits the ventilation of lung parenchyma served by the obstructed airways. Continuous bronchial narrowing and loss of elasticity, exacerbated by cigarette smoking, make it very difficult for the patient to exhale the stale air. The resulting air trapping and overinflation of the lung lead to alveolar distention and eventually to the rupture of alveolar septa. As the walls between alveoli are destroyed, these tiny air sacs become transformed into large air-filled spaces called **bullae.** With the loss of alveolar septa, the surface for gas exchange decreases, limiting the transfer of oxygen into the bloodstream. As the lungs become less efficient, the heart tries to compensate. This places excessive strain on the heart, which eventually enlarges. The large air sacs (bullae) may rupture, leading to air entering into the pleural space (spontaneous pneumothorax) and causing collapse of the lung (atelectasis).

Radiographic appearance

The major radiographic signs of emphysema are related to pulmonary overinflation, alterations in the pulmonary vasculature, and bullae formation.

The hallmark of pulmonary overinflation is flattening of the domes of the diaphragm (Figure 2-27). Another important sign seen on lateral chest radiographs is an increase in the size and lucency of the retrosternal air space, the distance between the posterior side of the sternum and the anterior wall of the ascending aorta. The anteroposterior (AP) diameter of the chest increases and the chest becomes more barrel shaped as the disease progresses. Air trapping may be detected fluoroscopically as a decrease in the normal movement of the diaphragm during respiration.

The major vascular change in patients with emphysema is a reduction in the number and size of the peripheral arteries. As the pressure in the pulmonary arteries increases, the main and central pulmonary arteries become more prominent, which further accentuates the appearance of rapid tapering of peripheral vessels.

Bullae appear as air-containing cystic spaces whose walls are usually of hairline thickness. They range in size from 1 to 2 cm in diameter up to an entire hemithorax (Figure 2-28). These large, radiolucent, air-filled sacs are found predominantly at the apices or at the bases and may become so large that they cause respiratory insufficiency by compressing the remaining relatively normal lung.

A less common radiographic appearance of emphysema is the increased-markings pattern. Instead of being narrowed, the vascular markings in this condition are more prominent than normal and tend to be irregular and indistinct, producing a "dirty chest" appearance.

Figure 2-28 Giant emphysematous bulla. Air-containing mass fills most of the left hemithorax.

Figure 2-29 Emphysematous blebs seen on CT scan show the destruction of lung parenchyma.

Emphysema occasionally occurs in young patients who have hereditary disorders of connective tissue (osteogenesis imperfecta). Striking lower lobe predominance develops in young patients who have a deficiency of the enzyme α-antitrypsin, which leads to destruction of elastic and connective tissue in the lungs.

When patients have advanced stages of pulmonary emphysema and have large amounts of air trapped in their lungs, the technologist should reduce exposure factors for chest radiography. CT demonstrates large blebs and destruction of the lung parenchyma, and it can detect any spontaneous pneumothorax (Figure 2-29).

Treatment

Currently there is no cure for emphysema. Treatment assists only in relieving symptoms and in preventing progressive destruction by the disease.

ASTHMA

Asthma is a very common disease in which widespread narrowing of the airways develops because of an increased responsiveness of the tracheobronchial tree to various stimuli (allergens). Common allergens include house dust, pollen, molds, animal dander, certain fabrics, and various foods **(extrinsic asthma)**. Exercise, heat or cold exposure, and emotional upset can also cause an asthma attack **(intrinsic asthma)**. The hypersensitivity reaction to one or more of these allergens leads to swelling of the mucous membranes of the bronchi, excess secretion of mucus, and spasm of the smooth muscle in the bronchial walls, all of which lead to severe narrowing of the airways. This makes breathing (especially expiration) difficult and results in the characteristic wheezing sound that is produced by air passing through the narrowed bronchial tubes. Untreated or uncontrolled asthma permanently scars the bronchial structure, causing progressive disease.

Radiographic appearance

Early in the course of the disease, chest radiographs obtained between acute episodes demonstrate no abnormalities. During an acute asthmatic attack, bronchial narrowing and difficulty in expiration lead to an increased volume of the hyperlucent lungs with flattening of the hemidiaphragms and an increase in the retrosternal air space. In asthma, unlike in emphysema, the pulmonary vascular markings remain normal. In patients with chronic asthma, especially those with a history of repeated episodes of superinfection, thickening of bronchial walls can produce prominence of interstitial markings and the "dirty chest" appearance (Figure 2-30). The results of the chest radiograph taken in the emergency room determine if the asthma has progressed to pneumonia.

Treatment

Those patients with allergy-induced asthma can use preventative and rescue bronchodilators. Allergy shots may build up natural antibodies. Asthmatics with exercise-induced problems may take Accolate, an oral medication to decrease bronchiomuscular spasm, in addition to preventative and rescue bronchodilators. Keeping airways open helps prevent infections, which

Figure 2-30   Asthma. Recurrent pulmonary infections have led to the development of diffuse pulmonary fibrosis and prominence of interstitial markings in lungs.

Figure 2-31   Chronic bronchiectasis. Severe coarsening of interstitial markings involves the bases and right upper lobe. Oval and circular cystic spaces, which produce a honeycomb-like pattern, are best seen in right upper lobe.

asthmatics are prone to contract. New inhaled steroid drugs help control the inflammatory process and decrease the potential for developing pulmonary infection.

BRONCHIECTASIS

Bronchiectasis refers to permanent abnormal dilatation of one or more large bronchi as a result of destruction of the elastic and muscular components of the bronchial wall. Bronchitis, a destructive process, is a common complication of bronchiectasis and is nearly always the result of a bacterial infection. The infection may be either a severe necrotizing pneumonia or a result of a local or systemic abnormality that impairs the body's defense mechanisms and promotes bacterial growth. Since the advent of antibiotic therapy and vaccines, the incidence of bronchiectasis has substantially decreased.

The patient with bronchiectasis typically has a chronic productive cough, often associated with recurrent episodes of acute pneumonia and hemoptysis. The disease usually involves the basal segments of the lower lobes, and it is bilateral in about half of the cases. Pulmonary function tests assist in the diagnostic process by determining any evidence of decreased gas exchange.

Radiographic appearance

Plain chest radiographs may show a coarseness and loss of definition of interstitial markings caused by peribronchial fibrosis and retained secretions (Figure 2-31). In more advanced disease, oval or circular cystic spaces can develop. These cystic dilatations can be up to 2 cm in diameter and often contain air–fluid levels. In very severe disease, coarse interstitial fibrosis surrounding local areas of dilatation can produce a honeycomb pattern.

Although plain radiographs may strongly indicate bronchiectasis, bronchography is necessary to fill the dilated cystic spaces with contrast material and to establish the diagnosis unequivocally (Figure 2-32).

Treatment

Vaccines prevent many of the bacterial and viral infections that led to bronchiectasis in the past. Treatment of bronchiectasis consists of therapy to decrease the symptoms and an antibiotic based on the specific bacterial cause.

Pneumoconiosis

Prolonged occupational exposure to certain irritating particulates can cause severe pulmonary disease and a spectrum of radiographic findings. Inhaled foreign substances retained permanently in the acini cause irreversible damage. These inhaled particles cause a chronic interstitial inflammation that leads to pulmonary fibrosis and a diffuse nonspecific radiographic pattern of linear streaks and nodules throughout the lungs. The inflammation initially causes injury

Figure 2-32   Chronic bronchiectasis. Bronchogram shows severe dilatation of the basal bronchi of the left lower lobe. (From Fraser RG, Paré JAP: *Diagnosis of diseases of the chest,* Philadelphia, 1979, Saunders.)

Summary of Findings for Diffuse Lung Disease

DISORDER	LOCATION	RADIOGRAPHIC APPEARANCE	TREATMENT
Chronic bronchitis	Bronchi/bronchioles Mucous gland hyperplasia	No image change in 50% Increased bronchovascular markings Hyperinflation and depressed diaphragm	Prophylactic antibiotics Bronchial dilators Expectorants No cure
Emphysema	Destroyed alveolar septa	Pulmonary hyperinflation Bulla formation Flattened diaphragm Radiolucent retrosternal space	Treat symptoms No cure
Asthma	Bronchi	No evidence unless during acute attack Bronchial narrowing/hyperlucent lungs Exclude other processes	Preventative and rescue bronchial dilators
Bronchiectasis	Basal segments of lower lobes	Coarseness and decreased interstitial markings	Antimicrobial or antibiotic drugs
Advanced bronchiectasis	Basal segments of lower lobes	Oval/circular cystic spaces	Bronchodilator to increase pulmonary function

to the mucosal lining; long-term exposure may injure the pulmonary parenchyma and even lead to the development of a malignant neoplasm. The severity of the pneumoconiosis depends on the size of the particles, the length of exposure, and the concentration of particulates in the atmosphere (type of exposure). The more severe the exposure, the more fibrotic the lung becomes and the greater the resultant shortness of breath. The most common of the pneumoconioses are silicosis, asbestosis, and anthracosis (coal worker's disease). Other causes include exposure to such dusts as tin, iron oxide, barium, and beryllium. As many as 40 minerals cause lung lesions when inhaled, although most do not cause morphologic or functional abnormalities.

SILICOSIS

Silicosis is the most common and best-known work-related lung disease. The inhalation of high concentrations of silicon dioxide (crystalline silica) primarily affects workers engaged in mining, foundry work, and sandblasting. Quartz dust, the most frequent cause of inhalation silicosis, is the second most common element in the earth's crust. The lung reacts to the silica by producing a fibroblast-stimulating factor that results in extensive fibrosis. Acute silicosis can develop within 10 months of exposure in workers exposed to sandblasting in confined spaces. Most radiographic changes are the result of 15 to 20 years of long-term, less intense exposure. As the disease process progresses, death occurs as a result of lung or heart failure.

Radiographic appearance

The classic radiographic pattern in silicosis consists of multiple nodular shadows scattered throughout the lungs. These nodules, usually fairly well circumscribed and of uniform density, may become calcified (Figure 2-33). As the pulmonary nodules increase in size, they tend to coalesce and form conglomerates of irregular masses in excess of 1 cm in diameter (progressive massive fibrosis) (Figure 2-34). These masses are usually bilateral and relatively symmetric, and they almost always occur in the upper lobes or segments of the lungs. Occasionally a single large homogeneous mass in the perihilar area of one lung may closely simulate bronchogenic carcinoma. Hilar lymph node enlargement is common. The deposition of calcium salts in the periphery of enlarged lymph nodes produces the characteristic eggshell appearance (Figure 2-35), which is virtually pathognomonic of silicosis.

ASBESTOSIS

Asbestosis may develop in improperly protected workers engaged in manufacturing asbestos products,

Figure 2-33 Silicosis. Calcification in miliary nodules is scattered throughout both lungs.

Figure 2-34 Progressive massive fibrosis in silicosis. Large, irregular nodules can be seen in both perihilar regions.

in handling building materials, or in working with insulation composed of asbestos. In the 1980s many public buildings, such as schools, with fireproof plasterboard and ceiling panels containing asbestos were reconstructed, removing the asbestos to prevent excessive public exposure to this particulate. Asbestos particles occur as long, thin fibers that cause little dust but produce major fibrosis in the lung. The disease presents as alveolitis, with asbestos deposits at the bifurcation of the alveolar ducts. These deposits activate the fibrogenic and growth factors and result in extensive

Figure 2-35 Silicosis. Chest tomogram demonstrates the characteristic eggshell lymph-node calcification associated with bilateral perihilar masses.

Figure 2-37 Asbestosis. CT scan shows calcified pleural plaques along lateral and posterior chest wall *(open arrows)* and adjacent to heart *(solid arrow)*.

Figure 2-36 Asbestosis. Frontal film shows en face pleural calcifications on right *(arrowheads)*, linear calcifications in profile in mediastinal reflection of pleura on right and in pericardium on left *(horizontal arrows)*, and linear calcification in left diaphragmatic pleura *(vertical arrow)*. (From Sargent EN, Jacobson G, Gordonson JS: *Semin Roentgenol* 12:287-297, 1977.)

fibrosis. The major complication of asbestosis is mesothelioma, a highly malignant pleural tumor.

Radiographic appearance

The radiographic hallmark of asbestosis is involvement of the pleura. Initially, pleural thickening appears as linear plaques of opacification, which are most often along the lower chest wall and diaphragm. Calcification of the pleural plaques is virtually pathognomonic of asbestosis, especially when the calcified plaques appear in the form of thin, curvilinear densities conforming to the upper surfaces of the diaphragm bilaterally (Figure 2-36). This pleural calcification generally does not develop until at least 20 years after the first exposure to asbestos (Figure 2-37). High-resolution CT best demonstrates the developing pleural plaques.

In the lungs, round or irregular opacities produce a combined linear and nodular pattern that may obscure the heart border, producing the so-called shaggy heart. Pleural mesothelioma appears as an irregular scalloped or nodular density within the pleural space. It is frequently associated with a large pleural effusion that may obscure the underlying tumor. CT demonstrates the precise tumor involvement of the lung tissue. In addition to mesothelioma, bronchogenic carcinoma is also unusually common in patients with asbestosis, especially those who are cigarette smokers.

ANTHRACOSIS (COAL WORKER'S PNEUMOCONIOSIS)

Coal miners, especially those working with anthracite (hard coal), have increased susceptibility to developing pneumoconiosis by inhaling high concentrations of coal dust. Anthracite collects in the walls of the respiratory bronchioles, causing weakened musculature

Figure 2-38 Coal worker's pneumoconiosis. Diffuse reticular pattern throughout both lungs is associated with ill-defined masses of fibrous tissue in the perihilar region that extend to the right base.

■ ■

Summary of Findings for Pneumoconiosis

DISORDER	LOCATION	RADIOGRAPHIC APPEARANCE	TREATMENT
Silicosis	Most often upper lobes Lung parenchyma	Multiple, well-defined, scattered nodules of uniform density	For all cases of pneumoconiosis:
Asbestosis	Pleural lining	Pleural thickening with calcified plaques	Prevent further exposure Breathe clean air
Anthracosis	Throughout lungs	Multiple less-well-defined nodules of granular density	Treat complications

■ ■

and dilatation. The deposition of anthracite particles changes the lung tissue to a dark color, leading to the term *black lung.*

Radiographic appearance

Initially, multiple small, irregular opacities produce a reticular pattern similar to that of silicosis (Figure 2-38). However, the nodules tend to be somewhat less well defined than those of silicosis, and they tend to have a granular density unlike the homogeneous density of silicosis nodules. With advanced disease, the pattern of progressive massive fibrosis can develop. In progressive massive fibrosis, one or more masses of fibrous tissue with smooth, well-defined lateral borders gradually migrate toward the hilum, leaving a zone of overinflated emphysematous lung between the fibrous mass and the chest wall. A single large ho-

mogeneous mass in the perihilar area of one lung may simulate bronchogenic carcinoma; an occupational history is necessary to make the proper diagnosis of pneumoconiosis.

Treatment

Today, there is no effective treatment for pneumoconiosis. Once the particles have embedded in the pulmonary tissue, the lungs deteriorate and lose the ability to remove them. The best available treatment is simply to avoid further exposure. Breathing clean air may assist in halting progression of the disease and reducing the severity of the symptoms. Treatment is limited to addressing complications of the disease. Patients who progress from asbestosis to mesothelioma may require lung resection to remove the cancerous tissue, radiation therapy to shrink the tumor, or chemotherapy.

Figure 2-39 Benign solitary pulmonary nodule (tuberculoma). Notice central calcification characteristic of this benign lesion.

Figure 2-40 Malignant solitary pulmonary nodule (bronchogenic carcinoma). Notice fuzzy, ill-defined margins.

■ Neoplasms

Solitary pulmonary nodule

The asymptomatic solitary pulmonary nodule seen as an incidental finding on a screening chest radiograph poses a diagnostic dilemma, since it could represent a benign granuloma or neoplastic process, a primary bronchogenic carcinoma, or a solitary metastasis. In persons under the age of 30, a small, round, sharply defined solitary pulmonary nodule is associated with a minimal risk of cancer (less than 1%). However, this risk rises to about 15% in individuals between the ages of 30 and 45, and to approximately 50% in those older than age 50.

Radiographic appearance

The presence of central dense or popcorn calcification is diagnostic of a benign process, and a low kilovolts-peak technique may be required to demonstrate the calcification to best advantage (Figure 2-39). Another sign of benignancy is the absence of growth of the lesion on serial chest films over 2 years (therefore comparison films must be eagerly sought).

A CT scan can demonstrate the size, density, position, and borders of the lesion, which helps determine the diagnosis. Although malignant tumors generally have ill-defined, irregular, or fuzzy borders (Figure 2-40) in contrast to the sharp margins of benign lesions (Figure 2-41), there are many exceptions to this rule. CT may best differentiate the smooth, sharp margins of a benign tumor (Figure 2-42) from the spiculated, ill-defined contour of a malignant nodule (Figure 2-43).

The growth rate (or doubling time) of a solitary pulmonary nodule has been used to determine the likelihood of its being malignant. A pulmonary nodule that doubles in volume in less than 1 month or more than 18 months is usually benign. However, the overlapping of growth rates of benign and malignant lesions, particularly among rapidly growing nodules, makes the use of doubling time unreliable as an absolute indicator of malignancy. In the patient older than 35 to 40 years of age, a solitary pulmonary nodule should be resected unless it can be unequivocally demonstrated to be benign. If the diagnosis is equivocal, CT is required. This modality may demonstrate additional nodules not visible on plain chest radiography (suggesting metastases), or it may detect hilar or mediastinal metastases (indicating a malignant process). Positron emission tomography (PET) may be employed to show increased metabolic activity of the lesion suggestive of malignancy (Figure 2-44). At times, percutaneous fine-needle aspiration biopsy (FNAB) may be required to provide a definitive diagnosis (Figure 2-45).

Bronchial adenoma

Bronchial adenomas are neoplasms of low-grade malignancy that constitute about 1% of all bronchial neoplasms. They are equally common in men and women. Bronchial adenomas appear in a younger age-group than bronchogenic carcinoma. Hemoptysis and recurring pneumonia are the most common presenting symptoms. They arise in the same glandular structures in the bronchi in which malignant neoplasms develop.

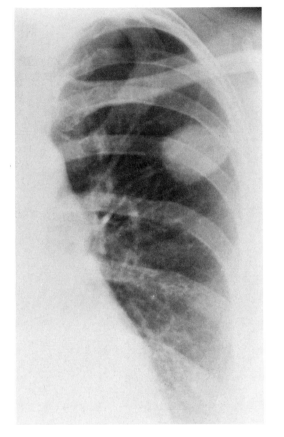

Figure 2-41　Benign solitary pulmonary nodule (tuberculoma). Notice sharp, well-defined borders of this left upper lobe mass.

Figure 2-42　Benign solitary pulmonary nodule (granuloma). CT scan demonstrates a discrete homogenous lobulated mass in the left lung periphery.

Figure 2-43　Malignant solitary pulmonary nodule (adenocarcinoma). CT scan demonstrates spiculated, ill-defined contour mass.

Figure 2-44   Pulmonary metastases. Images from PET with fluorodeoxyglucose (FDG) reveal foci demonstrating metastases. **A,** Intense radionuclide-labeled foci in each perihilar region. **B,** The posterior mediastinal focus was identified in conjunction with additional bilateral perihilar radionuclide-labeled foci. **C,** The thoracic vertebral radionuclide-labeled foci were identified in conjunction with a posterior right upper lobe focus that demonstrated a positive finding, noted by arrows on each image. PET confirmed the presence of metastasis; the patient was referred to the medical oncologist for consideration of chemotherapy.

Figure 2-45   CT-guided FNAB of peripheral lung nodule in left lower lobe. CT scan demonstrates the needle position. Cells were sent for cytologic testing, and the results indicated infiltrating, poorly differentiated adenocarcinoma.

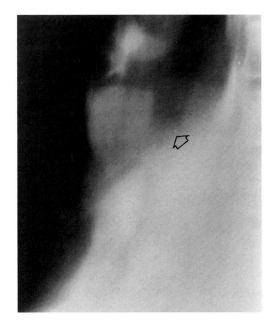

Figure 2-46   Central bronchial adenoma. Tomogram shows ill-defined mass causing high-grade obstruction of right lower lobe bronchus *(arrow)*.

Radiographic appearance

About 80% of bronchial adenomas occur centrally in major or segmental bronchi and cause obstruction. The most common radiographic findings are peripheral atelectasis and pneumonitis due to bronchial obstruction. This characteristically produces a homogeneous increase in density corresponding exactly to a lobe or one or more segments, usually with a substantial loss of volume. If large enough, a central bronchial adenoma that has caused peripheral atelectasis and pneumonia may be identifiable as a discrete, lobulated, soft-tissue mass. A tumor too small to obstruct the lumen may not be detectable on the chest radiograph. Tomography may demonstrate the rounded tumor mass within an air-filled bronchus (Figure 2-46). Peripheral bronchial adenomas do not cause bronchial obstruction and appear as nonspecific solitary pulmonary nodules (Figure 2-47).

Bronchogenic carcinoma

Primary carcinoma of the lung arises from the mucosa of the bronchial tree. The most common primary malignant lung neoplasm is bronchogenic carcinoma. Although its precise cause remains unknown, bronchogenic carcinoma has been closely linked to smoking and to the inhalation of cancer-causing agents (carcinogens) such as air pollution, exhaust gases, and industrial fumes. A major form of bronchogenic carcinoma is the solitary pulmonary nodule within the lung parenchyma.

Figure 2-47   Peripheral bronchial adenoma. Nonspecific solitary pulmonary nodule at the left base.

The most common type of lung cancer is **squamous carcinoma**, which typically arises in the major central bronchi and causes gradual narrowing of the bronchial lumen. **Adenocarcinomas** usually arise in the periphery of the lung rather than in the larger central bronchi. The least common type of lung tumor is **bronchiolar (alveolar cell) carcinoma.** Non–small cell lung cancers (i.e., the three types of lung cancer just listed) make up 80% of all lung cancers. **Small cell (oat cell) carcinomas** characteristically cause bulky enlargement of hilar lymph nodes, often bilaterally, and are responsible for the remaining 20% of primary pulmonary malignancies.

Although bronchogenic carcinoma may be diagnosed by detection of cancer cells in the sputum, a precise diagnosis usually requires biopsy of the tumor during bronchoscopy (i.e., direct visualization of the tracheobronchial tree using a tube inserted through the nose) or a needle biopsy in the radiology department under CT or fluoroscopic guidance.

Radiographic appearance

Bronchogenic carcinoma produces a broad spectrum of radiographic abnormalities that depend on the site of the tumor and its relationship to the bronchial tree. The tumor may appear as a discrete mass, or it may be undetectable and identified only by virtue of secondary changes resulting from an obstruction caused by the tumor within or compressing the bronchus.

Airway obstruction by bronchogenic carcinoma may cause atelectasis of a segment of lung and often leads to pneumonia that develops in the lung distal to the obstructed bronchus. An important radiographic sign differentiating this postobstructive pneumonia from simple inflammatory disease is the absence of an air bronchogram in the former, because the air bronchogram can be detected only if there is an open airway leading to the area of consolidation.

Unilateral enlargement of the hilum, best appreciated on serial chest radiographs, may be the earliest sign of bronchogenic carcinoma. The enlarged hilum represents either a primary carcinoma arising in the major hilar bronchus or metastases to enlarged pulmonary lymph nodes from a small primary lesion elsewhere in the lung (Figure 2-48). CT is far superior to plain radiographs in detecting hilar and mediastinal lymphadenopathy and bronchial narrowing resulting from bronchogenic carcinoma.

Cavitation commonly occurs in bronchogenic carcinoma. It most often involves upper lung lesions and represents central necrosis of the neoplasm. The cavities usually resemble acute lung abscesses and have thick walls with irregular, often nodular, inner surfaces (Figure 2-49).

Bronchiolar (alveolar cell) carcinoma has a spectrum of appearances, which can vary from a well-circumscribed, peripheral solitary nodule to a poorly defined mass simulating pneumonia or multiple nodules scattered throughout both lungs.

Treatment of pulmonary neoplastic diseases

For **bronchial adenomas**, the most common treatment involves surgical resection of the lobe.

Figure 2-48   Bronchogenic carcinoma. Tomography demonstrates bilateral bulky hilar adenopathy typical of oat cell carcinoma.

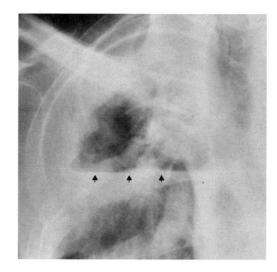

Figure 2-49   Bronchogenic carcinoma. Large cavitary right upper lobe mass with air-fluid level *(arrows)* and associated rib destruction.

The prognosis of **bronchogenic carcinoma** is poor, except when the tumor is in the form of a solitary pulmonary nodule that can be surgically removed. Direct lymphatic spread of a tumor can cause enlargement of hilar or mediastinal lymph nodes (Figure 2-50). Distant metastases most frequently involve the bones, where they cause osteolytic destruction. Metastases to the liver, brain, and adrenal glands commonly develop.

Squamous carcinoma, adenocarcinoma, and **bronchioalveolar carcinoma** grow more slowly than small cell carcinomas. Surgical resection has a cure rate of

Figure 2-50   Spread of bronchogenic carcinoma to mediastinum. **A,** CT scan shows enlarged lymph node *(n)* in pretracheal region, a finding consistent with the diagnosis of unresectable mediastinal spread. **B,** In another patient, CT scan shows obliteration of fat plane around descending aorta *(DA)* by adjacent neoplasm *(N)*. In addition, tumor extends deep into the mediastinum *(arrowheads)* behind the left main-stem bronchus and in front of the descending aorta. (From Lee JKT, Sagel SS, Stanley RJ, editors: *Computed body tomography,* New York, 1989, Raven Press.)

about 10%. Radiation therapy (which has a low cure rate) and chemotherapy are generally used for palliative treatment.

Pulmonary metastases

Up to one third of patients with cancer develop pulmonary metastases; in about half of these patients, the only demonstrable metastases are confined to the lungs. Pulmonary metastases may develop from hematogenous or lymphatic spread, most commonly from musculoskeletal sarcomas, myeloma, and carcinomas of the breast, urogenital tract, thyroid, and colon. Carcinomas of the breast, esophagus, or stomach may directly extend to involve the lungs because of anatomic proximity. Primary lung lesions may metastasize by spread through the bronchial tree.

Radiographic appearance

Hematogenous metastases typically appear radiographically as multiple, relatively well circumscribed, round or oval nodules throughout the lungs (Figure 2-51). The pattern may vary from fine miliary nodules (Figure 2-52) produced by highly vascular tumors (e.g., kidney or thyroid gland carcinomas, sarcoma of bone, trophoblastic disease) to huge, well-defined masses (cannonball lesions) caused by metastatic sarcomas. Carcinoma of the thyroid gland typically causes a snowstorm of metastatic deposits yet radiographically remains unchanged for a prolonged period because of a very low grade of malignancy.

Figure 2-51   Hematogenous metastases. Multiple, well-circumscribed nodules scattered diffusely throughout both lungs.

Solitary metastases, which occur in about 25% of cases, may be indistinguishable from primary bronchogenic carcinomas or benign granulomas (Figure 2-53). In such cases, CT may permit the detection of additional pulmonary masses that cannot be seen on standard chest radiographs but aid in determining the choice of treatment. The emerging technology of PET

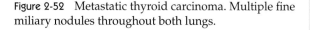

Figure 2-52   *Metastatic thyroid carcinoma. Multiple fine miliary nodules throughout both lungs.*

Figure 2-53   Pulmonary metastases. **A,** Solitary metastasis *(arrow).* **B,** Repeat examination 5 months later shows rapid growth of previous solitary nodule *(white arrow).* Second huge nodule *(black arrows)* was not appreciated on previous examination because it projected below the right hemidiaphragm.

scanning, which images cellular activity, has been used in the search for metastases when CT is inconclusive, as well as in determining whether a solitary pulmonary nodule is benign (when PET detects low cellular activity) or malignant (when PET detects high cellular activity) (Figure 2-54). Lymphangitic metastatic spread throughout the lungs is most commonly

a complication of carcinoma of the breast, stomach, thyroid, pancreas, larynx, cervix, or prostate. The radiographic appearance consists of coarsened interstitial markings that have an irregular contour and are poorly defined (Figure 2-55). These coarsened markings are most prominent in the lower lobes and may simulate interstitial pulmonary edema.

Figure 2-54   Non–small cell carcinoma. PET lung scan performed for initial staging. Following the injection of FDG, metabolically active metastases are suggested in the left hilum with lymphatic involvement (B) and in the right adrenal gland with hepatic involvement (A).

Figure 2-55 Lymphangitic metastases. Coarsened bronchovascular markings of irregular contour and poor definition are seen on the chest radiograph in this patient with metastatic carcinoma of stomach.

Summary of Findings for Pulmonary Neoplasms

DISORDER	LOCATION	RADIOGRAPHIC APPEARANCE	TREATMENT
Solitary pulmonary nodule	Throughout lungs	Solitary nodule Dense or popcorn calcification—benign Continued growth—malignancy	Depends on diagnosis (benign or malignant)
Bronchial adenoma	Glandular structure of major/segmental bronchi	Peripheral atelectasis (obstruction) Obstructive pneumonia	Surgical resection
Bronchogenic Carcinoma	Lung parenchyma	• Solitary lesion, ill-defined • Atelectasis with obstruction • Hilar enlargement • Cavitation in upper lung	Surgical resection (cure) Radiation therapy (cure and palliative) Chemotherapy (palliative)
Pulmonary metastases	Throughout lungs	Multiple nodules, sharp margins Miliary/snowstorm nodules Solitary nodule Coarsened interstitial markings	All treatments palliative Surgical resection Radiation therapy Chemotherapy

Treatment

The treatment of pulmonary metastases includes surgical resection, radiation therapy, and chemotherapy; however, these serve only a palliative purpose.

■ Vascular Diseases

Pulmonary embolism

Pulmonary embolism, a potentially fatal condition, is by far the most common pathologic process involving the lungs of hospitalized patients. In about 80% of patients with this disorder, the condition does not cause symptoms and thus remains unrecognized because the emboli are too small or too few to occlude blood flow to a substantial portion of the lung. Even when symptomatic, pulmonary embolism may be difficult to diagnose. More than 95% of pulmonary emboli arise from thrombi that develop in the deep venous system of the lower extremities because of venous stasis. The remainder come from thrombi that occur in the right side of the heart or in brachial or cervical veins and are trapped by the capillaries in the pulmonary artery circulation. Thrombi originating in the left side of the heart can embolize to the peripheral systemic arterial circulation, where they are trapped in the arterioles or capillaries before they can

Figure 2-56 Pulmonary embolism. Frontal **(A)** and lateral **(B)** projections of the chest demon-strate fairly well circumscribed shadow of homogeneous density occupying the posterior seg-ment of the right lower lobe. On lateral projection, the pleural-based density has the shape of a truncated cone and is convex toward the hilum (Hampton's hump; *arrow*). (From Fraser RG, Paré JAP: *Diagnosis of diseases of the chest,* Philadelphia, 1978, Saunders.)

return in the venous blood to the heart and the pul-monary circulation. Most embolic occlusions occur in the lower lobes because of the preferential blood flow to these regions.

The physiologic consequences of embolic occlusion of the pulmonary arteries depend on the size of the embolic mass and the general state of the pulmonary circulation. In young persons with good cardiovascu-lar function and adequate collateral circulation, the oc-clusion of a large central vessel may cause minimal, if any, functional impairment. In contrast, in patients with cardiovascular disease or severe debilitating ill-nesses, pulmonary vascular occlusion often leads to infarction.

Radiographic appearance

For most patients with thromboembolism without in-farction, the findings on the chest radiograph are nor-mal. Nevertheless, some subtle yet distinctive abnor-malities on plain radiographs can be strongly suggestive of this diagnosis. A large-vessel pulmonary embolism causes a focal reduction in blood volume without a sub-stantial change in air or tissue volume. This leads to fo-cal pulmonary oligemia and relative lucency of the in-volved portion of lung. Another sign of pulmonary embolism is enlargement of the ipsilateral main pul-monary artery caused by distention of the vessel by the bulk of the thrombus. Serial radiographs may demon-strate progressive enlargement of the affected vessel.

Pulmonary embolism with infarction appears radio-graphically as an area of lung consolidation. A highly characteristic, though somewhat uncommon, appear-ance of pulmonary infarction is the so-called Hamp-ton's hump (Figure 2-56). This pleura-based, wedge-shaped density has a rounded apex and is most commonly seen at the base of the lung, often in the costophrenic sulcus. In many instances an infarction merely produces a nonspecific parenchymal density that simulates acute pneumonia. A pleural effusion of-ten develops (Figure 2-57).

Because the findings on the chest radiograph are usually either normal or nonspecific, the radionuclide lung scan (or ventilation–perfusion ratio [V/Q] scan) is generally considered the most effective screening procedure for significant pulmonary embolism. On a radionuclide perfusion scan that measures blood flow to the lungs, the area of lung distal to an embolus ap-pears as a defect (Figure 2-58). Unfortunately, false-positive scan results may be recorded in portions of the lung that are poorly perfused because of impaired ventilation, even if no obstructing vascular lesion is present. Therefore ventilation lung scans are also per-formed to increase the diagnostic accuracy. The results of the ventilation scan are usually relatively normal in patients with pulmonary embolism, whereas they generally demonstrate defects corresponding to areas of decreased perfusion in patients with chronic pul-monary disease.

Figure 2-57 Pulmonary embolism. Plain chest radiograph demonstrates atelectasis at the right base; this is associated with elevation of the right hemidiaphragm and represents a large subpulmonic effusion.

Figure 2-58 Pulmonary embolism. **A,** Normal radionuclide perfusion lung scan with uniform uptake in both lungs. **B,** A different patient with multiple wedge-shaped areas without isotope uptake *(arrows).*

Continued

Figure 2-58, cont'd **C**, CT scan (correlating with lung scan in **B**) demonstrates pulmonary emboli in both right and left pulmonary arteries. Note that the emboli are connected—a "saddle" embolus.

Figure 2-59 Pulmonary embolism. A filling defect of the right pulmonary artery demonstrated on a high-resolution spiral CT scan.

High-resolution CT has now replaced lung scanning in many institutions as the preferred imaging modality for detecting and excluding pulmonary emboli. Following the injection of a contrast agent, cross-sectional images of the lung are obtained from the base of the heart to the top of the aortic arch. CT demonstrates pulmonary embolus either as a filling defect within the pulmonary artery (Figure 2-59) or as an abrupt cutoff indicating complete obstruction of a pulmonary vessel (Figure 2-60).

Pulmonary arteriography is the definitive technique for evaluating the patient with suspected pulmonary embolism (Figure 2-61). However, this invasive procedure carries a small but definite risk of morbidity and mortality. The unequivocal arteriographic diagnosis of pulmonary embolism requires the demonstration of an abrupt occlusion (cutoff) of a pulmonary artery or a persistent intraluminal filling defect within it. More recently, magnetic resonance imaging has been used to show a pulmonary embolus either as a moderate- to high-intensity signal within the black flow void of the normal pulmonary artery or as a generalized increased signal intensity caused by slow blood flow in an obstructed pulmonary vessel.

Treatment

The first line of treatment is anticoagulant therapy, which limits the extent of infarction of the affected lung tissue and decreases the likelihood of more emboli to the lung. The patient may be required to take the anticoagulants for an extended period. If the patient does not respond to anticoagulant therapy, thrombolytics can assist in dissolving the emboli. In

A   **B**

Figure 2-60   Pulmonary embolism. **A,** CT scan illustrates a filling defect in the right main pulmonary artery on a 41-year-old woman. **B,** The patient also has a thrombus located in the ascending aorta and aortic arch.

Figure 2-61   Pulmonary arteriogram shows virtually complete obstruction *(arrows)* of the right pulmonary artery.

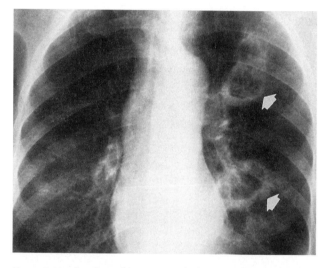

Figure 2-62   Septic pulmonary emboli. Large cavitary lesions *(arrows)* in the left lung of an intravenous drug abuser with septic thrombophlebitis.

patients with large clot burdens, thrombolytic therapy may be the first line of treatment. The most invasive treatment is the placement of a filter in the vena cava, which is indicated if the anticoagulant or thrombolytic therapy is contraindicated or ineffective.

Septic embolism

Septic embolism refers to a shower of bacteria that enter the pulmonary circulation and remain trapped within the lung. Septic emboli arise primarily from either the heart (bacterial endocarditis) or the peripheral veins (septic thrombophlebitis). Many patients have a clinical history of intravenous drug abuse.

Radiographic appearance

Septic emboli, almost always multiple, appear radiographically as ill-defined, round or wedge-shaped opacities in the periphery of the lung. They often present a migratory pattern, first appearing in one area and then in another as the older lesions resolve. Cavitation frequently develops (Figure 2-62).

Treatment

Patients with septic embolism require regimented doses of antibiotics to destroy the underlying bacterial infection.

Pulmonary arteriovenous fistula

Pulmonary arteriovenous fistula is an abnormal vascular communication from a pulmonary artery to a pulmonary vein. Pulmonary arteriovenous fistulas are multiple in about one third of patients; up to two thirds of patients with these pulmonary malformations have similar arteriovenous communications elsewhere (hereditary hemorrhagic telangiectasia). Very large or multiple fistulas can cause so much shunting of blood from the pulmonary arteries to the pulmonary veins that the blood cannot be adequately oxygenated and cyanosis results.

Radiographic appearance

A pulmonary arteriovenous fistula typically appears as a round or oval, lobulated soft-tissue mass that is most commonly situated in the lower lobes. A pathognomonic finding is a feeding artery and a draining vein (Figure 2-63, *A*). This may be difficult to demonstrate on plain radiographs and often requires tomography or angiography (Figure 2-63, *B*).

Treatment

Prior to surgical removal, a pulmonary angiogram can confirm the diagnosis and detect smaller, unsuspected vascular malformations that cannot be identified on routine radiographs. Another treatment for arteriovenous fistula is the placement of a detachable balloon (embolization) to block the flow of blood through the fistulous connection.

■ Miscellaneous Lung Disorders

Atelectasis

Atelectasis refers to a condition in which there is diminished air within the lung associated with reduced lung volume. Most commonly this results from bronchial obstruction, which may be attributable to a neoplasm, foreign body (e.g., peanut, coin, or tooth), or mucous plug. Mucoid obstruction may be attributable to an excessive secretion in patients with chronic bronchitis, or it may be a complication of abdominal surgery. As a result of surgery, mucus collects in the bronchi because of the irritative effect of anesthesia. Normal coughing, which would mobilize the secretions, is decreased because of the pain of the abdominal wound. Compression of the lung by pneu-

Figure 2-63 Pulmonary arteriovenous fistula. **A,** Radiographic film of right lung shows round soft-tissue mass *(straight arrows)* at the base. Feeding and draining vessels *(curved arrows)* extend to the lesion. **B,** Arteriogram clearly shows feeding artery and draining veins *(solid arrows)* associated with arteriovenous malformation *(open arrow).*

mothorax, pleural fluid, a tumor, a lung abscess, or a large emphysematous bulla may result in atelectasis. Regardless of the precise cause, air cannot enter that part of the lung supplied by the obstructed bronchus. As the air trapped in the lung is absorbed into the bloodstream, the lung collapses.

An important iatrogenic cause of atelectasis is the improper placement of an endotracheal tube below the level of the tracheal bifurcation. Because of geometric factors, the endotracheal tube tends to enter the right main-stem bronchus, effectively blocking the left bronchial tree and causing collapse of part or all of the left lung (Figure 2-64).

Radiographic appearance

The most common radiographic sign of atelectasis is a local increase in density caused by the airless lung,

Summary of Findings for Pulmonary Vascular Diseases

DISORDER	LOCATION	RADIOGRAPHIC APPEARANCE	TREATMENT
Pulmonary embolism	Most often lower lobes	Serial films demonstrating progressive enlargement of the affected vessel	Anticoagulants Thrombolytics Vena cava filter placement
Septic embolism	Lung periphery	Peripheral opacities	Regimented antibiotics until bacterial infection eradicated
Pulmonary arteriovenous fistula	Most often lower lobes	Defined soft-tissue mass	Surgical removal Embolization

Figure 2-64   Malpositioned endotracheal tube. Excessively low position of endotracheal tube in the bronchus intermedius causes collapse of right upper lobe and entire left lung.

Figure 2-65   Platelike atelectasis. Horizontal linear streaks of opacity (*arrows*) can be seen in lower portions of both lungs.

Figure 2-66   Right middle lobe and lingular collapse. **A,** Frontal chest radiograph demonstrates obliteration of right and left borders of the heart. **B,** Lateral projection demonstrates collapse of right middle lobe and lingula (*arrows*).

which may vary from thin platelike streaks (Figure 2-65) to lobar collapse (Figure 2-66). An important direct sign of atelectasis is displacement of interlobar fissures, which shift and become bowed, conforming to the contour of the collapsed segment. Indirect signs of atelectasis reflect an attempt by the remaining lung to compensate for the loss of the collapsed portion. These signs include elevation of the ipsilateral hemidiaphragm; displacement of the heart, mediastinum, and hilum toward the atelectatic segment; and compensatory overinflation of the remainder of the ipsilateral lung.

Treatment

The goal of the treatment of atelectasis is the removal of pulmonary secretions and reexpansion of the affected lung tissue. To accomplish this, positioning or incentive spirometry is employed. Positioning uses gravity to assist in expanding the affected lung tissue, and incentive spirometry directly increases lung volume by positive pressure.

Adult respiratory distress syndrome

The term **adult respiratory distress syndrome (ARDS)** describes a clinical picture of severe, unexpected, and life-threatening acute respiratory distress that develops in patients who have a variety of medical and surgical disorders but no major underlying lung disease. As it occurs most commonly in patients with nonthoracic trauma who develop hypotension and shock, it is often called "shock lung." Other conditions that may lead to ARDS include severe pulmonary infection, aspiration or inhalation of toxins and irritants, and drug overdose. Regardless of the cause, the structure of the lung completely breaks down, leading to massive leakage of cells and fluid into the interstitial and alveolar spaces. The structural breakdown results in severe hypoxemia caused by a pronounced respiratory impairment in the ability to oxygenate blood.

Radiographic appearance

Patchy, ill-defined areas of alveolar consolidation are scattered throughout both lungs (Figure 2-67). Unlike pulmonary edema caused by heart failure, in ARDS the size of the heart usually remains normal, and there is no evidence of redistribution of blood flow to the upper zones.

Treatment

The hypoxemia in ARDS may be fatal, even with intensive medical therapy. Drug treatment may consist of diuretics to decrease the fluid load and possible fluid build-up in the lung tissue. Oxygen therapy and ventilation may assist the patient in breathing, which helps prevent further capillary and alveolar destruction. Continuous positive-pressure ventilation may

Figure 2-67   ARDS. Ill-defined areas of alveolar consolidation scattered throughout the lungs.

cause air to enter the interstitium of the lung and lead to pneumothorax and pneumomediastinum. Diffuse interstitial and patchy air-space fibrosis may produce a coarse reticular pattern. If the patient recovers completely, the radiographic abnormalities may clear completely, and there may be only a mild decrease in pulmonary function.

Intrabronchial foreign bodies

The aspiration of solid foreign bodies into the tracheobronchial tree occurs almost exclusively in young children. Although some foreign bodies are radiopaque and easily detected on plain chest radiographs, most aspirated foreign bodies are not opaque and can be diagnosed only by observation of secondary signs in the lungs caused by partial or complete bronchial obstruction. Obstruction almost always involves the lower lobes, the right more often than the left.

Radiographic appearance

The complete obstruction of a major bronchus leads to resorption of trapped air, alveolar collapse, and atelectasis of the involved segment or lobe. Extensive volume loss causes a shift of the heart and mediastinal structures toward the affected side along with elevation of the ipsilateral hemidiaphragm and narrowing of the intercostal spaces.

Partial bronchial obstruction may produce air trapping as a result of a check-valve phenomenon. Air freely passes the partial obstruction during inspiration but remains trapped distally as the bronchus contracts normally during expiration (Figure 2-68). Hyperaeration of the affected lobes causes a shift of the heart and mediastinum toward the normal, contralateral side. This finding is accentuated during

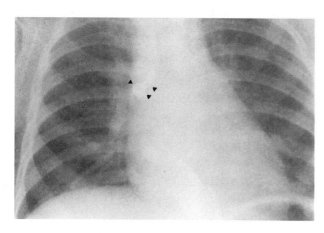

Figure 2-68   Intrabronchial foreign body. A nail *(arrows)* lies in the right main-stem bronchus. (From Cappitanio MA et al: *Radiology* 103:460-461, 1972.)

Figure 2-69   Mediastinal emphysema. Mediastinal pleura is displaced laterally and appears as a long linear opacity *(arrows)* parallel to the heart border but separated from it by gas.

forced expiration because the hyperaerated segment does not contract. This classic appearance of partial bronchial obstruction is dramatically demonstrated with fluoroscopy as the mediastinum shifts away from the affected side during deep expiration and returns toward the midline on full inspiration.

A malpositioned endotracheal tube can act as an intrabronchial foreign body. The tube tends to extend down the right main-stem bronchus, causing hyperlucency of the right lung and obstructive atelectasis of the left lung.

Treatment

The treatment of intrabronchial foreign bodies includes expectoration, intervention, and surgery. The simplest is expectoration, which requires the patient to cough hard enough to dislodge the foreign body and spit it out. More invasive interventional techniques employ a bronchoscope to retrieve the object blocking the airway. The most invasive procedure is direct surgical removal of the foreign body.

Mediastinal emphysema (pneumomediastinum)

Air within the mediastinal space may appear spontaneously, or it may result from chest trauma, from perforation of the esophagus or tracheobronchial tree, or from the spread of air along fascial planes in the neck, peritoneal cavity, or retroperitoneal space. Spontaneous pneumomediastinum usually results from a sudden rise in intraalveolar pressure (because of, e.g., severe coughing, vomiting, or straining) that causes alveolar rupture and the dissection of air along blood vessels in the interstitial space to the hilum and mediastinum. Air may also extend peripherally and rupture into the pleural space, causing an associated pneumothorax.

Radiographic appearance

On frontal chest radiographs, air causes lateral displacement of the mediastinal pleura, which appears as a long linear opacity that runs parallel to the heart border but is separated from it by the air (i.e., the bronchovascular sheath) (Figure 2-69). On lateral projections, air is typically seen to have collected behind the sternum, extending in streaks downward and anterior to the heart. Chest radiographs may also demonstrate air outlining the pulmonary arterial trunk and aorta, as well as dissecting into the soft tissues of the neck.

In infants, mediastinal air causes elevation of the thymus. Loculated air confined to one side produces an appearance similar to that of a windblown sail. Bilateral mediastinal air elevates both thymic lobes to produce an angel-wings configuration (Figure 2-70).

Subcutaneous emphysema

Subcutaneous emphysema is caused by penetrating or blunt injuries that disrupt the lung and parietal pleura and force air into the tissues of the chest wall. When palpating the skin, one might hear or feel crepitation (a crackling sound or sensation).

Radiographic appearance

The radiographic appearance is bizarre, with streaks of lucency outlining muscle bundles (Figure 2-71).

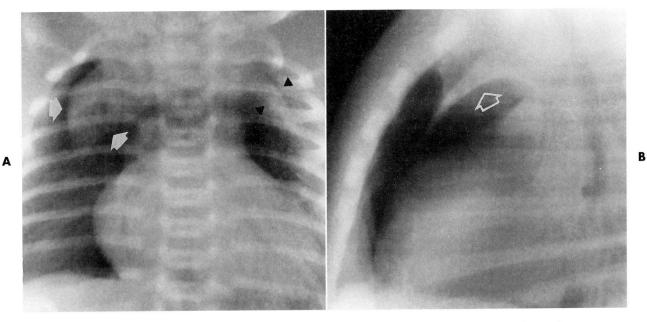

A

B

Figure 2-70 Mediastinal emphysema in an infant. **A,** Elevation of both lobes of thymus by mediastinal air *(arrows)* produces angel-wings sign. **B,** Lateral projection shows mediastinal air lifting thymus off pericardium and great vessels *(arrows* and *arrowheads).* (From Eisenberg R: *Atlas of signs in radiology,* Philadelphia, 1984, Lippincott.)

Figure 2-71 Subcutaneous emphysema. Frontal chest radiograph of severely injured patient shows streaks and bubbles of subcutaneous air *(black arrows)* in soft tissues along lateral borders of thorax, as well as broad lucencies outlining muscle bundles *(open arrows)* overlying the anterior chest wall. Note fracture of left scapula *(white arrows)* and multiple rib fractures.

Treatment of mediastinal and subcutaneous emphysema

If the emphysema appears minimal and does not progress, no treatment may be needed. If the air in the mediastinum or subcutaneous tissue does not absorb, or if it increases in amount, surgical resection to block off the source of air may be required.

■ Disorders of the Pleura

Pneumothorax

Pneumothorax, the presence of air in the pleural cavity, results in a partial or complete collapse of the lung (Figure 2-72). It most commonly results from rupture of a subpleural bulla, either as a complication of emphysema or as a spontaneous event in an otherwise healthy young adult. Other causes of pneumothorax include trauma (e.g., stabbing, gunshot, or fractured rib) and iatrogenic causes (e.g., after lung biopsy or the introduction of a chest tube for thoracentesis), or it may be a complication of neonatal hyaline membrane disease and require prolonged assisted ventilation. Regardless of the cause, the increased air in the pleural cavity compresses the lung and causes it to collapse. This may cause the patient to experience sudden, severe chest pain and dyspnea (difficulty in breathing).

Radiographic appearance

A pneumothorax appears radiographically as a hyperlucent area in which all pulmonary markings are absent. The radiographic hallmark of pneumothorax is the demonstration of the visceral pleural line, which is outlined centrally by air within the lung and peripherally by air within the pleural space. A large pneumothorax can cause collapse of an entire lung. Chest radiographs for pneumothorax should be taken with the patient in the upright position, as it may be

Figure 2-72   Spontaneous pneumothorax. Complete collapse of right lung.

Summary of Findings for Miscellaneous Lung Disorders

DISORDER	LOCATION	RADIOGRAPHIC APPEARANCE	TREATMENT
Atelectasis	Obstruction of segment/lobe or lung collapse	Local increased density; platelike streaks	Positioning of patient Incentive spirometry
Acute respiratory distress syndrome	Lung structure breakdown	Patchy, ill-defined areas of consolidation	Diuretics to decrease fluid build-up Oxygen therapy and ventilation
Intrabronchial foreign body	Lower lobes, most often right	Appears as atelectasis with possible shift	Removal of foreign body Expectoration, intervention, surgery
Mediastinal emphysema	Air in bronchovascular sheath	Radiolucency running parallel to heart border	If minimal, no treatment Surgical resection to prevent more air escape
Subcutaneous emphysema	Air in surrounding muscle bundles	Air streaks in muscle bundles	If minimal, no treatment Surgical resection to prevent more air escape

very difficult to identify this condition in the supine patient. In addition to routine full-inspiration films, a posteroanterior (PA) radiograph, or an AP radiograph, should be obtained with the lung in full expiration to allow identification of small pneumothoraces (Figure 2-73). This maneuver causes the lung to decrease in volume and become relatively denser, while the volume of air in the pleural space remains constant and is easier to detect. Very small pneumothoraces may be evident on lateral decubitus films. In this position, air rising to the highest point in the hemithorax is more clearly visible over the lateral chest wall than on erect views, in which a small amount of air in

the apical region may be obscured by overlying bony densities. Whenever an expiration radiograph is being obtained, the use of an automatic exposure control is *not* recommended, because the preset density may produce a radiographic film density capable of concealing a small pneumothorax. Using a manual technique, the exposure factor (in milliampere-seconds) for an expiration radiograph should be about one-third higher than that used for inspiration films.

Treatment

Small pneumothoraces usually reabsorb spontaneously. Larger pneumothoraces may require prompt chest tube

Figure 2-73 Pneumothorax. **A,** On routine frontal chest film, a faint rim of pleura *(arrows)* at the right apex is separated from the thoracic wall by an area containing air but no pulmonary vasculature. **B,** On expiratory film, right pneumothorax *(arrows)* is clearly seen.

Figure 2-74 Tension pneumothorax. Left hemithorax is completely radiolucent and lacks vascular markings. There is a dramatic shift of the mediastinum to the right. Left hemidiaphragm is greatly depressed, and there is spreading of the left ribs.

drainage with suction to remove the air and prevent recurrence. Tension pneumothorax is a medical emergency in which air continues to enter the pleural space but cannot exit. The accumulation of air within the pleural space causes complete collapse of the ipsilateral lung and depression of the hemidiaphragm (Figure 2-74). The heart and mediastinal structures shift toward the opposite side, severely compromising cardiac output because the elevated intrathoracic pressure decreases venous return to the heart. If a tension pneumothorax is not treated promptly, the resulting circulatory collapse may be fatal.

Pleural effusion

The accumulation of fluid in the pleural space is a nonspecific finding that may be caused by a wide variety of pathologic processes. The most common causes include congestive heart failure, pulmonary embolism, infection (especially tuberculosis), pleurisy, neoplastic disease, and connective tissue disorders. Pleural effusion can also be the result of abdominal disease, such as recent surgery, ascites, subphrenic abscess, and pancreatitis.

Radiographic appearance

The earliest radiographic finding in pleural effusion is blunting of the normally sharp angle between the diaphragm and the rib cage (the costophrenic angle) along with an upward concave border of the fluid level (or meniscus) (Figure 2-75). Because the costophrenic angles are deeper posteriorly than laterally, small pleural effusions are best seen on the routine lateral projection posteriorly. As much as 400 ml of pleural fluid may accumulate and still not produce blunting of the lateral costophrenic angles on erect frontal views of the chest. Larger amounts of pleural fluid produce a homogeneous radiolucency (or whiteness) that may obscure the diaphragm and adjacent borders of the heart. Massive effusions may compress the adjacent

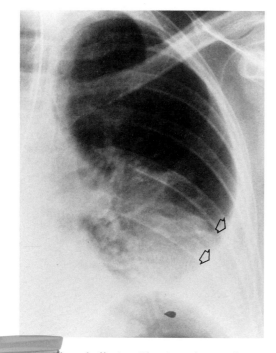

Figure 2-75 Pleural effusion. Blunting of normally sharp angle between diaphragm and rib cage *(arrows)* along with characteristic concave-upward fluid level (meniscus).

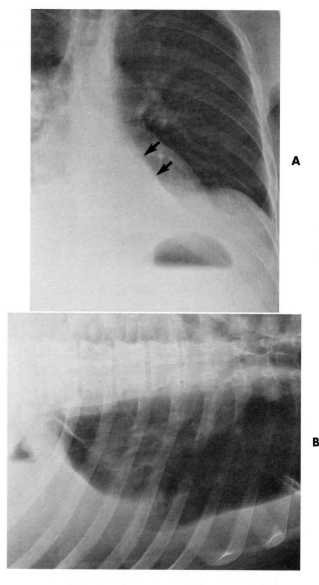

Figure 2-77 Pleural effusion. **A,** Frontal projection of chest demonstrates large distance between gastric air bubble and top of false left hemidiaphragm in this patient with large subpulmonic effusion. Note retrocardiac paraspinal density *(arrows)* that simulates left lower lobe infiltrate or atelectasis. **B,** Left lateral decubitus projection shows that retrocardiac density represents large amount of free pleural fluid. (From Vix VA: *Semin Roentgenol* 12:277-286, 1977.)

Figure 2-76 Pleural effusion causing shift of mediastinum. Left hemithorax is virtually opaque, and there is a shift of mediastinal structures to the right.

lung and even displace the heart and mediastinum to the opposite side (Figure 2-76).

Small pleural effusions may be difficult to distinguish from pleural thickening and fibrosis, which results from previous pleural inflammation and appears radiographically as a soft tissue density along the lateral chest wall. The diagnosis of a small pleural effusion is best made using a horizontal x-ray beam with

the patient in a lateral decubitus position with the affected side down. By placing the patient slightly in a slight lateral Trendelenburg position, as little as 5 ml of pleural fluid can be seen as a layer of linear opacification along the dependent chest wall. At times, however, a collection of pleural fluid may be loculated (i.e., fixed in place by fibrous adhesions) and therefore will not form this layer in decubitus views.

Figure 2-78   Empyema. Large soft-tissue mass fills much of left hemothorax. (From Eisenberg RL: *Diagnostic imaging in surgery,* New York, 1987, McGraw-Hill.)

Summary of Findings for Pleural Disorders

DISORDER	LOCATION	RADIOGRAPHIC APPEARANCE	TREATMENT
Pneumothorax	Air in pleural cavity	Peripheral radiolucency without pulmonary markings	Small—none (reabsorbed) Large—chest tube with suction
Pleural effusion	Fluid in pleural cavity	Fluid level—best seen on lateral decubitus	Thoracentesis to remove fluid
Empyema	Infected fluid in pleural cavity	Lesion—loculated fluid; possible air–fluid level	Needle aspiration with possible drain placement

Pleural effusions may produce less common appearances on chest radiographs. A pleural fluid collection that has become fixed by inflammatory fibrosis may mimic a solid mass. At times, pleural fluid may collect below the inferior surface of the lung (subpulmonic effusion) and give the radiographic appearance of an elevated hemidiaphragm (Figure 2-77). In patients with congestive heart failure, an effusion may develop in an interlobar fissure to produce a round or oval density resembling a solitary pulmonary nodule. As the patient's heart condition improves, repeat examinations demonstrate decreased size or complete resolution of these phantom tumors (see Figure 6-19).

Treatment

Thoracentesis is the procedure for removing fluid from the pleural cavity. Other treatments depend on the cause of the pleural effusion.

Empyema

Empyema refers to the presence of infected liquid or frank pus in the pleural space. Usually the result of the spread of an adjacent infection (e.g., bacterial pneumonia, subdiaphragmatic abscess, lung abscess, esophageal perforation), empyemas may also occur after thoracic surgery, trauma, or instrumentation of the pleural space. Since the development of antibiotics, empyemas are rare.

Radiographic appearance

Radiographically, an empyema is initially indistinguishable from pleural effusion. As the empyema develops, it becomes loculated and appears as a discrete mass that may vary in size from a large lesion filling much of the hemithorax (Figure 2-78) to a small mass along the chest wall or in an interlobar fissure. Air within a free or loculated empyema causes an

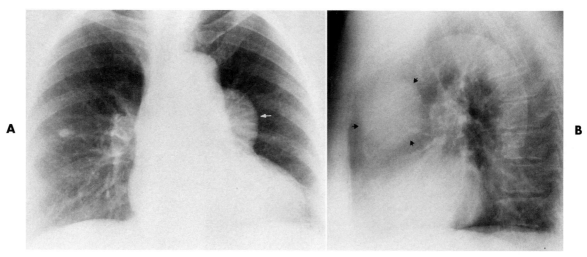

Figure 2-79   Anterior mediastinal mass. Frontal **(A)** and lateral **(B)** projections of chest demonstrate large mass (thymoma) in anterior mediastinum *(arrows)*.

Figure 2-80   Middle mediastinal mass. Frontal **(A)** and lateral **(B)** projections of chest demonstrate a smooth-walled, spherical mediastinal mass *(arrows)* projecting into left lung and left hilum (found to be a bronchogenic cyst).

air–fluid level and indicates communication with a bronchus or the skin surface.

Treatment

Needle aspiration of an empyema may be performed under fluoroscopic guidance; when the loculated mass is situated adjacent to the chest wall, ultrasound may be used to guide the aspiration needle. A sinus tract or fistula may require drainage tube placement.

■ Mediastinal Masses

Because various types of mediastinal masses tend to occur predominantly in specific locations, the mediastinum is often divided into anterior, middle, and posterior compartments. The anterior compartment extends from the sternum back to the trachea and the anterior border of the heart. The middle mediastinum contains the heart and great vessels, the central tracheobronchial tree and lymph nodes, and the phrenic nerves. The posterior compartment consists of the space behind the pericardium.

Major lesions of the anterior mediastinum include thymomas (Figure 2-79), teratomas, thyroid masses, lipomas, and lymphoma. The middle mediastinum involves lymph node disorders (e.g., lymphoma, metastatic carcinoma, granulomatous processes), bronchogenic cysts (Figure 2-80), vascular anomalies, and various masses situated in the anterior costophrenic angle (e.g., pericardial cysts, foramen of Morgagni hernia).

Figure 2-81   Posterior mediastinal mass. Frontal **(A)** and lateral **(B)** projections of chest demonstrate a large, oval, homogeneous mass in posterior mediastinum (neurenteric cyst). Note right hydropneumothorax *(arrows)* with long air–fluid level that developed as a complication of diagnostic needle biopsy.

The posterior mediastinum is the site of neurogenic tumors, neurogenic cysts (Figure 2-81), aneurysms of the descending aorta, and extramedullary hematopoiesis.

About one third of patients with mediastinal masses are asymptomatic, and the lesion is detected on a routine chest radiograph. Chest pain, cough, dyspnea, and symptoms caused by compression or invasion of structures in the mediastinum (e.g., dysphagia, hoarseness as a result of recurrent laryngeal nerve involvement, superior vena cava obstruction) are highly suggestive of malignancy.

The configuration of a mediastinal mass depends to a large extent on its consistency. Cystic masses, often compressed between blood vessels and the tracheobronchial tree, produce a multiloculated appearance. In contrast, solid masses tend to compress and displace adjacent structures.

In addition to plain chest radiographs, conventional tomography and contrast studies of the esophagus may be of value in defining the anatomic location and borders of the mass. CT of the chest after the intravenous injection of contrast material may help in distinguishing between vascular and nonvascular lesions, as well as in determining whether a lesion is cystic and thus most probably benign (Figures 2-82 and 2-83).

Treatment

For all masses found in the mediastinal region, surgical excision of the neoplasm is suggested because of the difficulty in differentiating the cause and the possible complications associated with these lesions.

Figure 2-82   CT of anterior mediastinal mass. Enormous soft-tissue mass (thymoma) causes posterior displacement of other mediastinal structures. No difference in density can be seen between the mass and the heart behind it.

■ Disorders of the Diaphragm

The diaphragm is the major muscle of respiration separating the thoracic and abdominal cavities. Radiographically, the height of the diaphragm varies considerably with the phase of respiration. On full inspiration, the diaphragm usually projects at about the level of the tenth posterior intercostal space. On

Figure 2-83 CT of posterior mediastinal mass. Contrast-enhanced scan at level just below carina shows large aneurysm of descending aorta. Large mural thrombus *(TH)* surrounds greatly dilated lumen of descending aorta *(L)*. Note also prominently dilated ascending aorta *(OA)*.

Summary of Findings for Mediastinal Masses

DISORDER	LOCATION	RADIOGRAPHIC APPEARANCE	TREATMENT
Thymoma Teratoma Thyroid mass Lipoma Lymphoma	Anterior mediastinum	Cystic masses—compress, producing multiloculated appearance Solid masses—compress and displace adjacent structures	Excision of lesion because of difficult differential diagnosis
Lymph node disorders Bronchogenic cysts Vascular anomalies	Middle mediastinum	Cystic masses—compress, producing multiloculated appearance Solid masses—compress and displace adjacent structures	Excision of lesion because of difficult differential diagnosis
Neurogenic tumors Neurogenic cysts Aneurysms Extramedullary hematopoiesis	Posterior mediastinum	Cystic masses—compress, producing multiloculated appearance Solid masses—compress and displace adjacent structures	Excision of lesion because of difficult differential diagnosis

expiration, it may appear two or three intercostal spaces higher. The average range of diaphragmatic motion with respiration is 3 to 6 cm, but in patients with emphysema this may be substantially reduced. The level of the diaphragm falls as the patient moves from a supine to an upright position. In an erect patient, the dome of the diaphragm tends to be about half an interspace higher on the right than on the left. However, in about 10% of normal individuals the hemidiaphragms are at the same height, or the left is higher than the right.

Diaphragmatic paralysis

Elevation of one or both leaves of the diaphragm can be caused by paralysis resulting from any process that interferes with the normal function of the phrenic nerve. The paralysis may be attributable to accidental surgical transection of the phrenic nerve, involvement of the nerve by primary bronchogenic carcinoma or metastatic malignancy in the mediastinum, or a variety of intrinsic neurologic diseases (Figure 2-84). Reduced lung volume results from this paralysis.

Figure 2-84 Paralysis of right hemidiaphragm caused by involvement of phrenic nerve by primary carcinoma of lung *(arrow)*.

Figure 2-85 Eventration of right hemidiaphragm.

Radiographic appearance

The radiographic hallmark of diaphragmatic paralysis is paradoxical movement of the diaphragm, which is best demonstrated at fluoroscopy by having the patient sniff. This rapid but shallow inspiration causes a quick downward thrust of a normal leaf of the diaphragm, whereas a paralyzed hemidiaphragm tends to rise with inspiration because of the increased intraabdominal pressure. During expiration, the normal hemidiaphragm rises and the paralyzed one descends. The demonstration of a pronounced degree of paradoxical motion is a valuable aid in differentiating paralysis of the diaphragm from limited diaphragmatic motion resulting from intrathoracic or intraabdominal disease.

Treatment

In most cases, diaphragmatic paralysis requires no treatment. If gravity does not provide enough lung volume, insertion of a diaphragmatic pacer may be necessary.

Eventration of the diaphragm

Eventration of the diaphragm, a rare congenital abnormality in which one hemidiaphragm (very rarely both) is poorly developed and too weak to permit the upward movement of abdominal contents into the thoracic cage. The condition is usually asymptomatic and occurs more frequently on the left.

Radiographic appearance

Eventration produces the radiographic appearance of a localized bulging or generalized elevation of the diaphragm (Figure 2-85). An eventration must be distinguished from a diaphragmatic hernia, through which abdominal contents are displaced into the chest. Oral administration of barium should permit the differentiation between the normal contours of the bowel below a diaphragmatic eventration and the crowding of these structures and narrowing of their afferent and efferent limbs when trapped in a hernia sac.

Treatment

Eventration rarely needs treatment. Infants in distress may require surgical plication to shorten the diaphragm by removing a fold.

Other causes of elevation of the diaphragm

Diffuse elevation of one or both leaves of the diaphragm can be caused by ascites, obesity, pregnancy, or any other process in which the intraabdominal volume is increased (Figure 2-86). Intraabdominal inflammatory diseases, such as subphrenic abscess, can lead to elevation of a hemidiaphragm with severe limitations of diaphragmatic motion. Cystic or tumor masses arising in the upper quadrants can cause localized or generalized bulging of the diaphragm. Acute intrathoracic processes (e.g., chest-wall injury,

Figure 2-86 Diffuse elevation of both leaves of the diaphragm caused by severe, acute gastric dilatation.

● ●

Summary of Findings for Diaphragmatic Disorders

DISORDER	LOCATION	RADIOGRAPHIC APPEARANCE	TREATMENT
Diaphragmatic paralysis	Diaphragm motion	Sniff test to distinguish normal from abnormal	No treatment in most cases Diaphragmatic pacer
Diaphragmatic eventration	Diaphragm poorly developed and elevated	Diaphragm elevation	No treatment in most cases Plication possible
Other causes of diaphragmatic elevation	Elevation due to extrinsic cause	Diaphragm elevation	Treatment varies on the basis of cause

● ●

atelectasis, pulmonary embolism) can produce diaphragmatic elevation caused by splinting of the diaphragm.

Radiographic appearance

An apparent elevation of a hemidiaphragm may be caused by a subpulmonic pleural effusion, which can be correctly diagnosed on a chest radiograph performed with a horizontal x-ray beam and the patient in a lateral decubitus position.

QUESTIONS

1. Describe the proper breathing instructions to be given to a patient for chest radiography.

2. In what portion of the respiratory system does the vital gas exchange take place?

3. The covering of the lungs is termed the _up_ _____.

4. _____ is a disease of newborns characterized by progressive underaeration of the lungs and a granular appearance.

5. _____ is a hereditary disease in which thick mucus is secreted by all the exocrine glands.

6. A necrotic area of pulmonary parenchyma containing purulent or puslike material is called a(n) _____.

7. What radiographic procedure is often required to confirm the diagnosis of bronchiectasis when the results of routine chest radiographs are inconclusive?

8. Flattening of the domes of the diaphragm, increased AP diameter of the chest, and increased lucency of the retrosternal air space are suggestive of a diagnosis of _emp_ _____.

9. The three most common pneumoconioses are _____, _____, and _____.

10. An abnormal vascular communication between a pulmonary artery and a pulmonary vein is termed a(n) _____.

11. What medical emergency has occurred when air continues to enter the pleural space and cannot escape, leading to complete collapse of a lung and shift of the heart and mediastinal structures? *tp*

12. Pus in the pleural space is called _____.

13. The major muscle of respiration is the _____ _____.

14. Describe why a true horizontal beam is desirable when one is performing any chest radiograph.

15. The Valsalva maneuver can cause the heart and major blood vessels to
    A. Appear enlarged   C. Appear elevated
    B. Appear smaller   D. Show no change

16. Place a "+" by those pathologic conditions that increase the attenuation of the x-ray and a "−" by those that cause a decrease in attenuation:
    ____ Pleural effusion   ____ Pneumonia
    ____ Empyema   ____ Lung abscess
    ____ Miliary tuberculosis   ____ Atelectasis
    ____ Asbestosis   ____ Pulmonary
    ____ Emphysema   effusion
                                ____ Bronchiectasis

17. Describe the pulmonary circulation of the lungs.

18. Describe the bronchial circulation of the lungs.

19. The lining of the thoracic cavity is called the _____.

20. A lung inflammation caused by bacteria or viruses is called a(n) _____.

21. Name two common types of pulmonary mycoses.

22. For the technologist's safety, it is important to remember that tuberculosis is spread mainly by _____, which produces infectious _____ _____.

23. What medical term is used to describe the entry of air into the pleural space? *pneumo*

24. An increased volume of air in the lungs is seen in ____ *emph* ____.

25. Inhalation of irritating dusts leading to chronic inflammation and pulmonary fibrosis is called _____.

26. A malignant pleural neoplasm that results from asbestosis is _____.

27. The trapping of bacteria in the pulmonary circulation that occurs in patients with a history of intravenous drug abuse is called _____.

28. Reduced air volume within a lung leading to collapse is termed ____ *atel* ____.

29. Why do intrabronchial foreign bodies occur more frequently in the lower right lung?

30. Blunt or penetrating trauma to the chest can produce _____, which appears as streaks of air that outline muscles of the thorax and sometimes the neck.

31. Name the two positions that are sometimes used to demonstrate a pneumothorax that are different from the routine chest radiograph positions.

32. To demonstrate a pneumothorax in an expiration film of the chest, the exposure factors should be increased. Why, and by how much?

33. At what costal interspace does the diaphragm lie when the lungs are fully inflated?
    A. Eighth   C. Tenth
    B. Ninth   D. Eleventh

34. What radiographic position is sometimes helpful in the diagnosis of very small pleural effusions?

35. Air collecting behind the sternum and dissecting up into the soft tissues of the neck is called _____.

36. An accumulation of fluid in the pleural space, sometimes caused by heart failure or pulmonary embolus, is called
    A. Empyema   C. Effusion
    B. Edema   D. Abscess

BIBLIOGRAPHY

Felson B: *Chest roentgenology*, Philadelphia, 1971, Saunders.
Heitzman ER: *The lung: radiologic-pathologic correlations*, St Louis, 1984, Mosby.

Paré JAP, Fraser RG: *Synopsis of diseases of the chest*, Philadelphia, 1983, Saunders.
Reed JC: *Chest radiology: patterns and differential diagnoses*, St Louis, 1981, Mosby.

CHAPTER 3

Skeletal System

■ **Prerequisite Knowledge**

The student should have a basic knowledge of the anatomy and physiology of the skeletal system. In addition, proper learning and understanding of the material will be facilitated if the student has some clinical experience in skeletal radiography and film evaluation, including a concept of the changes in technique required to compensate for density differences produced by the underlying pathologic conditions.

■ **Goals**

To acquaint the student radiographer with the pathophysiology and radiographic manifestations of all the common and some of the unusual disorders of the skeletal system.

■ **Objectives**

1. To be able to classify the more common diseases in terms of their attenuation of x-rays
2. To be familiar with the changes in technical factors required for obtaining optimal-quality radiographs in patients with various underlying pathologic conditions
3. To understand and be able to define or describe all bold-faced terms in this chapter
4. To be able to describe the physiology of the skeletal system
5. To be able to identify anatomic structures on both diagrams and radiographs of the skeletal system
6. To be able to describe the various pathologic conditions affecting the skeletal system, and their radiographic manifestations

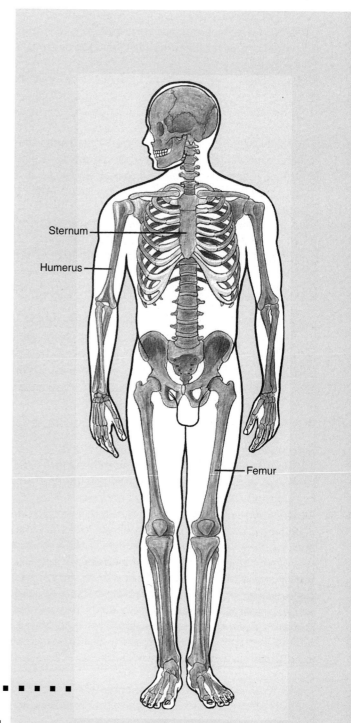

■ ■ ■ ■ ■ Radiographer Notes

Three factors are critical in radiography of the skeletal system: (1) proper patient positioning, (2) correct alignment of the radiographic tube, the body part being imaged, and the image receptor, and (3) exposure factors chosen to produce optimal contrast and visibility of detail. In patients with suspected fractures, two projections as close as possible to 90 degrees to each other must always be obtained to demonstrate fracture relationships. A variety of projections (e.g., oblique, tangential, coned-down) may be required to identify obscure fractures.

At times, the poor condition of a patient may require ingenuity on the part of the radiographer to obtain diagnostic radiographs when routine positioning methods cannot be accomplished. Patients with bone tumors, arthritis, or recent trauma are frequently in severe pain and extremely frightened of further injury or of suffering more discomfort. The radiographer must reassure the patient that positioning will be carefully accomplished with as little pain or discomfort as possible. Remember that a radiographer can easily cause further injury to the patient if the proper moving techniques are not used.

At times, the technologist may need to perform cross-table or tube-angulation projections to obtain the required films without moving the patient. In such cases, the radiographic tube must be perpendicular to the image receptor and the body part to prevent image distortion. Variations in this rela-

tionship can obscure pathologic bone conditions or lead to errors in interpretation of the alignment of fracture fragments.

Bone radiographs require a short scale of contrast to provide maximal visibility of detail. The periosteum, cortex, and internal bone structure (trabeculae) must be well demonstrated to detect the often subtle changes of fractures, demineralization, and bone destruction. For example, periosteal new bone formation may indicate underlying tumor, infection, or prior trauma, whereas minute juxta-articular erosions are often seen in arthritis. The scale of contrast must also allow visualization of the soft tissues and muscles, because soft-tissue swelling, calcifications, opaque foreign bodies, muscle wasting, and the presence of gas are all important radiographic findings.

It is recommended that lower to mid kilovolts-peak ranges be used in all skeletal radiography. To achieve the necessary scale of contrast, extremity radiographs should be exposed using an exposure in the 50 to 69 kVp range, whereas a range of 70 to 80 kVp is recommended for studies of the spine, pelvis, thoracic cage, and shoulder. Appropriate ratio grids, or Bucky devices, should be used for all body parts 10 cm or greater.

Special techniques such as magnification or tomography may be necessary to detect subtle fractures or other pathologic bone conditions. For example, the navicular bone of the wrist typically requires the use of the magnification technique. For

Continued

■ Physiology of the Skeletal System

The skeletal system is composed primarily of two highly specialized connective tissues: bone and cartilage. Bone consists of an organic matrix in which inorganic salts (primarily calcium and phosphate) are deposited. A fibrous membrane termed the **periosteum** covers the outer surfaces of bone, except at joint surfaces where articular cartilage covers the bone and acts as a protective cushion. The periosteum contains a network of blood vessels from which nutrient arteries penetrate into the underlying bone. The main shaftlike portion is termed the **diaphysis,** and the ends of the bone are called **epiphyses.** The hollow, tubelike structure within the diaphysis, known as the **medullary cavity,** or **marrow,** is lined by an inner membrane termed the **endosteum.**

There are two major types of bone. The outer layer consists of **compact bone,** which to the naked eye ap-

pears dense and structureless. Under the microscope, the matrix of compact bone consists of complex structural units called "haversian systems." **Cancellous (spongy) bone** is composed of a weblike arrangement of marrow-filled spaces separated by thin processes of bone, called **trabeculae,** which are visible to the naked eye. The relative amount of each type of bone depends on the degree of strength required and thus varies from bone to bone and in different portions of the same bone. For example, the shafts of long bones such as the femur and tibia have a thick outer layer of compact bone, whereas the layer of compact bone is relatively thin in irregular bones, such as vertebral bodies and facial bones, and in short bones, such as the carpal and tarsal bones.

Most bones form from models composed of hyaline cartilage (enchondral ossification). In a typical long bone, a primary ossification center appears in the

■ ■ ■ ■ ■ ■ ■ ■ ■ **Radiographer Notes—cont'd**

2× linear or 4× area magnification, the object must be an equal distance from the radiographic tube and the image receptor. For 3× linear or 9× area magnification, the body part must be twice as far from the image receptor as from the x-ray tube. Close collimation is extremely important to prevent undercutting the image. A radiographic tube with a fractional focal spot of 0.3 mm or less is mandatory for a magnification factor of 2× or more to compensate for the excessive penumbra (geometric blur) that results from the object image distance. Larger focal spot sizes cause excessive geometric blurred images that appear to have motion and lack recorded detail as a result of excessive penumbra.

Tomography may be required to make a definitive diagnosis if the plain radiographs are equivocal, or to delineate precisely the extent of bone involvement. For example, tomography is frequently needed in the evaluation of fractures of the tibial plateau and spine. CT is the modality of choice for spinal injuries, as it best demonstrates the vertebrae and fracture fragments that could impinge on the spinal cord or peripheral nerves. MRI better demonstrates nontraumatic disk herniation or tumor impingement.

In most cases, it is essential to prevent motion of the part of the body being radiographed. To accomplish this, make the patient as comfortable as possible, use immobilization devices when necessary, and use the shortest possible exposure times.

However, a few portions of the skeletal system are better visualized using a motion technique. For three such areas (the sternum and the lateral thoracic spine, and to obtain a transthoracic lateral projection of the upper humerus), a shallow breathing technique is used while the patient remains immobilized. A minimum exposure time of about 5 seconds and a very low milliamperage should be used. The patient is instructed to breathe rhythmically during the entire exposure to blur out overlying ribs and lung markings. An additional technique, the Ottonello (or "wagging jaw") method, is used to obtain an AP projection of the cervical spine. Movement of the jaw is used to blur out the image of the mandible, which otherwise would superimpose the upper portion of the cervical spine.

Certain pathologic conditions of the skeletal system require that the radiographer alter routine technical settings. Some disorders produce increased bone density (e.g., sclerosis, increased bone growth), which increases attenuation; others decrease the density of the bony structures (e.g., lytic bone destruction, loss of calcium from bone), and so they will attenuate x-rays less (see the box in Chapter 1 labeled Relative Attenuation of X-rays in Advanced Stages of Diseases). It is important to remember that the necessary technical changes may vary depending on the stage of the underlying condition.

---

center of the cartilage precursor in about the eighth week of intrauterine life, and bone formation extends so that the entire shaft is usually ossified before birth. Just before or after birth, secondary ossification centers appear in the epiphyses, the ends of developing long bones. Until the linear growth of bone is complete, the epiphysis remains separated from the diaphysis by a cartilaginous plate called the **epiphyseal cartilage.** The epiphyseal cartilage persists until the growth of the bone is complete. At that time, the epiphyseal plate ossifies, and the epiphysis and diaphysis fuse (at various ages depending on the specific bones). Where the diaphysis meets the epiphyseal growth plate is a slight flaring, known as the **metaphysis.**

The increase in length of a developing long bone occurs by growth of the epiphyseal cartilage followed by ossification. Bones grow in diameter by the combined action of two special types of cells called **osteoblasts** and **osteoclasts.** Osteoclasts enlarge the diameter of the medullary cavity by removing bone from the diaphysis walls. At the same time, osteoblasts from the periosteum produce new bone around the outer circumference. Osteoblasts and osteoclasts thus continuously resorb old bone and produce new bone. This constant process of remodeling occurs until the bone assumes its adult size and shape.

The radiographic determination of bone age is useful for evaluating physiologic age and growth potential, and for predicting adult stature. The most well known and widely accepted method of determining skeletal bone age (skeletal maturation) is that of Greulich and Pyle in their radiographic atlas compiled from thousands of examinations of American children at different ages. This atlas contains standard radiographs for age and sex that permit an assessment of bone age based on the presence or absence of ossification centers and their configuration and the fusion of epiphyses in various portions of the hand and wrist.

Throughout life, bone formation **(ossification)** and bone destruction **(resorption)** continues to occur. They are in balance during the early and middle years of adulthood. After about 40 years of age, however, bone loss at the inner or endosteal surface exceeds bone gain at the outer margins. Thus in long bones the thickness of compact bone in the diaphyses decreases, and the diameter of the medullary cavity increases. The bone eventually resembles a hollow shell and is less able to resist compressive and bending forces. This process may lead to collapse and loss of height of vertebral bodies and fractures of long bones after relatively mild injury.

Bones can also develop within a connective tissue membrane **(intramembranous ossification)**. The clavicles and flat bones of the skull have no cartilaginous stage and begin to take shape when groups of primitive cells differentiate into osteoblasts, which secrete matrix material and collagenous fibrils. Deposition of complex calcium salts in the organic bone matrix produces rodlike trabeculae that join in a network of interconnecting spicules to form spongy or cancellous bone. Eventually, plates of compact or dense bone cover the core layer of spongy bone. Flat bones grow in size by the addition of osseous tissue to their outer surfaces **(appositional growth)**. They cannot grow by expansion, as enchondral bone does.

Bones perform five basic functions:

1. They serve as the supporting framework of the body and protect the vital organs (e.g., skull protects the brain, rib cage protects the heart and lungs).
2. Bones serve as levers on which muscles can contract and shorten and thus produce movement at a joint.
3. Red bone marrow within certain bones (spinal column, upper humerus, and upper femur in the adult) is the major site of production of blood cells.
4. Bone serves as the major storehouse for calcium salts. The maintenance of a normal level of calcium, which is essential for survival, depends on a balance in the rates of calcium movement between the blood and bones.

■ Congenital/Hereditary Diseases of Bone

Vertebral anomalies

A **transitional vertebra** is one that has characteristics of vertebrae on both sides of a major division of the spine.

Radiographic appearance

Transitional vertebrae most frequently occur at the lumbosacral junction and contain expanded trans-

verse processes, which may form actual unilateral or bilateral joints with the sacrum (Figure 3-1). When unilateral, this process often leads to degenerative change involving the opposite hip and the intervertebral disk space above it. At the thoracolumbar junction, the first lumbar vertebra may have rudimentary ribs articulating with the transverse processes. The seventh cervical vertebra may also have a rudimentary rib (Figure 3-2).

Treatment

Most vertebral anomalies remain unnoticed and are incidental findings on radiographs. A **cervical rib** may compress the brachial nerve plexus (causing pain or numbness in the upper extremity) or the subclavian artery (decreasing blood flow to the arm) and therefore require surgical removal.

Figure 3-1 Transitional vertebrae. Expanded transverse process at the lumbosacral junction.

Figure 3-2 Bilateral cervical ribs (*arrowheads*).

Spina bifida

Spina bifida refers to a posterior defect of the spinal canal resulting from failure of the posterior elements to fuse properly. A mild, insignificant form is **spina bifida occulta,** in which there is a splitting of the bony neural canal at the L5 or S1 level (Figure 3-3). Large defects are associated with spinal cord abnormalities and may lead to a variety of muscular abnormalities and lack of bladder or bowel control. In many cases a slight dimpling of the skin or tuft of hair over the vertebral defect indicates the site of the lesion.

Large defects in the lumbar or cervical spine may be accompanied by herniation of the meninges **(meningocele),** or of the meninges and a portion of the spinal cord or nerve roots **(myelomeningocele).** A patient with a meningocele may be asymptomatic. Other malformations associated with a meningocele include clubfeet, gait disturbances, and bladder incontinence. The myelomeningocele has associated neurologic deficits at and below the site of protrusion. Almost all patients with myelomeningocele have the Chiari II malformation, with caudal displacement of posterior fossa structures into the cervical canal. Hydrocephalus is a frequent complication.

Radiographic appearance

These lesions are associated with large bony defects, absence of the laminae, and increased interpedicular distance (Figure 3-4). The herniated spinal contents are seen as a soft-tissue mass posterior to the spine. Myelography, computed tomography (CT), or magnetic resonance imaging (MRI) can demonstrate the presence of spinal cord or nerve roots within the herniated sac. Prenatal real-time ultrasound can now demonstrate this serious malformation in-utero.

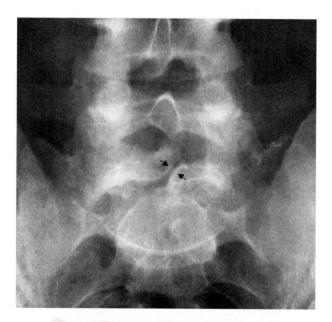

Figure 3-3 Spina bifida occulta *(arrows).*

Figure 3-4 Meningomyelocele. **A,** Frontal projection of abdomen shows greatly increased interpedicular distance of lumbar vertebrae. **B,** In another patient, lateral projection demonstrates large soft-tissue mass *(arrows)* situated posterior to spine. Notice absence of posterior elements in lower lumbar and sacral regions.

Treatment

Spina bifida occulta and meningoceles usually require no treatment. Sometimes a meningocele requires surgical repair, depending on the size and location of the protrusion. A myelomeningocele generally requires surgical repair. When this repair is being completed, a shunt is placed to prevent hydrocephalus.

Osteopetrosis

Osteopetrosis (marble bones) is a rare hereditary bone dysplasia in which failure of the resorptive mechanism of calcified cartilage interferes with the normal replacement by mature bone. This prevents the bone marrow from forming, so that the bones become very brittle and stress fractures occur often. The patient may also become anemic as a result of the lack of blood-producing bone marrow. Osteopetrosis varies in severity and age of clinical presentation from a fulminant, often fatal condition involving the entire skeleton at birth or in utero, to an essentially asymptomatic form that is an incidental radiographic finding.

Radiographic appearance

Osteopetrosis results in a symmetric, generalized increase in bone density (Figure 3-5). To produce a diagnostic image, the technologist must increase the ex-

posure factors (milliampere-seconds [mAs] and kilovolts [kV]) to compensate for the increase in bone formation. The image may appear blurred because of the structural changes; in some cases, a good film may be difficult to produce.

Treatment

Currently, no effective treatment exits for osteopetrosis. Bone marrow transplants help control the anemia in some cases. Transplantation of osteoclastic precursors may help control the balance of bone formation and resorption.

Osteogenesis imperfecta

Osteogenesis imperfecta (OI) is an inherited generalized disorder of connective tissue characterized by multiple fractures and an unusual blue color of the normally white sclera of the eye. Adult patients are generally wheel-chair bound because the skeletal structure does not support their body weight (Figure 3-6).

Radiographic appearance

Patients with this condition suffer repeated fractures caused by the severe osteoporosis and the thin, defective cortices (Figure 3-7, *A*). The fractures often heal with exuberant callus formation (often so extensive as

A   **B**

Figure 3-5   Osteopetrosis. **A,** Striking sclerosis of bones of hand and wrist. **B,** Generalized increased density of lower spine, pelvis, and hips.

Figure 3-6   Osteogenesis imperfecta of adult foot. Demineralization and the lack of bony cortices are demonstrated on AP and lateral projections.

A
B

Figure 3-7   Osteogenesis imperfecta. **A,** Generalized flattening of vertebral bodies associated with fractures of multiple ribs and long bones in an infant. **B,** Multiple wormian bones.

to simulate a malignant tumor), sometimes causing bizarre deformities. Because of the severe cortical bone loss, producing a good image may require lowering the kilovoltage to compensate for the loss of bone quality (only in advanced stages of disease). Ossification of the skull progresses slowly, leaving wide sutures and multiple juxtasutural accessory bones within a suture (wormian bones), which produce a mosaic appearance (Figure 3-7, B).

Treatment

The aim of treatment is to reduce fractures by using proper safety measures. Because of defective cortices in severe cases, the long bones become less supportive. Therefore in some instances extendable rods are surgically placed to provide more support, help prevent new fractures from occurring, and prevent bowing (Figure 3-8).

Achondroplasia

Achondroplasia is the most common form of dwarfism; it results from diminished proliferation of cartilage in the growth plate (decreased enchondral bone formation). This autosomal dominant condition does not affect membranous bone formation. Therefore, the individual has short limbs, which contrast

A

B

Figure 3-8   Osteogenesis imperfecta. AP **(A)** and lateral **(B)** projections of the lower leg show extension rod placement to strengthen bone and decrease fracture possibility.

with the nearly normal length of the trunk. Other characteristic physical features include a large head with frontal bulging, saddle nose, a prognathous (jutting) jaw, and prominent buttocks that give the false impression of lumbar lordosis.

Radiographic appearance

Typical radiographic findings include progressive narrowing of the interpedicular distances from above downward, the opposite of normal, and scalloping of the posterior margins of the lumbar vertebral bodies (Figure 3-9). The decreased enchondral bone formation may make the long bones appear short and thick with a widened metaphysis (Erlenmeyer flask deformity) (Figure 3-10).

Treatment

Achondroplasia has no cure, and treatments address complications or deformities associated with the disease process. Those afflicted live normal independent and productive lives. With today's technology the long bones can be surgically lengthened.

Congenital hip dysplasia (dislocation)

Congenital hip dysplasia results from incomplete acetabulum formation. Hip dysplasia is more common in females. Upon pediatric assessment of the hip, when the leg is flexed and abducted, the hip may "pop" out of joint and a "click" is felt or heard. The tendons and ligaments responsible for proper femoral head alignment are affected.

Radiographic appearance

Anteroposterior (AP) pelvis and bilateral Cleaves (frog-leg) views are required to make a diagnosis (Figure 3-11). In many cases the AP image appears almost normal with only a slightly larger joint space. On the bilateral Cleaves view, the hip is usually dislocated superiorly and posteriorly. Because the children will have a multitude of follow-up films to recheck development, it is very important to shield the gonadal anatomy.

Figure 3-10   Achondroplasia. View of the pelvis demonstrates femoral head deformity caused by decreased endochondral bone formation.

Figure 3-9   Achondroplasia. Posterior scalloping of multiple vertebral bodies *(arrowheads)*.

Figure 3-11   Hip dysplasia of the right hip in a 2-year-old child. Cleaves (frog-leg) view of the pelvis demonstrates superior and posterior displacement.

Treatment

Children not diagnosed and treated prior to walking may appear to "waddle like a duck." Immobilization of the femoral head is the most common treatment. To accomplish this, a pelvic cast is used. This allows the acetabulum to continue to form correctly before the infant begins to walk.

■ Inflammatory and Infectious Disorders

Rheumatoid arthritis

Rheumatoid arthritis is a chronic systemic disease of unknown cause that appears primarily as a nonsuppurative (noninfectious) inflammatory arthritis of the small joints of the hands and feet. Women are affected about three times more frequently than men, and the average age of onset in adults is 40 years.

Rheumatoid arthritis usually has an insidious origin and may either run a protracted and progressive course, leading to a crippling deformity of affected joints, or undergo spontaneous remissions of variable length. There is usually symmetric involvement of multiple joints, and the disease often progresses proximally toward the trunk until practically every joint in the body is involved.

Rheumatoid arthritis begins as an inflammation of the synovial membrane (synovitis) that lines the joints. The excessive exudate, a result of the inflammation, causes proliferation of the synovium. The resulting mass of thickened granulation tissue (pannus, meaning "covers like a sheet") causes erosion of the articular cartilage and underlying bony cortex, fibrous scarring, and even the development of ankylosis (bony fusion across a joint). The erosion occurs be-

Summary of Findings for Congenital/Hereditary Bone Diseases

DISORDER	LOCATION	RADIOGRAPHIC APPEARANCE	TREATMENT
Vertebral anomalies	Lumbar Cervical	Unilateral or bilateral, L5 expanded transverse process Rudimentary C7 rib	Cervical—may require surgical removal for compression of brachial plexus or subclavian artery
Spina bifida	Cervical, thoracic, or lumbar/sacral spine	Splitting of bony neural canal *lack of neural tube closure*	Nonfusion requires no treatment Myelomeningocele is removed surgically
Osteopetrosis	Entire skeleton	Generalized increased bone density *(marble bone disease)*	No efficacious treatment Possible transplant—bone marrow or osteoclastic precursors
Osteogenesis imperfecta	Long bones	Pathologic fracture, very thin cortical density *brittle bone disease*	Fracture alignment External fixation—casting or braces Internal fixation—extension rods for long-bone support to reduce deformities
Achondroplasia	Vertebrae (short stature), long bones *failure of cart. to form, dwarfism*	Progressive interpedicular distance from superior to inferior, and scalloping of posterior vertebral bodies Widened metaphysis (Erlenmeyer flask deformity)	Nonspecific
Hip dysplasia	Incomplete acetabulum formation	AP and Cleaves view of pelvis to demonstrate superior and posterior dislocation	Immobilization by casting

Figure 3-12 Mutilating rheumatoid arthritis. Severe, bilaterally symmetric destructive changes of hands and wrists with striking subluxations.

cause the inflammatory cells produce lytic enzymes. A combination of the fusion of joint surfaces and an inflammatory laxity of ligaments leads to the development of crippling deformities in the end stage of the disease (Figure 3-12).

Radiographic appearance

The earliest radiographic evidence of rheumatoid arthritis is fusiform periarticular soft-tissue swelling caused by joint effusion and hyperplastic synovial inflammation. Disuse and local hyperemia (increased blood flow) lead to periarticular osteoporosis that initially is confined to the portion of bone adjacent to the joint but may extend to involve the entire bone (Figure 3-13). Extension of the pannus from the synovial reflections onto the bone causes characteristic small foci of destruction at the edges of the joint, where articular cartilage is absent. These typical marginal erosions have poorly defined edges without a sclerotic rim and sometimes may be seen only on oblique or magnification views. Destruction of articular cartilage causes narrowing of the joint space. The laying down of bony trabeculae across a narrow joint space may completely obliterate the joint cavity and produce solid bony ankylosis, which most frequently involves the bones of the wrist.

Ligamentous involvement produces a variety of contractures and subluxations causing the common ulnar deviation of the hands. In the cervical spine, rheumatoid arthritis characteristically produces atlantoaxial subluxation (Figure 3-14), an increased distance between the anterior border of the odontoid and the superior border of the anterior arch of the atlas (normally less than 2.5 mm), which results from

Figure 3-13 Rheumatoid arthritis. Striking periarticular osteoporosis. (From Brown JC, Forrester DM: Arthritis. In Eisenberg RL, Amberg JR, editors: *Critical diagnostic pathways in radiology,* Philadelphia, 1981, Lippincott.)

weakening of the transverse ligaments from synovial inflammation.

Rheumatoid nodules are soft-tissue masses that usually appear over the extensor surfaces on the ulnar aspect of the wrist or the olecranon but occasionally are seen over other body prominences, tendons, or pressure points. These characteristic nodules, which develop in about 20% of patients with rheumatoid arthritis and do not occur in other diseases, aid in making the diagnosis.

Rheumatoid variants: ankylosing spondylitis, Reiter's syndrome, and psoriatic arthritis

Radiographic appearance of ankylosing spondylitis

Ankylosing spondylitis almost always begins in the sacroiliac joints, causing bilateral and usually symmetric involvement. Blurring of the articular margins and patchy sclerosis generally progress to narrowing

Figure 3-14   Subluxation of atlantoaxial joint in rheumatoid arthritis. **A,** Routine lateral film of cervical spine shows normal relationship between anterior border of odontoid process and superior portion of anterior arch of atlas *(arrowhead)*. **B,** With flexion, there is wide separation between the anterior arch of atlas *(solid arrow)* and the odontoid *(open arrow)*.

Figure 3-15   Ankylosing spondylitis. Bilateral, symmetric obliteration of sacroiliac joints and "bamboo spine."

Figure 3-16   Lumbar spine. Severe vertebral fusion illustrates "bamboo spine."

of the joint space and may lead to complete fibrous and bony ankylosis (Figure 3-15). The disease typically progresses from the lumbar spine upward.

Ossification in the paravertebral tissues and longitudinal spinal ligaments (poker spine) combines with extensive lateral bony bridges (syndesmophytes) between vertebral bodies to produce the characteristic "bamboo spine" of advanced disease (Figure 3-16, and see Figure 3-15). Limitation of activity leads to

generalized skeletal osteoporosis and a tendency to fracture in response to the stress of minor trauma (Figure 3-17).

Radiographic appearance of Reiter's syndrome

Reiter's syndrome (reactive arthritis) is characterized by arthritis, urethritis, and conjunctivitis. It primarily affects young adult men and appears to occur after certain types of venereal or gastrointestinal infections.

Figure 3-17   Ankylosing spondylitis. Oblique fracture of mid-cervical spine with anterior dislocation of superior segment is seen in patient who fell while dancing and struck his head. Fracture extends through lateral mass and lamina.

Figure 3-18   Reiter's syndrome. Striking bony erosion *(arrows)* at insertion of Achilles tendon on posterosuperior margin of calcaneus.

Reiter's syndrome most frequently involves the sacroiliac joints, heel, and toes (Figure 3-18). Unlike in ankylosing spondylitis, the sacroiliac involvement here is usually bilateral but asymmetric, and Reiter's syndrome tends to cause only minimal changes in the spine.

Although the radiographic changes in peripheral joints often mimic rheumatoid arthritis, Reiter's syndrome tends to be asymmetric and primarily involves the feet rather than the hands (Figure 3-19).

Figure 3-19   Reiter's syndrome. Erosive changes about the metatarsophalangeal joint of the fifth digit. Erosions involve juxtaarticular region, leaving articular cortex intact.

Radiographic appearance of psoriatic arthritis

Psoriatic arthritis refers to a rheumatoid-like destructive process involving peripheral joints that develops in patients with typical skin changes of psoriasis (Figure 3-20). Unlike rheumatoid arthritis, psoriatic arthritis predominantly involves the distal rather than the proximal interphalangeal joints of the hands and feet, produces asymmetric rather than symmetric destruction, and causes little or no periarticular osteoporosis.

Characteristic findings include bony ankylosis of the interphalangeal joints of the hands and feet and resorption of the terminal tufts of the distal phalanges (Figure 3-21). Common characteristics of Reiter's syndrome and psoriatic arthritis include erosions and hypertrophic changes occurring in the origin and insertion of the tendons and ligaments.

Osteoarthritis (degenerative joint disease)

Osteoarthritis is an extremely common generalized disorder characterized pathologically by loss of joint cartilage and reactive new bone formation. Part of the wear and tear of the aging process, degenerative joint disease tends to predominantly affect the weight-

Figure 3-20   Psoriatic arthritis. Bizarre pattern of asymmetric bone destruction, subluxation, and ankylosis. Notice the particularly severe pencil-in-cup deformity of third proximal interphalangeal joint, and the bony ankylosis involving wrist and phalanges of second and fifth digits.

Figure 3-21   Psoriatic arthritis. Severe mutilating arthritis of foot and ankle. There is extreme pencil-like destruction of metatarsals and phalanges, with ankylosis of almost all tarsal joints.

bearing joints (spine, hip, knee, ankle) and the interphalangeal joints of the fingers. A secondary form of degenerative joint disease may develop in a joint that has been repeatedly traumatized or subjected to abnormal stresses because of orthopedic deformities, or it may be a result of a septic or inflammatory arthritis that destroys cartilage.

Radiographic appearance

The earliest radiographic findings in degenerative joint disease are narrowing of the joint space, caused by thinning of the articular cartilage, and development of small bony spurs (osteophytes) along the margins of the articular edges of the bones. In contrast to the smooth, even narrowing of the joint space in rheumatoid arthritis, the joint space narrowing in degenerative joint disease is irregular and more pronounced in that part of the joint where weight-bearing stress is

greatest and where degeneration of the articular cartilage is most noticeable. The articular ends of the bones become increasingly dense (periarticular sclerosis). Erosion of the articular cortex may produce typical irregular, cystlike lesions with sclerotic margins in the subchondral bone near the joint. Calcific or ossified loose bodies may develop, especially at the knee. With advanced disease, relaxation of the joint capsule and other ligamentous structures may lead to subluxation. Local osteoporosis does not occur unless pain causes prolonged disuse of the joint.

In the fingers, degenerative joint disease involves primarily the distal interphalangeal joints (Figure 3-22). Marginal spurs produce well-defined bony protuberances that appear clinically as the palpable and visible knobby thickening of Heberden's nodes. In the hip, the most prominent finding is asymmetric narrowing of the joint space that involves predominantly

Figure 3-22   Osteoarthritis of fingers. Note narrowing of interphalangeal joints with spurring and erosions.

Figure 3-23   Osteoarthritis of the hip.

Figure 3-24   Osteoarthritis of the knee.

the superior and lateral aspects of the joint, where the greatest stress of weight bearing exists (Figure 3-23). Joint space narrowing is also asymmetric in the knee, where it predominantly involves the medial femoro-tibial compartment (Figure 3-24).

Infectious arthritis

Pyogenic (pus-forming) organisms may gain entry into a joint by the hematogenous route, by direct extension from an adjacent focus of osteomyelitis, or from trauma to the joint (e.g., after surgery, needling). The onset of bacterial arthritis usually presents abruptly with a high fever, shaking chills, and one or a few severely tender and swollen joints. The most common type today is a migratory arthritis from Lyme disease.

Radiographic appearance

Soft-tissue swelling is the first radiographic sign of acute bacterial arthritis. In children, fluid distention of the joint capsule may cause widening of the joint space and actual subluxation, especially about the hip and shoulder. Periarticular edema displaces or obliterates

adjacent tissue fat planes (Figure 3-25, *A*). Rapid destruction of articular cartilage causes joint space narrowing early in the course of the disease. The earliest bone changes, which tend to appear 8 to 10 days after the onset of symptoms, are small focal erosions in the articular cortex. Because of the delay in bone changes, detection of the characteristic soft-tissue abnormalities is essential for early diagnosis. Severe, untreated infections cause extensive destruction and a loss of the entire cortical outline (Figure 3-25). With healing, sclerotic bone reaction results in an irregular articular surface. If the articular cartilage has been completely destroyed, bony ankylosis usually follows.

Figure 3-25 Acute staphylococcal arthritis. **A,** Several days after instrumentation of shoulder for joint pain, there is separation of humeral head from glenoid fossa caused by fluid in joint space. **B,** Six weeks later, pronounced cartilage and bone destruction are evident, with sclerosis on both sides of the glenohumeral joint. **C,** Septic arthritis. On a radionuclide bone scan, a focal area of increased activity in the right shoulder correlates with the clinical history of septic arthritis.

Radiographic appearance of tuberculous arthritis

Tuberculous arthritis is a chronic, indolent infection that has an insidious onset and a slowly progressive course (Figure 3-26). It usually involves only one joint, and it affects primarily the spine, hips, and knees. Most patients have a focus of tuberculosis elsewhere in the body, most commonly in the lungs.

A distinctive early radiographic feature of tuberculous arthritis is the extensive juxtaarticular osteoporosis that precedes bone destruction; this is in contrast to bacterial arthritis, in which osteoporosis is a relatively late finding. Joint effusion leads to a nonspecific periarticular soft-tissue swelling. Cartilage and bone destruction occur relatively late in the course of tuberculous arthritis and tend to initially involve the periphery

Figure 3-26 Tuberculous arthritis of the elbow with complete destruction of the joint space. A large chronic granulomatous mass can be seen in the antecubital region. (*From Forrester DM, Brown JC, Nesson JW: The radiology of joint disease, Philadelphia, 1978, Saunders.*)

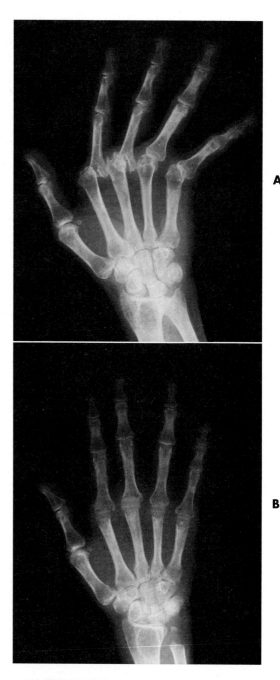

Figure 3-27 Rheumatoid arthritis. **A,** This posteroanterior (PA) image of the hand demonstrates dislocation and joint destruction of the second through fifth metacarpophalangeal joints. **B,** Postoperative image, with digits fully extended, illustrates joint implants.

of the joint, sparing the maximal weight-bearing surfaces that are destroyed in pyogenic arthritis. Therefore joint space narrowing occurs late in tuberculous arthritis in contrast to the early narrowing with bacterial infections. As in pyogenic arthritis, the earliest evidence of bone destruction is usually erosion at the margins of the articular ends of bone. With progressive disease, there is ragged destruction of the articular cartilage and subchondral cortex and disorganization of the joint, often with preservation of necrotic fragments of bone (sequestra) that may involve opposing surfaces ("kissing sequestra").

Treatment of Arthritis

Arthritis therapy should protect affected joints, maintain mobility, and strengthen muscles. For this to occur, lifestyle changes, use of support devices, drugs, and surgery may be necessary. For those with rheumatoid arthritis and osteoarthritis, which make up 90% of all cases diagnosed, rest and exercise are recommended to minimize inflammation and preserve the range of motion. The first-line medications are nonsteroidal anti-inflammatory drugs (NSAIDs), which decrease the inflammatory response but do not affect the disease process. Prostaglandin inhibitors, such as aspirin and ibuprofen (salicylates), fall into this category of drugs that reduce the triggering of inflammation. A more aggressive group of drugs, disease-modifying antirheumatic drugs, are used in advanced stages to reduce symptoms. The antimetabolite methotrexate, a cytoxic

drug, tempers cell division in the synovial joint. Invasive surgery includes replacing joints with new artificial joints (Figure 3-27) to increase joint mobility. For infectious arthritis, antibiotics usually eradicate the infection and cure the arthritis. Aspiration may be needed if fluid accumulates in the bursa.

Bursitis

Bursitis refers to an inflammation of the bursae, small fluid-filled sacs located near the joints that reduce the friction caused by movement. Repeated physical activity commonly causes bursitis, but trauma, rheumatoid arthritis, gout, or infections also can cause this inflammation. Bursitis or tenosynovitis is usually not visualized on plain radiographs but disorders of the bursa and synovium can be seen on ultrasound images (Figure 3-28). Plain films may exclude other disorders that cause similar symptoms.

Radiographic appearance

The major radiographic manifestation of bursitis is the deposition of calcification in adjacent tendons, which is a common cause of pain, limitation of motion (frozen joints), and disability about a joint. Calcific tendinitis most commonly involves the shoulder, and calcification may be demonstrated radiographically in about half the patients with persistent pain and disability in the shoulder region (Figure 3-29). However, calcification may also be detected in asymptomatic persons, and severe clinical symptoms may occur without evidence of calcification. Calcific tendinitis appears as amorphous calcium deposits that most frequently occur about the shoulder in the supraspinatus tendon, where they are seen directly above the greater tuberosity of the humerus. The deposits vary greatly in size and shape, from thin curvilinear densities to large calcific masses.

Treatment

First-line treatments for bursitis include application of heat, rest, and immobilization. NSAIDs are taken to reduce inflammation and relieve pain, as necessary. If the inflammation results from an infection, a regimen of antibiotics is appropriate. In recurring or severe bursitis, corticosteroid injections into the affected bursa may reduce the inflammation.

Rotator cuff tears

The rotator cuff of the shoulder is a musculotendinous structure composed of the teres minor, infraspinatus, supraspinatus, and subscapularis muscles. Rupture of the rotator cuff produces a communication between the shoulder joint and the subacromial bursa that can be demonstrated by arthrography (the injection of contrast material directly into the shoulder joint) (Figure 3-30). Currently, MRI is considered the modality of choice for demonstrating a rotator cuff disorder. The normal rotator cuff appears as a black structure, but tears cause it to have high signal intensity (Figure 3-31). However, ultrasound may be the preferred initial modality to demonstrate the tear of the tendon (Figure 3-32) because of its wider availability and lower cost.

Figure 3-28 Bursitis. Transverse scan of the posterior aspect of the elbow shows the thick-walled, fluid-containing olecranal bursa. Power-mode color Doppler imaging shows the bursa's activity. (From Rumack C, Wilson S, Charboneau JW, editors: *Diagnostic ultrasound,* ed 2, St Louis, 1998, Mosby.)

Figure 3-29 Calcific tendinitis. Frontal projection of shoulder demonstrates amorphous calcium deposits *(arrows)* in supraspinatus tendon.

Tears of the menisci of the knee

Meniscal tears are a common cause of knee pain. Although occasionally the result of acute trauma, meniscal tears more frequently reflect a degenerative process caused by the chronic trauma inherent in human knee function. In the past, meniscal tears were

Figure 3-30　Shoulder arthrography of rotator cuff tear. Opacification of subacromial and subdeltoid bursae indicates abnormal communication between them and the glenohumeral joint cavity, thus confirming the diagnosis. (From Greenspan A: *Orthopedic radiology*, Philadelphia, 1988, Lippincott.)

best demonstrated by arthrography, which is invasive; now, MRI is clearly the imaging modality of choice, as it is noninvasive and has an accuracy of 90% to 98%.

MRI demonstrates a tear as a sharply marginated line of high signal intensity (Figure 3-33) that crosses the normally dark, triangular meniscus. In addition, this modality can show the often-associated tears of the anterior and posterior cruciate ligaments as well as changes in the underlying bone. Ultrasound may demonstrate tenosynovitis of related tendons, which appears as a thickened synovial sheath (Figure 3-34).

Treatment for intraarticular components

Antiinflammatory medications and immobilization of the joint are the first line of treatment if the damage will repair itself. When the component is not completely destroyed, this treatment may result in cure (30% to 90% of patients respond to nonsurgical treatment). When irreparable joint damage has occurred, the orthopedist performs arthroscopic surgery to remove a complete or nonhealing tear, or to attempt suture repair.

Osteomyelitis—bacterial

Bacterial osteomyelitis is an inflammation of the bone (osteitis) and bone marrow (myelitis) caused by a broad spectrum of infectious (most often gram-

Figure 3-31　MR image of rotator cuff tear. **A,** Normal shoulder. Notice the low signal intensity of the supraspinatus tendon *(ss)*. *A,* Acromion; *C,* clavicle; *D,* deltoid muscle; *G,* glenoid fossa; *H,* humeral head; *IG,* inferior glenohumeral ligament; *L,* glenoid labrum. **B,** Degenerative tear. A high signal intensity *(arrow)* can be seen within the rotator cuff. (From Stark DD, Bradley WG Jr: *Magnetic resonance imaging*, ed 2, St Louis, 1991, Mosby.)

positive) organisms that reach bone by hematogenous spread, by extension from an adjacent site of infection, or by direct introduction of organisms (after trauma or surgery). Acute hematogenous osteomyelitis tends to involve bones with rich red marrow. In infants and children, the metaphyses of long bones, especially the femur and tibia, are most often affected; staphylococci and streptococci are the most common organisms. Patients with acute osteomyelitis experience fever and localized warmth, swelling, and tenderness. In adults, acute hematogenous osteomyelitis primarily occurs in the vertebrae, causing localized back pain and muscle spasm, and it rarely involves the long bones. Although the incidence and severity of osteomyelitis have decreased since the advent of antibiotics, this disease has recently become more prevalent as a complication of intravenous drug abuse (in which case,

Figure 3-32 Horizontal full-thickness tear. The longitudinal ultrasound image through the supraspinatus tendons, *S*, shows 2-cm retraction of the torn tendon (the distance between the calipers [x]). Bursa and peribursal fat *(curved arrow)* rest directly on the irregular bone surface of the greater tuberosity, *gt. E*, Humeral epiphysis. (From Rumack C, Wilson S, Charboneau JW, editors: *Diagnostic ultrasound*, ed 2, St Louis, 1998, Mosby.)

Figure 3-33 Meniscal tear. Sagittal MR scan of knee shows horizontal line of high signal intensity *(arrow)* crossing dark posterior horn of medial meniscus. (From Stark DD, Bradley WG Jr: *Magnetic resonance imaging,* ed 2, St Louis, 1991, Mosby.)

gram-negative organisms are found). In diabetic patients and those with other types of vascular insufficiency, a soft-tissue infection may spread from a skin abscess or a decubitus ulcer, usually in the foot, to cause cellulitis and eventually osteomyelitis in adjacent bones.

Osteomyelitis begins as an abscess of the bone. Pus produced by the acute inflammation spreads down the medullary cavity and outward to the surface. Once the infectious process has reached the outer margin of the bone, it raises the periosteum from the bone and may spread along the surface for a considerable distance.

Because the earliest changes of osteomyelitis are usually not evident on plain radiographs until about 10 days after the onset of symptoms, radionuclide (gallium) bone scanning is the most valuable imaging modality for the early diagnosis of osteomyelitis. Increased nuclide uptake, reflecting the inflammatory process and increased blood flow, is evident within hours of the onset of symptoms (Figure 3-35).

Radiographic appearance

On plain radiographs the earliest evidence of osteomyelitis in a long bone is a localized, deep soft-tissue swelling adjacent to the metaphysis. The inflammation causes displacement or obliteration of the normal fat planes adjacent to and between the deep

Figure 3-34 Acute patellar tendinitis. Longitudinal ultrasound scan shows thickening and decreased echogenicity of the upper two thirds of the tendon *(arrows). F,* Femoral condyle; *P,* patella. (From Rumack C, Wilson S, Charboneau JW, editors: Diagnostic ultrasound, ed 2, St Louis, 1998, Mosby.)

muscle bundles, unlike in skin infections, where the initial swelling is superficial. The initial bony change appears as subtle areas of metaphyseal lucency reflecting resorption of necrotic bone. Soon, bone destruction becomes more prominent, producing a ragged, moth-eaten appearance (Figures 3-36 and

Figure 3-35 Osteomyelitis. Radionuclide bone scan (posterior projection) demonstrates increased uptake of radionuclide in trochanteric portion of right femur *(arrow)*. Plain film of pelvis and hips obtained at the same time showed no detectable abnormality.

Figure 3-36 Osteomyelitis. Patchy pattern of bone destruction involves much of the shaft of the radius. Notice early periosteal new bone formation *(arrows)*.

3-37). The more virulent the organism, the larger is the area of destruction. Subperiosteal spread of inflammation elevates the periosteum and stimulates the deposition of layers of new bone parallel to the shaft. This results in a layered periosteal reaction that is characteristic of benign diseases, especially infection. Eventually, a large amount of new bone surrounds the cortex in a thick, irregular bony sleeve (involucrum). Disruption of cortical blood supply leads to bone necrosis. Segments of avascular dead bone (sequestra) remain as dense as normal bone and are clearly differentiated from the demineralized bone, infected granulation tissue, and pus around them (Figure 3-38).

After the acute infection has subsided, a pattern of chronic osteomyelitis develops. The bone appears thickened and sclerotic with an irregular outer margin. The cortex may become so dense that the medullary cavity is difficult to demonstrate. Reactivation of infection may appear as the recurrence of deep soft-tissue swelling or periosteal calcification, or the development of lytic abscess cavities within the bone. However, plain radiographs are often inadequate to determine whether an active infection is present. Radionuclide scanning is much more sensitive and accurate for establishing recurrence.

The earliest sign of vertebral osteomyelitis is subtle erosion of the subchondral bony plate with loss of the sharp cortical outline. This may progress to total destruction of the vertebral body associated with a paravertebral soft-tissue abscess (Figure 3-39). Unlike neoplastic processes, osteomyelitis usually affects the intervertebral disk space and often involves adjacent vertebrae. Depending on the site of disease, anterior extension of osteomyelitis may cause retropharyngeal abscess, mediastinitis, empyema, pericarditis, subdiaphragmatic abscess, psoas muscle abscess, or peritonitis; posterior extension of inflammatory tissue can compress the spinal cord or produce menin-

Figure 3-37 Staphylococcal osteomyelitis. **A,** Initial film of first metatarsophalangeal joint shows soft-tissue swelling and periarticular demineralization caused by increased blood flow to region. **B,** Several weeks later, severe bony destruction about metatarsophalangeal joint can be seen.

gitis if the infection penetrates the dura to enter the subarachnoid space.

CT can be of value in the diagnosis of osteomyelitis, especially that involving the spine. This modality can precisely define the size of the surrounding soft-tissue mass, its relation to nearby vital structures (aorta, spinal cord), and the presence of abscess cavities requiring surgical drainage (see Figure 3-38, *B*).

MRI can assist in determining whether an abscess has formed and in excluding cellulitis. Bone marrow changes caused by inflammatory exudate result in decreased signal intensity on T1-weighted images and increased signal intensity on T2-weighted images (see Figure 3-38, *C*).

Treatment

Antibiotics to eradicate gram-negative or gram-positive organisms should be taken for 4 to 8 weeks to prevent recurrence. Surgery may be required for debridement of necrotic tissue or for drainage placement into an abscess. Bone grafts, usually of bone marrow, are placed to fill bony defects or to help bones heal. After surgery, the patient must continue to take antibiotics for approximately 3 weeks.

Osteomyelitis—tuberculous

Tuberculous osteomyelitis (which is rare today) most commonly involves the thoracic and lumbar spine. **Pott's disease** (tuberculosis of the spine) occurs in the mid-thoracic spine and thoracolumbar region. Irregular, poorly marginated bone destruction within the vertebral body is often associated with a characteristic paravertebral abscess, an accumulation of purulent material that produces a fusiform soft-tissue mass about the vertebra. The spread of tuberculous osteomyelitis causes narrowing of the adjacent intervertebral disk and the extension of infection and bone destruction across the disk to involve the adjacent vertebral body. Unlike bacterial infection, tuberculous osteomyelitis is rarely associated with periosteal reaction or bone sclerosis.

Radiographic appearance

The infection tends to begin in the anterior part of the vertebral body adjacent to the intervertebral disk (Figure 3-40, *A).* Caseous necrosis of the vertebral marrow produces a slow resorption of bony trabeculae, with bone destruction appearing 2 to 5 months after onset of infection. In the untreated patient, progressive vertebral collapse and anterior wedging lead

A   **B**   **C**

Figure 3-38 Chronic osteomyelitis. **A,** Involucrum *(straight arrows)* surrounds sequestra *(curved arrows).* **B,** After knee surgery, multiple foci can be seen to be lacking trabeculation in both femoral condyles in this 33-year-old woman. **C,** Sagittal MRI on the patient in **B** shows decreased signal intensity from the femoral condyle extending into the femoral shaft.

Figure 3-39 Bacterial vertebral osteomyelitis. Narrowing of intervertebral disk space with irregularity of end plates and reactive sclerosis.

Figure 3-40 Tuberculous osteomyelitis. **A,** Initial film demonstrates vertebral collapse and anterior wedging of adjacent mid-thoracic vertebrae *(arrow)*. Residual intervertebral disk space can barely be seen. **B,** Several months later there is virtual fusion of collapsed vertebral bodies, producing characteristic sharp kyphotic angulation (gibbous deformity).

to a characteristic sharp kyphotic angulation (gibbous deformity) (Figure 3-40, *B*). A radionuclide bone scan may demonstrate early activity but cannot distinguish tumors or fractures. The gallium bone scan can help to define the total tissue involvement and determine therapy response in tuberculous osteomyelitis. CT also may delineate the extent of soft-tissue involvement and illustrate osseous destruction. Soft tissue calcifications identified on CT aid in distinguishing tuberculous osteomyelitis from other conditions. MRI scans demonstrate changes in the bone marrow but are no more specific than the radionuclide bone scans.

Tuberculosis can, rarely, involve a low-grade chronic infection of the long bones that appears radiographically as a generally destructive lytic process with minimal or no periosteal reaction. The spectrum of radiographic appearances is wide, varying from localized, well-circumscribed, expansile lesions to diffuse, uniform, honeycomb-like areas of destruction that are often associated with pathologic fractures. Chronic draining sinuses may develop, especially in children.

Treatment

Nonoperative treatments for tuberculous osteomyelitis include a regimen of antibiotics, antituberculous drug therapy, and possible bracing. Antibiotics help prevent abscess development, antituberculous drug therapy eradicates the tuberculosis bacilli, and bracing provides support. With this treatment combination, most patients do not require surgery. If the pain, neurologic deficits, and deformities progress, surgical intervention may be necessary. Spinal fusion or Harrington rod placement for stability may be performed.

■ Metabolic Bone Disease

Osteoporosis

Osteoporosis is a generalized or localized deficiency of bone matrix in which the mass of bone per unit volume is decreased in amount but normal in composition. Bone is a living, constantly changing tissue, and normally a balance exists between the amount of old bone being removed (an osteoclastic process) and the amount of new bone replacement (an osteoblastic process). Osteoporosis is usually caused by accelerated resorption of bone, although decreased bone formation may lead to osteoporosis in some situations, for example in Cushing's syndrome, after prolonged steroid administration, and after prolonged disuse or immobilization as in a casted extremity (Figure 3-41).

Loss of mineral salts causes osteoporotic bone to become more lucent than normal. This may be difficult to detect, because about 50% to 70% of the bone density must be lost before it can be demonstrated as a lucent area on routine radiographs. For patients with osteoporosis it is essential to use the lowest practical kilovolts peak (kVp). This technique provides the extremely short scale of contrast necessary

Summary of Findings for Inflammatory and Infectious Disorders

DISORDER	LOCATION	RADIOGRAPHIC APPEARANCE	TREATMENT
Rheumatoid arthritis	Small joints	Periarticular soft-tissue swelling Symmetric joint destruction and deformity	NSAIDs Surgery is last resort Possible joint implants or replacements
Osteoarthritis	Weight-bearing joints	Irregular narrowing of joint space	NSAIDs (timed release and coated)
Infectious arthritis	Any joint	Early joint narrowing with focal erosions	Antibiotics
Bursitis	Shoulder most common	Radiograph—calcific tendinitis in 50% US—thickened synovium or dense synovial fluid	Antibiotics if infection related Immobilization NSAIDs Corticosteroid injection
Rotator cuff tear Meniscal tear of the knee	Shoulder Knee	US—tear in bursa and inflamed synovium MRI—tears have a high signal intensity (normal—black)	Nonsurgical: physical therapy, immobilization, and NSAIDs Surgery: rotator cuff repair or meniscus removal
Osteomyelitis—bacterial	Child—long bones high in red marrow Adult—vertebra or bone associated with decubitus ulcer	Radiograph—soft tissue swelling with periosteal elevation CT—defines tissue involvement MRI—demonstrates changes in bone marrow signal intensity	Antibiotics first-line treatment Surgery for debridement
Osteomyelitis—tuberculous	Vertebra (Pott's disease)—thoracic and lumbar most common	Lytic lesion without periosteal elevation Collapsed vertebra with kyphosis	Nonoperative: antibiotics, antituberculous drug therapy, and bracing Surgical: spinal fusion and Harrington rod placement for stability

NSAIDs, Nonsteroidal antiinflammatory drugs; *US*, ultrasound.

to visualize the demineralized osteoporotic bones. Today, quantitative CT, single-photon absorptiometry, and dual-energy x-ray absorptiometry (DEXA bone densitometry—qualitative) provide data that measure bone mineral content. A quantitative CT scan accurately demonstrates levels of bone mass and determines the rate of bone decay, which represents bone quantity. CT scans, because of their high radiation dose, are not done as frequently as bone densitometry.

DEXA bone densitometry is used to image the hip and spine, assisting in determining bone quality. The patient's history is entered into the computer system and two images, usually an AP lumbar spine and an AP hip, are taken (Figure 3-42). The image data are compared to those of other individuals of the same race, age, and weight to determine a bone-quality value. This value indicates whether the patient has normal bone (T-score greater than −1.0 standard deviation (SD), osteopenia (T-score between −1.0 and −2.5 SD), or osteoporosis (T-score less than −2.5 SD).

The major causes of generalized osteoporosis include aging and postmenopausal hormonal changes. With increasing age, bones lose density and become more brittle, fracturing more easily and healing more slowly. Two factors contribute to this: elderly persons may become less active and they may have poor diets, often deficient in protein. In post-

Figure 3-41   Disuse osteoporosis. Severe periarticular demineralization after prolonged immobilization of the hand.

menopausal women there is a deficiency in the gonadal hormonal levels that stimulate bone formation. This decreased bone formation plus an increase in bone resorption by a factor of three to five times result in a loss in density.

Radiographic appearance

Regardless of the cause, the radiographic appearance is somewhat similar in all conditions producing osteoporosis. The most striking change is cortical thinning, with irregularity and resorption of the endosteal (inner) surfaces (Figure 3-43). These findings are most evident in the spine and pelvis. As the bone density of a vertebral body decreases, the cortex appears as a relatively dense and prominent thin line producing the typical picture-frame pattern. Because of the severe loss of bone density, anterior wedging or compression fractures of one or more vertebral bodies may result, most commonly in the middle and lower thoracic and upper lumbar areas. The intervertebral disk may expand into the weakened vertebral bodies and produce characteristic concave contours of the superior and inferior disk surfaces. In the skull, the calvaria may show a spotty loss of density, and there is commonly deossification (bone loss) of the floor of the sella turcica and dorsum sellae.

Figure 3-42   Osteoporosis. Results of DEXA bone mineral densitometry (BMD) of the spine. **A,** A T-score average of 3.3 demonstrates osteoporosis. **B,** The dual femur of this 65-year-old woman has a T-score average of 2.3, indicating osteopenia.

Treatment

To help prevent osteoporosis, weight-bearing exercises help build bone density and muscle mass. For postmenopausal osteoporosis, hormonal replacement therapy and dietary supplements of calcium and vitamin D may reduce development of the disease process.

Osteomalacia

Osteomalacia refers to insufficient mineralization of the adult skeleton. The lack of a balance between osteoid formation and mineralization influencing

Figure 3-43   Osteoporosis of aging. Generalized demineralization of spine in postmenopausal woman. Cortex appears as a thin line that is relatively dense and prominent (picture-frame pattern).

bone quality results in either excessive osteoid formation or, more frequently, insufficient mineralization. Proper calcification of osteoid requires that adequate amounts of calcium and phosphorus be available at the mineralization sites. In osteomalacia, failure of calcium and phosphorus deposition in bone matrix may be attributable to an inadequate intake of, or to a failure of absorption of, calcium, phosphorus, or vitamin D. Vitamin D is necessary for intestinal absorption of calcium and phosphorus and may have a direct effect on bone. At times, the level of vitamin D is sufficient but is not used because of resistance to the action of the vitamin at end organs, such as the kidneys. Other nonnutritional causes of osteomalacia include chronic kidney failure and certain renal diseases in which calcium is lost to the urine and then bone breaks down as the body attempts to maintain a normal calcium level in the blood.

Radiographic appearance

Regardless of the cause, osteomalacia appears radiographically as a loss of bone density because of the presence of nonmineralized osteoid. Although the cortex is thinned, it may stand out more prominently than normal because of the uniform deossification of medullary bone (Figure 3-44). In contrast to the situation in osteoporosis, the cortical borders in osteomalacia often appear indistinct. Fine-detail radiographs of the hands in patients with osteomalacia often demonstrate intracortical lines caused by local resorption or lack of mineralization, a finding not seen in osteoporosis.

Bones that are softened by osteomalacia may bend or give way as a result of weight bearing. Bowing deformities primarily involve the pelvis, vertebral column, thorax, and proximal extremities. In the pelvis, there may be a characteristic inward bending of the sidewalls with deepening of the acetabular cavities (protrusio acetabuli) (Figure 3-45).

Rickets

Rickets is a systemic disease of infancy and childhood that is the equivalent of osteomalacia in the mature skeleton. In this condition, calcification of growing skeletal elements is defective because of a deficiency of vitamin D in the diet or a lack of exposure to ultraviolet radiation (sunshine), which converts sterols in the skin into vitamin D. Rickets, most common in premature infants, usually develops between the ages of 6 months and 1 year.

Radiographic appearance

The early radiographic changes in rickets are best seen in the fastest-growing portions of bone, such as the sternal ends of the ribs, the proximal ends of the tibia and humerus, and the distal ends of the radius and ulna. An overgrowth of noncalcified osteoid tissue appears radiographically as a characteristic increase in distance between the ossified portion of the epiphysis and the end of the shaft. In response to the pull of muscular and ligamentous attachments, the metaphyseal ends of the bone become cupped and frayed, and the normally sharp metaphyseal lines disappear (Figure 3-46). Lack of calcification leads to a delayed appearance of the epiphyseal ossification centers. Because of poor mineralization, bowing of weight-bearing bones (especially the tibia) develops once the infant begins to stand or walk. Extensive osteoid tissue in the sternal ends of the ribs produces a characteristic beading (rachitic rosary).

Softening of the vertebral bodies leads to the development of kyphosis. In females, narrowing of the pelvic inlet may make normal delivery impossible in later life.

Figure 3-44   Osteomalacia. Striking prominence of cortices of vertebral bodies with increased trabeculation of spongy bone.

Figure 3-45   Protrusio acetabuli, as seen in osteomalacia and also in Paget's disease.

Treatment for osteomalacia and rickets

Treatment consists of doses of vitamin D with calcium supplements. Other treatments are required if the calcium loss has a nonnutritional cause.

Gout

Gout is a disorder in the metabolism of purine (a component of nucleic acids) in which an increase in the

Figure 3-46   Rickets. **A,** Initial film of this wrist shows characteristic cupping and fraying of metaphyseal ends of the radius and ulna, with disappearance of normally sharp metaphyseal lines. **B,** After therapy with vitamin D, there is remineralization of metaphyseal ends of the radius and ulna, increased sharpness of metaphyseal lines, and a return of epiphyseal centers to normal density and sharpness of outline.

blood level of uric acid leads to the deposition of uric acid crystals in the joints, cartilage, and kidney. Several inherited enzyme defects can cause overproduction of uric acid (primary gout). In secondary gout, hyperuricemia can be caused by an overproduction of uric acid, which in turn may be caused by increased turnover of nucleic acids (e.g., as in metastatic carcinoma, myeloma, hemolytic anemia),

Figure 3-47   Gout. Effusion with tophi deposits at the first, fourth, and fifth metatarsophalangeal joints.

drugs (chemotherapy, thiazides used to treat hypertension), or a decrease in the excretion of uric acid resulting from kidney failure.

Radiographic appearance

Acute gout primarily manifests as an exquisitely painful arthritis that initially attacks a single joint, primarily the first metatarsophalangeal joint (Figure 3-47). Radiographic changes develop late in the disease and only after repeated attacks. Therefore negative radiographs do not exclude gout and thus do not aid in early diagnostic evaluation.

Deposition of nonopaque urate crystals in the joint synovial membrane and on the surface of articular cartilage incites an inflammatory reaction that produces the earliest radiographic signs of joint effusion and periarticular swelling (Figure 3-48). Clumps of urate crystals (tophi) form along the margins of the articular cortex and erode the underlying bone, producing small, sharply marginated, punched-out defects at the joint margins of the small bones of the hand and foot. These erosions often have the appearance of cystlike lesions with thin sclerotic margins and characteristic overhanging edges ("rat-bite" erosions) (Figure 3-49). In advanced disease, severe destructive lesions are associated with joint space narrowing and even fibrous ankylosis. Because patients are relatively free of symptoms between acute exacerbations of the disease, the bone density remains relatively normal, and diffuse osteoporosis is not part of the radiographic appearance.

Continued deposition of urate crystals in the periarticular tissues causes the development of the characteristic large, lumpy soft-tissue swellings representing gouty tophi. In addition to the first metatarsophalangeal

Figure 3-48   Gout. Severe joint effusion and periarticular swelling of proximal interphalangeal joint of finger. Note associated erosion of articular cartilage.

joints, other common sites of tophi include the ear, the olecranon bursa, and the insertion of the Achilles tendon. Tophi consisting of only sodium urate appear as a soft-tissue density. Deposition of calcium in these urate collections causes the tophaceous periarticular masses to become radiopaque (Figure 3-50).

Although some renal dysfunction occurs in almost all patients with gouty arthritis, no radiographic abnormalities in the urinary tract can be demonstrated unless uric acid stones form. Nonradiopaque pure uric acid stones can be demonstrated only on excretory urograms, where they appear as filling defects in the pelvocalyceal system or ureter. Stones containing the calcium salts of uric acid can be detected on plain abdominal radiographs, where they appear radiopaque.

MRI produces various patterns, although regions of persistent low signal intensity are characteristic.

Figure 3-49 Two examples of typical "rat-bite" erosions about first metatarsophalangeal joint *(arrows)*. The cystlike lesions have thin sclerotic margins and characteristic overhanging edges.

Treatment

Patients receiving doses of antihyperuricemic drugs rarely experience tophi. Untreated gout may lead to decreased renal excretion because of renal damage resulting from crystal deposits in the interstitial tissue. Eventually, this causes obstruction of the renal tubules and renal failure.

Paget's disease

Paget's disease (osteitis deformans) is one of the most common chronic metabolic diseases of the skeleton. Destruction of bone, followed by a reparative process, results in weakened, deformed, and thickened bony structures that tend to fracture easily. The disease, seen most commonly during middle life, affects men twice as often as women and has been reported to occur in about 3% of all persons older than 40 years of age. Although the destructive phase often predominates initially, there is more frequently a combination of destruction and repair in the pelvis and weight-bearing bones of the lower extremities. The reparative process may begin early and may be the prominent feature, often involving multiple bones. Paget's disease affects particularly the pelvis, femurs, skull, tibias, vertebrae, clavicles, and ribs. The radionuclide bone scan is the most efficient method to visualize multicentric lesions (Figure 3-51, *A*).

Radiographic appearance

In the skull, Paget's disease begins as an area of sharply demarcated radiolucency (osteoporosis circumscripta) that represents the destructive phase of the disease (see Figure 3-51, *B*). During the reparative process, the development of irregular islands of sclerosis and cortical thickening results in a mottled,

Figure 3-50 Gout. Massive deposition of calcium in long-standing tophaceous lesion about elbow.

cotton-wool appearance (see Figure 3-51, *C*). In the spine, Paget's disease characteristically causes enlargement of the vertebral body. Increased trabeculation, which is most prominent at the periphery of the bone, produces a rim of thickened cortex and a picture-frame appearance. Uniform dense sclerosis of one or more vertebral bodies (ivory vertebrae) may occur.

The pelvis is the most common and often the initial site of Paget's disease. A distinctive early sign is coarsening of the trabeculae along the iliac margins, which produces thickening of the pelvic brim (Figure 3-52).

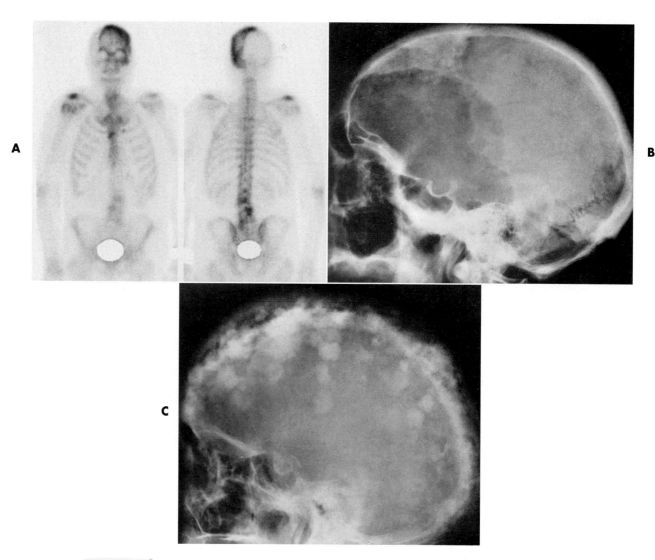

Figure 3-51 Paget's disease of the skull. **A,** Nuclear medicine bone scan demonstrating a "cold spot" within a "hot spot" in the skull. The cold spot represents the initial destructive phase, whereas the hot spot is a result of the reparative process. **B,** Radiograph obtained during the destructive phase of the disease demonstrates an area of sharply demarcated radiolucency (osteoporosis circumscripta) that involves primarily the frontal portion of the calvaria. **C,** During reparative phase in another patient, irregular areas of sclerosis produce the characteristic cotton-wool appearance of the skull.

In the long bones, the destructive phase almost invariably begins at one end of the bone and extends along the shaft for a variable distance before ending in a typical, sharply demarcated, V-shaped configuration (blade of grass appearance). In the reparative stage the bone is enlarged, with an irregularly widened cortex and coarse, thickened trabeculae (Figure 3-53). Although dense, the bones are soft and weakened, and deformities are common.

Paget's disease may lead to severe clinical complications. The downward thrust of the heavy head on the softened bone of the spine may compress the brainstem and cause numerous cranial nerve deficits. Expansion and distortion of softened vertebral bodies, sometimes with pathologic fractures, may compress the spinal cord and produce nerve root deficits. Multiple microscopic arteriovenous malformations in pagetoid bone may result in high-output cardiac failure. The most serious complication of Paget's disease, the development of osteosarcoma, fortunately occurs in less than 1% of patients with this condition. MRI and CT provide the most accurate imaging if osteosarcoma is suspected.

Treatment

No known cure exists for Paget's disease; however, administration of calcitonin may reduce the rate of

Figure 3-52 Paget's disease of the pelvis. Diffuse sclerosis with cortical thickening involves the right femur and both iliac bones. Note characteristic thickening and coarsening of the iliopectineal line *(arrow)* on the involved right side.

bone resorption. Sometimes antiinflammatory drugs reduce the inflammation caused by cell breakdown.

■ Fibrous Dysplasia

Fibrous dysplasia, a disorder that usually begins during childhood, is characterized by the proliferation of fibrous tissue within the medullary cavity. This proliferation causes loss of trabecular markings and widening of the bone. The disease may be confined to a single bone (monostotic) or the bones of one extremity, which is the most common form when it occurs in adults. The other form, in which the disease is widely distributed throughout the skeleton (polyostotic—among patients with this form, 25% have involvement of half the skeleton), presents in children and occurs most often in females. Fibrous dysplasia involves primarily the long bones (especially the femur and tibia), ribs, and facial bones.

Radiographic appearance

Fibrous replacement of the medullary cavity typically produces a well-defined radiolucent area, which may vary from completely radiolucent to a homogeneous ground-glass density, depending on the amount of fibrous or osseous tissue deposited in the medullary cavity (Figure 3-54). Irregular bands of sclerosis may cross the cystlike lesion, giving it a multilocular appearance (Figure 3-55). The bone is often locally expanded (suggesting a balloon), and the cortex may be eroded from within, predisposing to pathologic fractures. In severe and

Figure 3-53 Paget's disease of knee. Note characteristic cortical thickening, destruction of fine trabeculae, and accentuation of secondary trabeculae.

long-standing disease, affected bones may become bowed or deformed.

Fibrous dysplasia is the most common cause of an expansile focal rib lesion, which usually has a ground-glass or soap-bubble appearance.

Treatment

Treatment consists of curettage, repair of fractures, and prevention of deformities.

■ Ischemic Necrosis of Bone

Ischemic necrosis of bone results from loss of the blood supply, which in turn can result from such varied conditions as thrombosis, vasculitis, disease of surrounding bone, or single or repeated episodes of trauma. Among the many conditions associated with ischemic necrosis are acute trauma (fracture or dislocation), steroid therapy or Cushing's disease, hemolytic anemia (especially sickle cell disease), chronic alcoholism and

Summary of Findings for Metabolic Bone Disease

DISORDER	LOCATION	RADIOGRAPHIC APPEARANCE	TREATMENT

Osteoporosis	Loss of bone mass in entire skeleton (accelerated bone resorption)	Cortical thinning appears as a relatively dense and prominent thin line ↓ bone density
		DEXA BMD T-scores:
		  Normal, ≥ −1.0 SD
		  Osteopenia, −1.0 to −2.25 SD
		  Osteoporosis, ≤ −2.5 SD
			Weight-bearing exercise
			Postmenopausal—hormonal replacement therapy
			Vitamin D and calcium supplements

Osteomalacia	Insufficient mineralization of adult skeleton (deossification of medullary bone)	Loss of bone density Cortex becomes thin and often indistinct	Vitamin D supplements with calcium
Rickets	Insufficient mineralization of immature skeleton	Cupped and frayed metaphysis in long bones vitamin def.	Vitamin D with calcium supplements
Gout	1st metatarsophalangeal joint May attack any joint	Joint inflammation (effusion) Urate crystals (tophi) in joint space deposit of uric acid	Antihyperuricemic drugs
Paget's	Destruction and reparative process in pelvis, weight-bearing bones, and skull	Radiolucencies in destructive phase Cotton-wool appearance in reparative phase	No known cure Calcitonin to slow bone resorption Antiinflammatory drugs

BMD, Bone mineral density; *DEXA*, dual-energy x-ray absorptiometry; *SD*, standard deviation.

chronic pancreatitis, Gaucher's disease, radiation therapy, and caisson disease (a complication of underwater diving, the so-called bends).

Radiographic appearance

The femoral head is the most frequent site of ischemic necrosis. Initially, the ischemic bone may appear denser than adjacent viable bone. The first sign of structural failure is the development of a radiolucent subcortical band (the crescent sign) representing a fracture line (Figure 3-56, *A*). As the disorder progresses, fragmentation, compression, and resorption of dead bone, along with proliferation of granulation tissue, revascularization, and production of new bone, produce a pattern of lytic and sclerotic areas with flattening of the femoral head and periosteal new bone formation (Figure 3-56, *B*). Mechanical distortion about the hip leads to uneven weight bearing and accelerated secondary osteoarthritis.

It is often necessary to obtain two radiographs in patients with ischemic necrosis. The first is taken with normal density, whereas the second is made with increased kilovolts peak to allow for adequate penetration of the more opaque ischemic bone.

Radionuclide bone scanning is more sensitive than plain radiography for detecting changes of ischemic necrosis. In the initial stages of infarction, nuclide activity is absent in the area of involvement. As the disease progresses, this area of decreased activity may become rimmed by a zone of increased activity as a result of the reparative process.

MRI may be even more sensitive than radionuclide bone scanning for detecting ischemic necrosis. Infarction at the end of a bone causes changes in the fatty marrow, sharply reducing the normally intense T1-weighted signal from the marrow so that the infarcted area becomes gray or black (Figure 3-57).

In addition to ischemic changes in the subchondral areas of bone, infarction may involve the shaft of a long bone. In many cases this type of bone infarction is asymptomatic and is detected only on radiographs obtained for another purpose. A mature

Figure 3-54   Fibrous dysplasia. Note smudgy, ground-glass appearance of medullary cavities with failure of normal modeling.

Figure 3-55   Fibrous dysplasia. An expansile lesion of the humerus contains irregular bands of sclerosis, giving it a multilocular appearance.

A

B

Figure 3-56   Ischemic necrosis of femoral head. **A,** An arclike radiolucent cortical band (the crescent sign) *(arrow)* in the femoral head represents the fracture line. **B,** Eventually there is combination of lytic and sclerotic areas with severe flattening of the femoral head.

Figure 3-57   Ischemic necrosis. On this T1-weighted image, the ischemic left femoral head has lost its normal bright signal intensity and appears dark.

Figure 3-58   Bone infarct. Densely calcified area in medullary cavity of humerus with dense streaks extending from central region.

infarct in the shaft of a bone appears as a densely calcified area in the medullary cavity (Figure 3-58). It may be sharply limited by a dense sclerotic zone or associated with dense streaks extending from the central region. Bone infarction must be differentiated from a calcified enchondroma, which contains amorphous, spotty calcific densities, is not surrounded by a sclerotic rim, and may expand the bone.

Treatment

Immobilization is accomplished with braces (pelvic for femoral head necrosis) to prevent further erosion and necrosis. Antibiotics may be useful if the necrosis results from infection. Analgesics are appropriate if inflammation is caused by vasculitis or trauma.

▪ Benign Bone Tumors

Benign bone neoplasms generally displace soft tissue, whereas malignant bone tumors produce true soft-tissue swelling. When there is bone expansion, an intact cortex with a sclerotic margin usually indicates a benign lesion. Benign bone neoplasms occur much less often than bone metastases.

Radiographic appearance of osteochondromas

Osteochondroma (exostosis) is a benign projection of bone with a cartilaginous cap that arises in childhood or the teen years, especially about the knee. The exostosis occurs in the epiphyseal plate (the ring

of Ranvier) and grows laterally from the epiphysis. A true osteochondroma must exhibit the cortex and medullary portion as continuous bone growth. The cartilaginous cap may convert to a malignancy (chondrosarcoma or osteosarcoma). A hereditary form of osteochondroma (autosomal dominant) produces multiple lesions and has an increased risk of malignancy.

The cortex of an osteochondroma blends with that of normal bone, and the long axis of the tumor characteristically runs parallel to the parent bone and points away from the nearest joint (Figure 3-59). The best modality to demonstrate the thickness of the cartilagenic cap and thus rule out malignant conversion is MRI with long TR pulses (increased signal).

Radiographic appearance of enchondromas

Enchondromas begin as slow-growing benign cartilaginous tumors arising in the medullary canal. They are most frequently found in children and young adults, and they involve primarily the small bones of the hands and feet. Enchondromas are often multiple.

As the well-demarcated tumor grows, it expands bone locally, causing thinning and endosteal scalloping of the cortex. This often leads to a pathologic fracture with only minimal trauma (Figure 3-60). A characteristic finding of enchondroma is stippled, speckled, and ring or arclike calcifications within the lucent matrix.

Summary of Findings for Fibrous Dysplasia

DISORDER	LOCATION	RADIOGRAPHIC APPEARANCE	TREATMENT
Fibrous dysplasia	Monostotic—single bone or entire extremity Polyostotic—widely distributed	Well-defined radiolucent area, homogeneous ground-glass density, possible soap-bubble appearance	Curettage Repair of fractures Prevention of deformities
Ischemic necrosis	Femoral head most common	Crescent sign, lytic/sclerotic areas with flattening of femoral head	Immobilization Antibiotics Analgesics

Figure 3-59 Osteochondroma. The long axis of the tumor is parallel to that of the femur and points away from the knee joint.

Radiographic appearance of giant cell tumors

Giant cell tumor (osteoclastoma) typically arises at the end of the distal femur or proximal tibia of a young adult after epiphyseal closure. It begins as an eccentric lucent lesion in the metaphysis, and it characteristically extends to the immediate subarticular cortex of the bone but does not involve the joint (Fig-ure 3-61). A few giant cell tumors may be premalignant or actually malignant.

As the tumor expands toward the shaft, it produces the characteristic radiographic appearance of multiple large bubbles separated by thin strips of bone.

Radiographic appearance of osteomas

Osteomas most often arise in the outer table of the skull, the paranasal sinuses (especially frontal and ethmoid), and the mandible. Diagnosis of this tumor may be incidental on radiographs taken because of the pain produced by bone expansion.

Osteomas appear radiographically as well-circumscribed, extremely dense, round lesions that are rarely larger than 2 cm in diameter (Figure 3-62).

Radiographic appearance of osteoid osteomas

Osteoid osteoma usually develops in teenagers or young adults and produces the classic clinical symptom of local pain that is worse at night and is dramatically relieved by aspirin. Most osteoid osteomas occur in the femur and tibia and originate from osteoblastic cells. A radionuclide bone scan can help differentiate osteoid osteoma from osteomyelitis; osteoid osteoma presents as a double density, whereas osteomyelitis demonstrates only an outline because of the avascularity of the inner structure.

The tumor is typically seen as a small, round or oval, lucent center (the nidus), less than 1 cm in diameter, that is surrounded by a large, dense sclerotic zone of cortical thickening (Figure 3-63). The nidus may not be visualized depending on the bone structure involved (cortical versus cancellous). Because this dense reaction may obscure the nidus on conventional radiographs, overpenetrated films or tomography (conventional or computed) may be necessary to demonstrate it. CT is commonly used if there is need to demonstrate the central radiolucent nidus.

Figure 3-60 Enchondroma. **A,** Well-demarcated tumor *(arrow)* expands bone and thins cortex. **B,** Pathologic fracture *(arrow).*

Figure 3-61 Giant cell tumor. Typical eccentric lucent lesion in distal femoral metaphysis extends to the immediate subarticular cortex. Surrounding cortex, although thinned, remains intact.

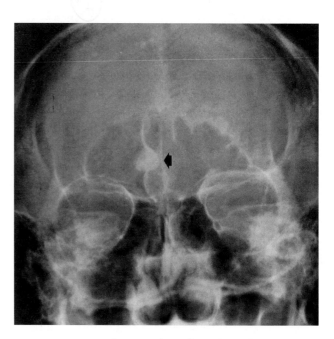

Figure 3-62 Osteoma *(arrow)* in a frontal sinus.

Figure 3-63 Osteoid osteoma. Full **(A)** and coned **(B)** projections of the mid shaft of the femur demonstrate a dense sclerotic zone of cortical thickening laterally, which contains a small oval lucent nidus *(arrowhead)*.

Radiographic appearance of simple bone cysts

A **simple bone cyst (unicameral)** is a true fluid-filled cyst with a wall of fibrous tissue that most often occurs in the proximal humerus or femur. Although not a true neoplasm, a simple bone cyst may resemble one radiographically and clinically. Solitary bone cysts are asymptomatic and often discovered either incidentally or after pathologic fracture.

The simple bone cyst appears as an expansile lucent lesion that is sharply demarcated from adjacent normal bone and may have a thin rim of sclerosis around it. It has an oval configuration, with its long axis parallel to that of the host bone (Figure 3-64).

Radiographic appearance of aneurysmal bone cysts

An **aneurysmal bone cyst,** rather than being a true neoplasm or cyst, consists of numerous blood-filled arteriovenous communications.

In long bones, an aneurysmal bone cyst is an expansile, eccentric, cystlike lesion that causes pronounced ballooning of the thinned cortex (Figure 3-65). In some cases, the cystlike lesion may present with internal separations. At times, the cortex may be so thin that it is invisible on plain radiographs, and thus this benign lesion may be mistaken for a malignant bone tumor. A CT scan may assist in defining the

Figure 3-65 Aneurysmal bone cyst. This expansile, eccentric, cystic lesion of the tibia has multiple fine internal septa. Because severely thinned cortex is difficult to detect, the tumor resembles a malignant process.

Figure 3-64 Simple bone cyst. This cyst in the proximal humerus has an oval configuration, with its long axis parallel to that of host bone.

Figure 3-66 Bone island (arrow) in femoral head.

well-lobulated lesion, but MRI better shows the internal loculations and fluid levels.

Bone islands are solitary, sharply demarcated areas of dense compact bone that occur most commonly in the pelvis and upper femur. They appear in every bone except the skull (Figure 3-66). Although almost half of the bone islands enlarge over a period of years and many show activity on radionuclide scans, bone islands are asymptomatic and completely benign and must be distinguished from osteoblastic metastases.

Treatment of benign bone tumors

An **osteochondroma** requires treatment only when mechanical friction (joint mobility) impinges on nerves, blood vessels, or muscles. For an **enchondroma**, curettage of the lesion is the common treatment. The treatment for **giant cell tumor** includes curettage of the bone and local resection. About 50% of giant cell tumors recur. Surgical excision of the nidus of an **osteoid osteoma** is essential for cure; it is not necessary to remove the reactive calcification, although it may form the major part of the lesion.

∎ ∎

Summary of Findings for Benign Bone Tumors (Neoplasia)

DISORDER	LOCATION	RADIOGRAPHIC APPEARANCE	TREATMENT
Osteochondroma	Epiphyseal plate growing laterally in long bones	Tumor runs parallel to long bone and points away from nearest joint	Surgical removal only when mechanical impingement occurs
Enchondroma	Arises in the medullary canal of hands and feet	Cortical thinning and endosteal scalloping. Calcifications within lesion appear stippled, speckled, ringlike, or arclike	Curettage of lesion
Giant cell tumor (osteoclastoma)	Metaphysis extends into subarticular cortex; does not involve the joint	Multiple large bubbles separated by stripes of bone	Curettage and local resection
Osteoma	Outer table of the skull	Extremely dense round lesions less than 2 cm in diameter	No treatment required
Osteoid osteoma	Femur and tibia, osteoblastic cells	Round or oval lesion with lucent center (nidus), sometimes surrounded by dense sclerotic zone; less than 1 cm	Surgical removal includes nidus to be successful
Simple bone cyst	Most common in proximal humerus and femur	Expansile lucent lesion with a thin rim of sclerosis	Many require no treatment. Curettage with implantation of bone chips
Aneurysmal bone cyst	Metaphysis or long bones	Pronounced ballooning with thinned cortex (internal separations)	Curettage
Bone island	Every bone except the skull	Sharply defined, dense compact lesion	No treatment required

(handwritten note: Benign Bone prog. w/ cartilaginous cap)

∎ ∎

CT-guided percutaneous radiofrequency ablation (destruction) may provide the best treatment. **Simple bone cyst** treatment depends on the size and location of the cyst. If the cyst continues to develop, surgical curettage and implantation of bone chips is performed. **Aneurysmal bone cysts** require curettage to prevent further destruction from occurring. **Bone islands** require no treatment.

∎ Malignant Bone Tumors

Malignant bone neoplasms generally cause soft-tissue swelling and cortical bone erosion that has a poorly defined or absent margin. The neoplasm extends into the soft tissue through spiculations (fingerlike projections). Plain radiographs may identify a single lesion. A radionuclide bone scan or positron emission tomography (PET) scan can detect silent lesions when minimal cellular destruction has occurred. Discover-

ing additional lesions determines the treatment and prognosis. CT and MRI can precisely define the location of a malignant bone tumor, as well as its extension into the medullary cavity and spread to surrounding structures (Figures 3-67 and 3-68).

Radiographic appearance of osteogenic sarcoma

Osteogenic sarcoma generally occurs in the end of a long bone in the metaphysis (especially about the knee). This tumor consists of osteoblasts, which produce osteoid and spicules of calcified bone. Most osteogenic sarcomas arise in persons between 10 and 25 years old, although a smaller peak incidence is seen in older persons who have a preexisting bone disorder, particularly Paget's disease. The usual initial complaints are local pain and swelling, sometimes followed by fever, weight loss, and secondary anemia. Pulmonary metastases develop early, and a plain

Figure 3-67 Osteogenic sarcoma. CT scan through the level of the femoral heads shows destruction of the left ischium, which was seen on plain radiographs. In addition, CT scan demonstrates large soft-tissue mass *(arrows)* in area covered by gluteus maximus muscle and separated from rectum. Mass was not clinically palpable. (From deSantos LA, Bernardino ME, Murray JA: Computed tomography in the evaluation of osteosarcoma: experience with 25 cases. *AJR Am J Roentgenol* 132:535-540, 1979.)

Figure 3-68 Magnetic resonance image of osteogenic sarcoma. Coronal image shows the intramedullary and soft-tissue extent of the mass. (From Stark DD, Bradley WG Jr: *Magnetic resonance imaging,* ed 2, St Louis, 1991, Mosby.)

Figure 3-69 Osteogenic sarcoma. **A,** Predominantly destructive lesion with irregular periosteal reaction. **B,** Classic sunburst pattern with bony spicules extending outward in radiating fashion.

chest radiograph should be obtained to exclude this unfavorable prognostic sign. If no metastases to the lung are detected by this modality, CT or a PET scan should be performed.

The typical radiographic appearance of osteogenic sarcoma is a mixed destructive and sclerotic lesion associated with a soft-tissue mass, irregular periosteal reaction, and reactive new bone formation (Figure 3-69, A). In the classic sunburst pattern, horizontal bony spicules extend in radiating fashion into the soft-tissue mass (Figure 3-69, B). A characteristic finding is elevation of the periosteum at the periphery of a lesion, with subsequent new bone formation (Codman's triangle) (Figure 3-70).

Radiographic appearance of chondrosarcoma

Chondrosarcoma is a malignant tumor of cartilaginous origin that may originate anew or within a preexisting cartilaginous lesion (e.g., osteochondroma, enchondroma). Tumor grading of this particular neoplasm depends on the maturity and differentiation of the cells. Chondrosarcomas commonly occur in long bones but often originate in a rib, scapula, or vertebra. The tumor is about half as common as osteogenic sarcoma; it develops at a later age (peak incidence in 35- to 60-year-olds), grows more slowly, and metastasizes later.

In addition to the bone destruction seen with all malignant tumors, chondrosarcoma often contains punctate or amorphous calcification within its cartilaginous matrix (Figure 3-71).

Radiographic appearance of Ewing's sarcoma

Ewing's sarcoma is a primary malignant tumor arising in the bone marrow of long bones. A tumor of children and young adults, Ewing's sarcoma has a peak incidence in the mid teens and is rare in persons over 30 years of age. The major clinical complaint is local pain, often of several months' duration, that persistently increases in severity and may be associated with a tender soft-tissue mass. Patients with this tumor characteristically have malaise and appear sick, often with fever and leukocytosis, suggestive of osteomyelitis.

The classic radiographic appearance of Ewing's sarcoma is an ill-defined permeative area of bone destruction that involves a large central portion of the shaft of a long bone (underlying medullary destruction) and is associated with a fusiform layered periosteal reaction (onionskin appearance) parallel to the shaft (Figure 3-72). Tumor cells invade the cortical bone and spread into the soft tissue.

Radiographic appearance of multiple myeloma

Multiple myeloma is a disseminated (widespread) malignancy of plasma cells that may be associated

Figure 3-70 Codman's triangle. Thin periosteal elevation and subsequent new bone formation at periphery of this neoplastic lesion.

Figure 3-71 Chondrosarcoma. Prominent dense calcification in large neoplastic mass.

with bone destruction, bone marrow failure, hypercalcemia, renal failure, and recurrent infections. The disease affects primarily persons between 40 and 70 years of age. This frequently occurring primary bone tumor attacks the intramedullary canal of the di-

Figure 3-72   Ewing's sarcoma. Diffuse permeative destruction with mild periosteal response involving distal half of femur.

Figure 3-73   Multiple myeloma. Diffuse punched-out osteolytic lesions scattered throughout skull.

aphysis. Typical laboratory findings include an abnormal spike of monoclonal immunoglobulin and the presence of Bence Jones protein in the urine.

The classic radiographic appearance of multiple myeloma is multiple punched-out osteolytic lesions scattered throughout the skeletal system and best seen on lateral views of the skull (Figures 3-73 and 3-74). Because the bone destruction is attributable to the proliferation of plasma cells distributed throughout the bone marrow, the flat bones containing red marrow (vertebrae, skull, ribs, pelvis) are primarily affected. The appearance may be indistinguishable from that of a metastatic carcinoma, although the lytic defects in multiple myeloma tend to be more discrete and uniform in size. Extensive plasma cell proliferation in the bone marrow with no tendency to form discrete tumor masses may produce generalized skeletal deossifications simulating postmenopausal osteoporosis. In the

spine, decreased bone density and destructive changes in multiple myeloma are usually limited to the vertebral bodies, sparing the pedicles (which lack red marrow and are frequently destroyed by metastatic disease). The severe loss of bone substance in the spine often results in multiple vertebral compression fractures (Figure 3-75).

Because multiple myeloma causes little or no stimulation of new bone formation, radionuclide bone scans may be normal even with extensive skeletal infiltration. On T1-weighted MR images, low-intensity tumor tissue replaces the normal high-intensity fatty marrow.

Treatment of malignant bone tumors

The treatment of **osteogenic sarcoma** includes surgical removal with or without chemotherapy and/or radiation therapy. Although osteogenic sarcoma is usually fatal, about 30% of patients receiving chemotherapy are cured. For **chondrosarcoma** lesions, the treatment usually includes surgical excision and radiation therapy. The more differentiated the involved cells, the higher the survival rate. Chondrosarcoma tumors are not sensitive to chemotherapy. **Ewing's sarcoma** and **multiple myeloma** are treated with radiation therapy and chemotherapy. Chemotherapy for Ewing's sarcoma increases the survival rate to about 30%. Multiple myeloma (Figure 3-76) patients have a grim prognosis, most dying within 3 to 4 years.

■ Bone Metastases

Metastases are the most common malignant bone tumors, spreading by means of the bloodstream or lym-

Figure 3-75   Multiple myeloma. Diffuse myelomatous infiltration has caused generalized demineralization of vertebral bodies and compression fracture of L2.

Figure 3-74   Diffuse destructive bone lesion that has led to pathologic fracture of femur.

phatic vessels or by direct extension. The most common primary tumors are carcinomas of the breast, lung, prostate, kidney, and thyroid. Favorite sites of metastatic spread are bones containing red marrow, such as the spine, pelvis, ribs, skull, and the upper ends of the humerus and femur. Metastases distal to the knees and elbows are infrequent but do occur, especially with bronchogenic (lung) tumors.

The detection of skeletal metastases is critical in the management of patients with known or suspected neoplastic disease, both at the time of initial staging and during the period of continuing follow-up care. The presence of metastases may exclude some patients from the radical "curative" therapy that is offered to those without disseminated disease, thus sparing them from fruitless, high-morbidity procedures for a nonremediable condition.

The best screening examination for the detection of asymptomatic skeletal metastases is the radionuclide bone scan (Figure 3-77) or the PET scan (Fig-

ure 3-78), which is unquestionably more sensitive than the radiographic skeletal survey. Because almost half the mineral content of a bone must be lost before the loss is detectable on plain radiographs, the skeletal survey should be abandoned as a general screening examination for the detection of asymptomatic skeletal metastases. False-negative findings on bone scans occur only with aggressively osteolytic lesions, especially in patients with multiple myeloma. The role of plain radiographs in screening for metastases is to further evaluate focal abnormalities detected on radionuclide scanning, because a variety of lesions (e.g., infections, benign tumors, fibrous dysplasia, bone islands) can also show positive findings on bone scans. Because the presence of multiple focal abnormalities is typical of metastatic disease, it is necessary to radiographically examine only a single lesion or area to confirm the diagnosis. In addition, because of the occasional false-negative results on a bone scan, it is imperative that all *symptomatic* sites in patients with neoplastic disease be examined by plain radiographs unless the radionuclide bone scan unequivocally demonstrates diffuse metastatic disease.

Figure 3-76 Multiple myeloma. The PET oncologic survey is positive with a pattern of extensive metabolically active tumor metastases demonstrated throughout the axial skeleton and in both lower lung fields on coronal **(A)** and transverse **(B)** images. After 4 months, when the patient is in his last cycle of chemotherapy, the survey images **(C** and **D)** still demonstrate persistent, viable, metabolically active neoplasm. However, a dramatic improvement in the overall pattern is seen when compared to the earlier scan.

Figure 3-78   PET scan showing metastases. Arrows point to metabolic activity in the skeletal system (ribs) on the fluorodeoxyglucose-PET scan.

Radiographic appearance

Metastatic disease may produce a broad spectrum of radiographic appearances. Osteolytic metastases cause destruction without accompanying bone proliferation. They develop from tumor embolic deposits in the medullary canal and eventually extend to destroy cortical bone. The margins of the lucent lesions are irregular and poorly defined, rarely sharp and smooth. The most common primary lesions causing osteolytic metastases are carcinomas of the breast, kidney, and thyroid. Metastases from carcinomas of the kidney and thyroid typically produce a single large metastatic focus that may appear as an expansile trabeculated lesion (a "blow-out") (Figure 3-79). Metastases from breast carcinoma are most often multiple when first detected.

In the spine, osteolytic metastases tend to involve not only the vertebral bodies but also the pedicles and posterior arches. Destruction of one or more pedicles may be the earliest sign of metastatic disease and may help in differentiating this process from multiple myeloma, in which the pedicles are much less often involved. Because cartilage is resistant to invasion by metastases, preservation of the intervertebral disk space may help to distinguish metastases from an inflammatory process. Pathologic collapse of vertebral bodies frequently occurs in advanced disease.

Figure 3-77   Screening radionuclide bone scan. Multiple focal areas of radionuclide uptake in axial skeleton, representing metastases from prostate carcinoma.

Figure 3-79 Blow-out metastases. **A,** Lytic expansile destruction of left ilium *(arrows)* in metastatic thyroid carcinoma. **B,** Osteolytic metastasis to humerus from carcinoma of kidney.

Osteoblastic metastases are generally considered evidence of slow growth in a neoplasm that has allowed time for a proliferation of reactive bone. In men, osteoblastic metastases are usually a result of carcinoma of the prostate gland; carcinoma of the breast is the most common primary site of osteoblastic metastases in women. These lesions initially appear as ill-defined areas of increased density that may progress to complete loss of normal bony architecture. They may vary from small, isolated round foci of sclerotic density to a diffuse sclerosis involving most or all of a bone (Figure 3-80). In the spine, this may produce the characteristic uniform density of an "ivory" vertebral body (Figure 3-81).

The combination of destruction and sclerosis in the mixed type of metastasis causes the affected bone to have a mottled appearance, with intermixed areas of lucency and increased density.

Bone destruction by metastases and associated extension of tumor in the adjacent soft tissues can be well demonstrated by CT and MRI (Figure 3-82). A PET scan can quickly determine if the patient has a solitary metastatic lesion or multiple lesions. New fusion technology (superimposition of two imaging modality scans, such as PET and MRI) can further define the number, size, and location of metastatic lesions, influencing the type of treatment best suited for the patient.

Figure 3-80 Osteoblastic metastases. Multiple areas of increased density involving pelvis and proximal femurs representing metastases from carcinoma of urinary bladder.

Treatment

Radiation therapy and chemotherapy are the most common types of treatment, but they are generally only palliative because patients diagnosed with bone metastasis have a poor prognosis.

Figure 3-81　Ivory vertebra. Diffuse sclerosis of L4 vertebral body from metastatic carcinoma of prostate.

Figure 3-82　**A,** MR image of metastases. Sagittal scan shows gross metastatic destruction and replacement of the body of T2, which has collapsed. The metastasis has a lower signal intensity than that of vertebral marrow or the spinal cord. The spinal cord is focally indented and displaced posteriorly by the tumor. Also, a low-signal-intensity lytic metastasis involves the anterior portion of T3. **B,** Vertebral metastasis of breast carcinoma. Many lytic lesions are evident on this MRI scan of the lumbar region. (**A** from Stark DD, Bradley WG Jr: *Magnetic resonance imaging,* ed 2, St Louis, 1991, Mosby.)

Summary of Findings for Malignant Bone Tumors (Neoplasia)

DISORDER	LOCATION	RADIOGRAPHIC APPEARANCE	TREATMENT
Osteogenic sarcoma	Metaphysis of long bone Most common in knee	Mixed destructive/sclerotic lesion with soft-tissue mass "Sunburst" pattern Codman's triangle	Surgical excision, with/without chemotherapy or radiation therapy
Chondrosarcoma	Metaphysis of long bone or flat bones	Punctate or amorphous calcification in cartilaginous matrix	Surgical excision Radiation therapy
Ewing's sarcoma	Bone marrow of long bones	Medullary destruction with "onionskin" periosteal reaction	Radiation therapy Chemotherapy
Multiple myeloma	Intramedullary and diaphysis of the bone	Multiple punched-out lesions	Radiation therapy Chemotherapy
Bone metastases	Entire skeleton	Irregular, poorly defined lucent lesions or poorly defined increased densities depending on site of origin	Radiation therapy Chemotherapy

▪ Fractures

Fractures are the most common skeletal abnormality seen in a general radiology practice. A fracture is defined as a disruption of bone caused by mechanical forces applied either directly to the bone or transmitted along the shaft of a bone. Although often obvious, some fractures are subtle and difficult to detect. A fracture typically appears as a radiolucent line crossing the bone and disrupting the cortical margins. However, the fracture line may be thin and easily overlooked, whereas overlap of fragments may produce a radiopaque line. Secondary signs of an underlying fracture include joint effusion, soft-tissue swelling, and interruption of the normal pattern of bony trabeculae.

Types of fractures

Fractures are described and classified by their extent, direction, and position; the number of fracture lines; and the integrity of the overlying skin (Figure 3-83). A fracture that results in discontinuity between two or more fragments is **complete;** an **incomplete** fracture causes only partial discontinuity, with a portion of the cortex remaining intact. In **closed** fractures, the overlying skin is intact; if the overlying skin is disrupted, the fracture is **open,** or **compound.** Although it is a clinical distinction, the radiographic demonstration of bone clearly protruding through the skin

and the presence of air and soft tissues about the fracture site on radiographs obtained immediately after the injury are findings highly suggestive of an open fracture.

The direction of a fracture is determined by its relationship to the long axis of long and short bones and to the longest axis of irregular bones (e.g., the talus or carpal navicular). A **transverse** fracture runs at a right angle to the long axis of a bone and most commonly results from a direct blow or is a fracture within pathologic bone. An **oblique** fracture runs a course of approximately 45 degrees to the long axis of the bone and is caused by angulation or by both angulation and compression forces. A **spiral** fracture encircles the shaft, is generally longer than an oblique fracture, and is caused by torsional forces. **Avulsion** fractures are generally small fragments torn from bony prominences; they are usually the result of indirectly applied tension forces within attached ligaments and tendons rather than direct blows.

A **comminuted** fracture is composed of more than two fragments. A **butterfly** fragment is an elongated triangular fragment of cortical bone generally detached from two other larger fragments of bone. A **segmental** fracture consists of a segment of the shaft isolated by proximal and distal lines of fracture.

A **compression** fracture results from a compression force that causes compaction of bone trabeculae and re-

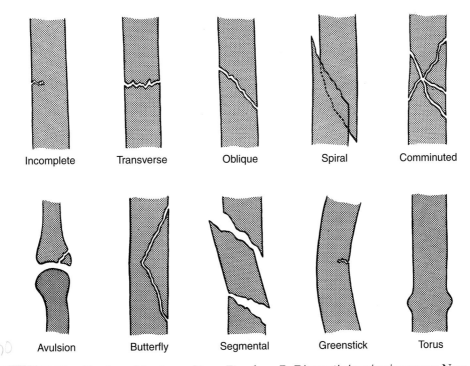

Incomplete   Transverse   Oblique   Spiral   Comminuted

Avulsion   Butterfly   Segmental   Greenstick   Torus

Figure 3-83   Classification of fractures. (From Eisenberg R: *Diagnostic imaging in surgery,* New York, 1987, McGraw-Hill.)

sults in decreased length or width of a portion of a bone. Compression fractures most commonly occur in the vertebral body as a result of flexion of the spine; they may also be seen as impacted fractures of the humeral or femoral heads. A **depressed** fracture occurs in the skull or tibial plateau. In the skull, a small object with great force can produce a comminuted fracture, with portions of the fracture fragments driven inward. In the knee, the relatively hard lateral femoral condyle may impact on the relatively soft lateral tibial plateau with sufficient force to push the cortical surface of the tibia into the underlying cancellous bone.

A **stress,** or **fatigue,** fracture is the response of bone to repeated stresses, no one of which is sufficient to cause a fracture. The earliest pathologic process in a stress fracture is osteoclastic resorption, followed by the development of periosteal callus in an attempt to repair and strengthen the bone. A **pathologic** fracture occurs in bone at an area of weakness, caused by such processes as tumor, infection, or metabolic bone disease.

A **greenstick** fracture is an incomplete fracture with the opposite cortex intact. Greenstick fractures are found almost exclusively in infants and children because of the softness of their cancellous bone. A **torus (buckle)** fracture is one in which one cortex is intact with buckling or compaction of the opposite cortex. A **bowing** fracture is a plastic deformation

caused by a stress that is too great to permit a complete recovery of normal shape but is less than the stress required to produce a fracture.

An **undisplaced** fracture occurs when a plane of cleavage exists in the bone without angulation or separation. **Displacement** refers to separation of bone fragments; the direction of displacement describes the relationship of the distal fragment with respect to the proximal fragment and is usually measured in terms of the thickness of the shaft. **Angulation** indicates an angular deformity between the axes of the major fragments and also describes the position of the distal fragment with respect to the proximal one. **Dislocation** refers to the displacement of a bone that is no longer in contact with its normal articulation. If there is only partial loss of continuity of the joint surfaces, the displacement is called a **subluxation.**

Radiographic appearance

Radiographs are essential in the diagnosis and management of fractures. Initially, a radiograph documents the clinically suspected fracture and determines whether the underlying bone is normal or whether the fracture is pathologic and has occurred in abnormal bone. After the orthopedic reduction of a fracture, repeat radiographs determine whether the fracture fragments are in anatomic position. Over the next several weeks or months, additional radiographs are obtained to assess fracture healing and to exclude possible complications.

In all cases of trauma, it is essential to have at least two projections of the injured part, preferably taken at 90 degrees to each other to determine fracture continuity or displacement in the anterior or posterior, medial or lateral, and superior or inferior direction. It is also important to demonstrate the joint above and below the fracture to search for a dislocation or a second fracture that may have resulted from transmission of the mechanical force. An example of this mechanism is the fracture or dislocation of the head of the fibula that frequently occurs with a fracture of the distal part of the tibia at the ankle.

Fracture treatment

The overall goal of fracture treatment is to restore function and stability with an acceptable cosmetic result and a minimum of residual deformity. In **external,** or **closed,** reduction the fracture is treated by manipulation of the affected body part without surgical incision. **Open reduction** is a surgical procedure utilizing direct or indirect manipulation of the fracture fragments and usually involving the application or insertion of some type of appliance or device to achieve and maintain the reduction (Figure 3-84). **External fixation** is accomplished by the use of splints or casts; **internal fixation** uses metal plates and screws, wires, rods, or nails, either alone or in combination, to maintain the reduction.

Most reduced fractures are immobilized or protected by an overlying cast. Fiberglass casting material causes less attenuation than plaster and thus produces less artifact. The radiopaque cast causes some obscuration of fine bony detail and, in severely osteoporotic bone, may make it difficult to visualize the fracture site. Therefore if there is a question of healing that requires the demonstration of early callus formation or if there is a possibility of osteomyelitis, it is essential that the cast be removed by the physician before obtaining radiographs so that there is sufficient visibility of bone detail to resolve these questions.

Fracture healing

The radiographic evidence of fracture healing is a continuous external bridge of callus (calcium deposition) that extends across the line of fracture and unites the fracture fragments (Figure 3-85). The callus uniformly ossifies and approaches the density of normal bone. It is essential that at least two views be taken (preferably 90 degrees to each other) to ensure that there is callus about the fracture line in all directions. Proper expo-

Figure 3-84 Open reduction with internal fixation. Intramedullary rod has been placed across a fracture of the femoral shaft. Note extensive callus formation about fracture site.

sure of the radiograph is required because underexposed films may produce the illusion of obliteration of the fracture line by bony trabeculae, whereas a properly exposed film would demonstrate the continued presence of the fracture line and a lack of healing. If the findings are equivocal, either computed or conventional tomography may be required to determine the degree of union. "Stress" films, a series of radiographs obtained with the injured part in the neutral position and during the application of stress by a physician or designated assistant on the distal frag-

Figure 3-85   Normal union of a fracture. There is dense callus formation bridging the previous fracture of the mid shaft of the femur. The original fracture line is completely obliterated.

Figure 3-86   Malunion. Healing of proximal phalangeal fracture in poor position led to impairment of normal function.

ment or part in the plane of suspected motion, may demonstrate a change in the alignment of the fragment, which indicates a lack of union.

Malunion is the healing of fracture fragments in a faulty position. This leads to impairment of normal function or a cosmetic appearance that may require surgical correction (Figure 3-86).

Delayed union is an ill-defined term arbitrarily applied to any fracture that takes longer to heal than the average fracture at that anatomic location. Delayed union may result from infection, from inadequate im-

mobilization, from limited blood supply, or from loss of bone at the fracture site.

Nonunion refers to a condition in which the fracture healing process has completely stopped and the fragments remain ununited even with prolonged immobilization. Radiographically, nonunion characteristically appears as smooth, well-defined sclerosis about the fracture margins with occlusion of the medullary canal by sclerotic bone (Figure 3-87). A persistent defect, consisting of fibrous tissue and cartilage, appears between the fragments. Nonunion

Figure 3-87 Nonunion of fracture of carpal navicular bone. Twenty years after initial injury, there is a smooth, well-defined line of sclerosis *(arrows)* about the fracture margin.

Figure 3-88 Pathologic fracture. A transverse fracture crosses the large benign tumor *(arrows)* of the distal femur.

occurs predominantly in adults, is rare in children, and requires operative intervention to reinitiate the healing process.

Pathologic fractures

Pathologic fractures are those occurring in bone that has been weakened by a preexisting condition. The most common underlying process is metastatic malignancy or multiple myeloma. In children, developmental diseases such as osteogenesis imperfecta or osteopetrosis, or nutritional deficiencies (rickets, scurvy) may result in pathologic fractures. Pathologic fractures also may occur when there is a benign cause of weakened bone, such as simple bone cyst, enchondroma, aneurysmal bone cyst, and fibrous dysplasia. Metabolic disorders causing a diffuse loss of bone substance (osteoporosis, osteomalacia, hyperparathyroidism) also make the skeleton more susceptible to injury.

Radiographic appearance

Clinically, pathologic fractures arise from minor trauma that would not affect normal bone. Radiographically, the fracture crosses an area of abnormal thinning, expansion, or bone destruction (Figure 3-88). The most frequent sites of pathologic fractures are the spine, femur, and humerus, areas in which metastatic disease is most common. In the spine, a pathologic fracture results in collapse of the vertebral body; indeed, a compressed vertebra in a patient older than 40 years should indicate underlying myeloma or metastatic disease.

CT or MRI scanning may detect a subtle change in the abnormal bone that is obscured by an abnormal lytic area or by sclerotic changes on plain radiographs.

Remember that patients with suspected pathologic fractures must be handled with extreme care lest the radiographer cause either further injury to the bone in question or an additional pathologic fracture in another area.

Treatment

Treatment of a pathologic fracture varies depending on the cause. Patients with malignant causes of fracture receive palliative therapy with possible surgery to place an orthotic fixation device, joint replacement, or amputation. For benign lytic lesions (cysts), surgical bone grafts or implantation of bone chips may be required to increase bone strength and structure.

Stress fractures

Stress (fatigue) fractures are the result of repeated stresses to a bone that would not be injured by isolated forces of the same magnitude. The type of stress fracture and the site where it occurs vary with

Figure 3-89 Stress fracture of third metacarpal. Initial radiograph was within normal limits. **A,** Radiograph obtained 14 days after onset of symptoms demonstrates thin oblique lucency *(arrow)* interrupting one cortex, and a small amount of fluffy periosteal callus formation *(arrowhead)* along the opposite cortex. There is no evidence of complete fracture line. **B,** Repeat radiograph 3 weeks later shows dense callus formation *(arrows)* about fracture site.

the activity. Regardless of location, the activities resulting in stress fractures are usually strenuous, often new or different, and repeated with frequency before producing pain. Stress fractures frequently occur in soldiers during basic training ("march" fracture). The most common sites are the shafts of the second and third metatarsals, the calcaneus, the proximal and distal shafts of the tibia and fibula, the shaft and neck of the femur, and the ischial and pubic rami.

Radiographic appearance
Initially, plain radiographs of the symptomatic area are within normal limits (Figure 3-89). The stress fracture is first visualized 10 to 20 days after the onset of symptoms as either a thin line of transverse or occasionally oblique radiolucency or as fluffy periosteal callus formation without evidence of a fracture line. When this radiographic appearance is detected at a site common to stress fractures, a history of athletic or other unusual activity should be elicited as the underlying cause.

Radionuclide bone scans using a triple-phase technique to maximize specificity can demonstrate a stress fracture before it can be detected on plain radiographs (Figure 3-90). MRI, used only for cases with indeterminate radiographic findings, is highly sensitive for detecting stress fractures. In some cases, MRI has higher specificity than radionuclide bone scans. Early stress fractures produce low signal intensity on T1-weighted images; there is a progressive increase in signal intensity with increased T2-weighting. A fat saturation (fat-suppressing) technique may demonstrate associated medullary edema or hemorrhage, which produces a high signal compared to the fat-suppressed background.

Treatment
Immobilization of the injured area prevents further injury and gives the stressed area time to heal.

Battered-child syndrome
The battered-child syndrome refers to multiple, repeated, physically induced injuries in young children caused by parents or guardians. The facility treating the suspected battered child, also known as suspected nonaccidental trauma (SNAT), has a legal responsibility to report suspicious cases to child protective services. While the child is being evaluated, diagnosed, and treated, the environment must be protective for the child.

Shaken-baby syndrome, Münchausen's syndrome by proxy, and sudden infant death syndrome are all situations investigated to prove or disprove abusive injury. A skeletal series is performed in such instances and includes an AP view of each extremity and the pelvis. AP and lateral projections of the chest and skull are also required.

Figure 3-90 Radionuclide bone scan of stress fracture. Greatly increased radionuclide uptake in femoral neck *(open arrow)* and intertrochanteric region *(solid arrow)*, with lack of uptake at actual fracture site *(thin arrow)*. Plain radiograph and tomograms showed only minimal trabecular disruption and slight callus formation. (From Dorne HL, Lander PH: Spontaneous stress fractures of the femoral neck. *AJR Am J Roentgenol* 144:343-347, 1985.)

Radiographic appearance

The radiographic findings in this syndrome include multiple fractures of varying age in various stages of healing, fractures of the corners of metaphyses with or without associated epiphyseal displacement, and exuberant subperiosteal new bone formation along the shafts of long bones (Figure 3-91). Skull fractures or widening of the cranial sutures are commonly associated. Another highly suggestive finding is one or more fractures at otherwise unusual sites (usually fractured only by direct blows), such as the ribs, scapula, sternum, spine, or lateral ends of the clavicles (Figure 3-92).

Treatment

Prompt and accurate diagnosis of battered-child syndrome is essential to minimize the extent of physical and psychological damage and sometimes to prevent a fatal injury.

Common fractures and dislocations

Colles' fracture is a transverse fracture through the distal radius with dorsal (posterior) angulation and often overriding of the distal fracture fragment (Figure 3-93). In more than half the cases, there is an associated avulsion fracture of the ulnar styloid process. Colles' fracture is usually caused by a fall on the outstretched hand and is the most common fracture of the wrist.

Navicular (scaphoid) fractures are the most common fractures involving the carpal bones. They are usually transverse and occur through the central part (the waist) of the bone. Although most navicular fractures can be identified on routine frontal projections of the wrist, subtle fractures may require specific oblique and angulated projections or films made using magnification techniques. In some cases, a navicular fracture cannot be detected on the initial examination despite strong clinical suspicion (Figure 3-94, *A*). In this situation, the wrist should be placed in a cast or plaster splint and reexamined (out of plaster) in 7 to 10 days. At this time, resorption of bone at the margins of the fracture widens the fracture line and makes it more apparent radiographically (Figure 3-94, *B*).

Nonunion is a serious complication of navicular fractures (see Figure 3-87). Its incidence increases with motion or displacement of the fracture fragments resulting from either poor immobilization or neglect. Because the blood supply to the navicular bone comes primarily from the distal portion, the proximal fragment may become avascular and undergo ischemic necrosis. This is seen as an increase in bone density associated with collapse of bone or loss of volume in the affected fragment (Figure 3-95).

A **boxer's** fracture is a transverse fracture of the neck of the fifth metacarpal with volar (palmar) angulation of the distal fragment (Figure 3-96). This injury is typically the result of a blow struck with the fist.

In the detection of fractures about the elbow, a valuable clue is displacement of the normal elbow fat pads (the fat pad sign). On lateral projections of the elbow, the anterior fat pad normally appears as a radiolucency closely applied to the anterior surface of the distal end of the humerus. The posterior fat pad, normally hidden in the depths of the olecranon fossa, should not be visible on standard lateral projections of the elbow. Any process producing synovial or hemorrhagic effusion within the elbow joint displaces the fat pads. The normally hidden posterior fat pad, posteriorly displaced, becomes visible as a crescentic lucency behind the lower end of the humerus (Figure 3-97). The anterior fat pad becomes more rounded and further separated from the underlying bone. The posterior fat pad is by far the more sensitive indicator of an elbow joint effusion. Its presence on the lateral projection of the patient with elbow trauma strongly suggests an underlying fracture, especially of the radial head, and indicates the need for oblique projections if no fracture is seen on standard projections. If no fracture is identified, a repeat radiograph obtained 2 weeks or more after appropriate immobilization often shows a fracture by demonstrating a fracture line or callus formation indicating healing.

Figure 3-91 Battered-child syndrome. **A,** Frontal radiograph of right arm demonstrates corner fracture *(arrow)* of proximal humerus. **B,** Frontal radiograph of left arm shows healing displaced fracture of distal humerus. (From Sty JR, Starshak RJ: The role of bone scintigraphy in the evaluation of the suspected abused child. *Radiology* 146:369-375, 1983.)

Figure 3-92 Bone scan of upper body with multiple hot-spots indicating fracture sites in the humerus, clavicle, and scapula.

Summary of Findings for Fractures

FRACTURE TYPE	LOCATION	RADIOGRAPHIC APPEARANCE	TREATMENT
Trauma	All skeletal bones	Fragments, bone separation, and/or discontinuity	Reduction with immobilization—external/cast, internal/surgical fixation
Pathologic	Diseased bone	Vertebral collapse	Treat cause
		Bone destruction—radiolucency due to underlying cause	Immobilization
Stress	Site of increased stress activity	Bone discontinuity	Immobilization
		Radiolucent, transverse or oblique line	Reduce cause of stress
		Fluffy periosteal callus formation without fracture line	
Battered-child syndrome	Skull, long bones, flat bones	Multiple fractures of varying age and at various stages of healing	Minimize physical and psychological damage

Figure 3-93 Colles' fracture. Frontal **(A)** and lateral **(B)** projections of the wrist show overriding and dorsal displacement of distal fragment. There is also a displaced fracture of the distal ulna.

Figure 3-94   Navicular fracture. **A,** On a radiograph obtained immediately after injury, fracture cannot be detected. **B,** On the repeat radiograph obtained 3 weeks later, fracture is clearly identified by sclerotic band *(arrow)* of opaque internal callus. (From Silverman FN: *Caffey's pediatric x-ray imaging,* St Louis, 1985, Mosby.)

Figure 3-95   Avascular necrosis of navicular fracture. Increased bone density is seen in the avascular proximal fragment *(arrow)*.

Figure 3-96   Boxer's fracture. There is fracture at neck of fifth metacarpal *(arrow)* with volar angulation of distal fragment.

Figure 3-97 Fat pad sign in the elbow. Anterior fat pad *(solid arrow)* is clearly lifted from its fossa as a result of a large joint effusion in this child with a supracondylar fracture of the distal humerus. The normally hidden posterior fat pad is posteriorly displaced by effusion *(open arrow)*.

Figure 3-99 Bimalleolar fracture of ankle. A transverse fracture of the medial malleolus *(broad arrow)* is associated with a low oblique fracture of distal fibula *(thin arrow)*.

Figure 3-98 Monteggia fracture. Displaced fracture of ulnar shaft is associated with anterior dislocation of radial head.

Most fractures of the forearm involve both the radius and the ulna. If only one bone fractures, it is essential to examine both the elbow and the wrist to exclude the possibility of proximal or distal joint dislocation. A **Monteggia** fracture (Figure 3-98) is an isolated fracture of the shaft of the ulna associated with anterior dislocation of the radius at the elbow. A **Galeazzi** fracture is the combination of a fracture of the shaft of the radius and a dorsal (posterior) dislocation of the ulna at the wrist.

Pott's fracture involves both malleoli (i.e., of tibia and fibula) with dislocation of the ankle joint. A bimalleolar fracture is one involving both the medial and the lateral malleoli (Figure 3-99). Because of the mechanism of injury, the fracture on one side is transverse, whereas the fracture on the opposite side is oblique or spiral. Trimalleolar fractures involve the posterior lip of the tibia in addition to the medial and lateral malleoli and usually represent fracture dislocations.

One of the most frequent injuries to the foot is a transverse fracture at the base of the fifth metatarsal (a **Jones** fracture) (Figure 3-100). This fracture represents an avulsion injury that results from plantar flexion and inversion of the foot, as occurs when stepping off a curb or falling while walking on stairs. It is important to distinguish this fracture from the longitudinally oriented apophysis that is normally found in children at the lateral margin of the base of the fifth metatarsal.

The shoulder is by far the most commonly dislocated joint in the body (Figure 3-101). About 95% of shoulder dislocations are anterior, resulting from external rotation and abduction of the arm. As the anterior displacement occurs, the posterolateral surface

Figure 3-100   Jones fracture of base of fifth metatarsal. Note that the fracture line is transverse *(black arrow)* on the base of the fifth metatarsal whereas the normal apophysis in this child has vertical orientation *(white arrow).*

Figure 3-101   Dislocation of shoulder. Anterior **(A)** dilocation seen with inferior and medial displacement of the humeral head and posterior **(B)** dislocation demonstrated by the increased distance between the anterior glenoid rim and the humeral head.

of the humeral head impacts against the anterior or anteroinferior surface of the glenoid fossa and may result in a compression fracture of the humeral head, a fracture of the glenoid rim, or both. In most cases, the humeral head is displaced medially and anteriorly and comes to rest beneath the coracoid process.

Dislocations of the hip, with or without associated fracture of the acetabulum, are caused by severe injuries such as automobile collisions, pedestrian accidents, or falls from a great height. Unlike in the shoulder, posterior dislocations of the hip are far more common than anterior dislocations and account for 85% to 90% of the cases (Figure 3-102).

■ Fractures and Dislocations of the Spine

Fractures and dislocations of the spine may be the result of direct trauma, hyperextension–flexion injuries (whiplash), or normal stresses in abnormal bone (osteoporosis, metastatic destruction). In the patient with spinal injury, the major goal of the radiographic evaluation is to determine whether a fracture or dislocation is present and whether the injury is stable or unstable. The spine can be considered as consisting of two major columns. The anterior column consists of the verte-

bral bodies, intervertebral disks, and anterior and posterior longitudinal ligaments. The facets, apophyseal joints, pedicles, laminae, spinous processes, and all the intervening ligaments form the posterior column. If one of the two columns remains intact, the injury is considered **stable.** If both columns are disrupted, the injury is considered **unstable.**

If there is a strong suspicion of injury to the cervical spine, the initial radiograph should be a horizontal-beam lateral projection with the patient supine. This cross-table lateral radiograph *must* be checked by the physician before obtaining any other projections. It is essential to include all seven cervical vertebrae on the film lest the relatively common injuries of C6 and C7 be overlooked (Figure 3-103). This may require

Figure 3-102 Dislocations of hip. Frontal radiograph of teen-aged girl injured in motor vehicle collision demonstrates right posterior dislocation and left anterior dislocation of hip. Right posterior dislocation is characterized by typical superolateral displacement of femoral head, fixed adduction, and internal rotation (lesser trochanter superimposed on femoral shaft). Left anterior dislocation is manifested by characteristic inferomedial displacement of femoral head, which has come to overlie obturator foramen; fixed abduction; and external rotation (lesser trochanter depicted in profile). (From Bassett LW, Gold RH, Epstein HC: Anterior hip dislocation: atypical superolateral displacement of the femoral head. *AJR Am J Roentgenol* 141:385-386, 1983.)

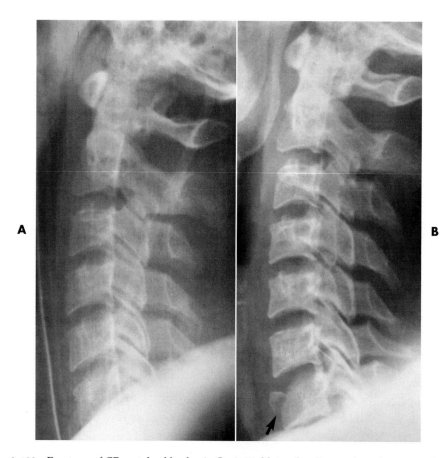

Figure 3-103 Fracture of C7 vertebral body. **A,** On initial lateral radiograph, only upper six cervical vertebrae can be seen. Patient's shoulders overlie seventh cervical vertebra. **B,** With shoulders pulled down to expose seventh cervical vertebra, anterosuperior fracture *(arrow)* is clearly identified.

supine oblique projections or films made in the swimmer's position, in which one arm of the patient is extended over the head while the other arm remains by the side so as to slightly oblique the upper torso and permit visualization of the cervicothoracic junction. A frontal projection of the spine and an open-mouth projection of the atlas and axis (C1 and C2) should be obtained next. In an acutely injured patient, oblique or flexion and extension projections should be performed *only* under the direct supervision of the attending physician. Computed or even conventional tomography may be used to confirm the presence or absence of a fracture (especially of the posterior elements) and to visualize otherwise obscured areas of the spine such as the craniovertebral and cervicothoracic junctions. CT can precisely localize fracture fragments in relation to the spinal canal and detect otherwise obscure fractures of the posterior elements. Myelography may be performed in patients with a spinal cord injury in the absence of an obvious fracture or dislocation to identify a condition amenable

to surgical removal or repair (e.g., a herniated disk fragment or an epidural hematoma of the spinal cord).

Several types of fractures are peculiar to the cervical spine. A **Jefferson fracture,** a comminuted fracture of the ring of the atlas, involves both the anterior and the posterior arches and causes displacement of the fragments. The characteristic appearance on frontal radiographs or tomograms is a bilateral offset or spreading of the lateral articular masses of C1 in relation to the opposing articular surfaces of C2 (Figure 3-104).

Fractures of the odontoid process are usually transverse and located at the base of the dens at its junction with the body (Figure 3-105). On an open-mouth view, a lucency between the upper central

Figure 3-104 Jefferson fracture. **A,** On frontal projection, there is lateral displacement of lateral masses of C1 bilaterally *(white lines).* **B,** CT scan in another patient shows unilateral break in arch of C1 *(arrow).* D, dens.

Figure 3-105 Fracture of odontoid process. **A,** Open-mouth frontal projection shows combined oblique and transverse fracture at base of dens *(arrows).* There is also separate cortical fragment on left *(arrowhead),* which most likely remains attached to alar ligament. **B,** In another patient, frontal tomogram shows low fracture *(arrows)* through body of C2.

Figure 3-106   Hangman's fracture. Neural arch fracture *(solid arrow)* associated with complete C2-3 subluxation *(open arrow)*. (From Osborn AG: Head trauma. In Eisenberg RL, Amberg JR, editors: *Critical diagnostic pathways in radiology,* Philadelphia, 1981, Lippincott.)

incisor teeth often overlaps the dens; this must be differentiated from a rare vertical fracture of the dens.

The **hangman's fracture** is the result of acute hyperextension of the head on the neck. This appears as a fracture of the arch of C2 anterior to the inferior facet and is usually associated with anterior subluxation of C2 on C3 (Figure 3-106). Although originally described in patients who had been hanged, this injury is now far more commonly the result of motor vehicle accidents.

Clay shoveler's fracture is an avulsion fracture of a spinous process in the lower cervical or upper thoracic spine. The fracture is difficult to demonstrate on emergency cross-table lateral radiographs because the shoulders frequently obscure the lower cervical region. The diagnosis can be made on the frontal view by noting the double shadow of the spinous processes caused by the caudal displacement of the avulsed fragment (Figure 3-107). This double–spinous-process sign must be differentiated from a bifid spinous process, which usually lies at a higher level and on a more horizontal plane.

Most fractures of the thoracolumbar spine are attributable to compressive forces that cause anterior wedging or depression of the superior end plate of a

Figure 3-107   Clay shoveler's fracture. **A,** Frontal projection of cervical spine shows characteristic double-spinous-process sign resulting from caudal displacement of avulsed fragment *(open arrow)* with respect to normal position of major portion of spinous process *(solid arrow).* **B,** Lateral projection clearly shows avulsed fragment *(arrow).*

vertebral body (Figure 3-108). The **seat belt fracture** is a transverse fracture of a lumbar vertebra that is often associated with significant visceral injuries (Figure 3-109). In this condition, a horizontal fracture of the vertebral body extends to involve some or all of the posterior elements.

■ Herniation of Intervertebral Disks

The intervertebral disks act as shock absorbers between the vertebrae, cushioning the movements of the spine. They consist of a fibrous outer cartilage (annu-

Figure 3-108 Vertebral body fracture. Characteristic anterior wedging of superior end plate of L1 vertebral body.

Figure 3-110 Degenerative disk disease. Hypertrophic spurring, intervertebral disk space narrowing, and reactive sclerosis. Note linear lucent collections (vacuum phenomenon) overlying several intervertebral disks.

Figure 3-109 Seat belt fracture. CT scan shows fracture of lumbar vertebral body (black arrows) associated with lamina fracture at the same level (white arrow).

lus) surrounding a central nucleus pulposus, which is the essential part of the disk. The nucleus pulposus is a highly elastic, semifluid mass compressed like a spring between the vertebral surfaces. In youth, it contains a large amount of fluid to cushion the motion of the spine. With increasing age, the fluid and elasticity gradually diminish, leading to degenerative changes and back pain. Protrusion, or herniation, of a lumbar intervertebral disk is the major cause of severe acute, chronic, or recurring low back and leg pain. It most frequently involves the L4-5 and L5-S1 levels in the lumbar region, where it often causes sciatica, pain that radiates down the sciatic nerve to the back of the thigh and lower leg. Other major sites are the C5-6 and C6-7 levels in the neck and the T9 through T12 levels in the thoracic region.

Radiographic appearance

Although plain radiographs show characteristic narrowing of the intervertebral disk spaces with hypertrophic spur formation, bony sclerosis, spurs impinging on the neural foramina, and the vacuum phenomenon (lucent collections overlying the intervertebral disks), these findings are nonspecific and frequently occur in patients with minimal symptoms (Figure 3-110). The diagnosis of herniation of an intervertebral disk requires CT, MRI, or myelography to demonstrate impression of the disk on the spinal cord or individual nerve roots (Figures 3-111 to 3-116).

Treatment

Patients with symptoms suggestive of disk herniation are initially treated conservatively with bed rest, muscle relaxants, and analgesics before being subjected to radiographic studies. If conservative treatment is

Figure 3-111 Lumbar disk herniation. Myelogram shows extradural lesion *(arrow)* at level of intervertebral disk space. Note amputation of nerve root by disk compression.

Figure 3-112 CT of normal lumbar disk *(D)*. The normal lumbar intervertebral disk has a concave posterior border *(arrowheads)*. Note normal epidural fat *(F)* surrounding the thecal sac *(T)*.

Figure 3-113 Central bulging of intervertebral disk. CT scan shows convex posterior border of the disk *(arrowheads)*. Note preservation of epidural fat.

Figure 3-114 Disk herniation at L5-S1 level. CT shows herniation of disk *(arrowheads)* to the left with obliteration of epidural fat. (From Eisenberg RL: *Diagnostic imaging in surgery,* New York, 1987, McGraw-Hill.)

no

Figure 3-115 MR image of intervertebral disk herniation in cervical region. Note extradural impression on spinal cord *(arrowhead)*.

A   **B**

Figure 3-116 Lumbar disc herniation. MRI illustrating a torn annulus fibrosis and nucleus pulposus of L5-S1 *(arrows)* in sagittal **(A)** and transverse **(B)** planes. (Courtesy Bartram J. Pierce, RT [R] [MR], Good Samaritan Regional Medical Center, Corvallis, Ore.)

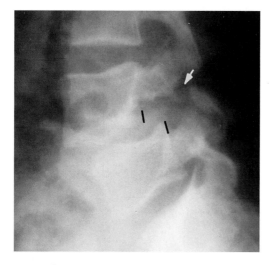

Figure 3-117 Spondylolisthesis. Lateral view of lower lumbar spine shows break in pars interarticularis *(arrow)*, with resultant anterior slippage of L4 with respect to L5. Vertical black lines indicate posterior margins of vertebral bodies.

Figure 3-118 Spondylolysis. **A,** Diagram of Scotty dog sign. **B,** Oblique projection of lumbar spine demonstrates a defect in the pars interarticularis, which appears as a fracture through the neck of the Scotty dog *(arrow)*.

unsuccessful, surgery may be necessary to remove the cause of impingement and alleviate the pain and symptoms.

■ Spondylolysis and Spondylolisthesis

Spondylolysis refers to a cleft in the pars interarticularis that is situated between the superior and inferior articular processes of a vertebra. Occurring in about 5% of the population, these clefts are usually bilateral, most commonly involve the fifth lumbar vertebra, and predispose to the forward displacement of one vertebra on the other that may cause chronic back pain. *Spondylolysis* is the term for a defect in the pars interarticularis without displacement; if displacement occurs, the condition is called **spondylolisthesis.**

Radiographic appearance

A plain lateral radiograph of the lower lumbar spine clearly shows any spondylolisthesis and may demonstrate the lucent cleft in the pars interarticularis even if no displacement has occurred (Figure 3-117). In grading spondylolisthesis of the lumbosacral junction on the lateral projection, the superior surface of the sacrum is divided into four equal parts. A forward displacement of the fifth lumbar vertebra up to one-fourth the thickness of the sacrum is called a first-degree spondylolisthesis; half the thickness, a second-degree spondylolisthesis, and so on.

The diagnosis of spondylolysis without displacement may require an oblique projection of the lumbar spine, on which the appearance of the posterior elements has been likened to that of a Scotty dog (Figure 3-118). The pedicle and transverse process form the eye and nose; the superior and inferior articular processes form the ear and leg; and the pars interarticularis forms the neck, which is "fractured" in a patient with spondylolysis.

Treatment

Passive treatment includes bracing, physical therapy, restricted activity, and nonnarcotic analgesics to control pain to a tolerable level. Conservative therapy works for the majority of patients. Surgical treatment is needed only when passive treatment is unsuccessful for controlling pain. A complete laminectomy, usually with spinal fusion, is performed to free the peripheral nerves and stabilize spinal movement.

- -

Summary of Findings for Common Spinal Disorders

DISORDER	LOCATION	RADIOGRAPHIC APPEARANCE	TREATMENT
Disk herniation	Cervical and lumbar spine regions	CT and MRI—disk impingement on nerve or spinal cord	Conservative—bed rest, muscle relaxants, and analgesics Aggressive—surgical removal of disk
Spondylolysis Spondylolisthesis	Fifth lumbar vertebra, lumbosacral junction	Defect in pars interarticularis without displacement Forward displacement with pars interarticularis defect	Nonoperative—bracing, physical therapy, restricted activity, and nonnarcotic analgesics Surgical—complete laminectomy with spinal fusion

[handwritten note: rupture of nucleus pulposous most freq. L4-L5]

- -

QUESTIONS

1. The shaft of any long bone is termed the
   - A. Epiphysis
   - B. Diaphysis
   - C. Metaphysis
   - D. Periosteum

2. The end of a long bone is referred to as the
   - A. Epiphysis
   - B. Diaphysis
   - C. Metaphysis
   - D. Periosteum

3. The special types of cells responsible for the diameter growth of bones are
   - A. Osteoblasts
   - B. Osteoclasts
   - C. Chondroblasts
   - D. Both A and B

4. The common area(s) of the body radiographed to determine bone age is/are
   - A. Skull
   - B. Wrist
   - C. Hand
   - D. Both B and C

5. What pathologic condition is present if the posterior elements of one or more vertebrae fail to unite?
   - A. Meningocele
   - B. Spina bifida
   - C. Myelomeningocele
   - D. Spondylolisthesis

6. In patients with advanced osteoporosis, what type of radiographic technique is preferred?
   - A. Low kVp; short scale of contrast
   - B. High kVp; short scale of contrast
   - C. Low kVp; long scale of contrast
   - D. High kVp; long scale of contrast

7. Aging and postmenopausal hormonal changes are the major causes of generalized
   - A. Osteogenesis imperfecta
   - B. Osteoporosis
   - C. Osteopetrosis
   - D. Osteomalacia

8. An inherited generalized disorder of connective tissue characterized by multiple fractures and a bluish color of the sclera of the eye is
   - A. Osteogenesis imperfecta
   - B. Osteoporosis
   - C. Osteopetrosis
   - D. Osteomalacia

9. Lack of vitamin D in the diet of infants and children can cause a systemic disease called
   - A. Achondroplasia
   - B. Rickets
   - C. Osteomalacia
   - D. Osteopetrosis

10. A disorder of metabolism causing an increased blood level of uric acid is called
    - A. Achondroplasia
    - B. Rickets
    - C. Gout
    - D. Urasia

11. A benign projection of bone with a cartilage-like cap occurring around the knee in children or adolescents is
    - A. Osteochondroma
    - B. Enchondroma
    - C. Achondroplasia
    - D. Osteoma

12. An example of a malignant bone tumor is
    - A. Osteogenic sarcoma
    - B. Chondrosarcoma
    - C. Ewing's sarcoma
    - D. All of the above

13. The form of noninfectious arthritis characterized by osteoporosis, soft-tissue swelling, and erosions of the metacarpophalangeal joints and ulnar styloid processes is
    - A. Reiter's
    - B. Rheumatoid
    - C. Psoriatic
    - D. Osteoarthritis

14. The extremely common form of arthritis that is characterized by loss of joint cartilage and reactive new bone growth and is part of the normal wear of aging is
    A. Reiter's　　C. Psoriatic
    B. Rheumatoid　D. Osteoarthritis

15. Inflammation of the small fluid-filled sacs that are located around joints and reduce friction is termed
    A. Tendinitis　C. Bursitis
    B. Arthritis　D. Both A and C

16. In what type of fracture is the skin broken?
    A. Open　　C. Comminuted
    B. Compound　D. Both A and C

17. What type of fracture consists of more than two fragments?
    A. Open　　C. Comminuted
    B. Compound　D. Both A and C

18. What term applies to the new calcium deposits that unite fracture sites?
    A. Bone　　C. Periosteum
    B. Callus　D. Both A and C

19. What type of fracture occurs in bone weakened by some preexisting condition such as a metastatic lesion or multiple myeloma?
    A. Stress　C. Pott's
    B. Colles'　D. Pathologic

20. What is the name for the type of fracture that can occur from falling on the outstretched hand and involves the distal portion of the radius?
    A. Stress　C. Pott's
    B. Colles'　D. Pathologic

21. What name is applied to a fracture involving both malleoli?
    A. Stress　C. Pott's
    B. Colles'　D. Pathologic

22. What is the name applied to the fracture resulting from acute hyperextension of the head on the neck that usually affects C2 and C3?
    A. Hangman's　C. Boxer's
    B. Jefferson　D. Monteggia

23. What area of the spine does a clay shoveler's fracture involve?
    A. Lower thoracic and upper lumbar
    B. Lumbar only
    C. Lower cervical and upper thoracic
    D. Cervical only

24. Diagnosis of an intervertebral disk herniation requires which radiographic procedure(s)?
    A. Myelography　C. MRI
    B. CT　　D. A or B or C

25. What medical term refers to a cleft in the pars interarticularis commonly involving the fifth lumbar vertebra?
    A. Spondylolisthesis　C. Spondylitis
    B. Spondylolysis　D. A or B or C

26. What pathologic condition sometimes occurs after trauma, causing an interrupted blood supply to a bone?
    A. Vasculitis　　C. Cushing's
    B. Ischemic necrosis　D. Stress fracture

27. Place an "I" by those pathologic conditions that have an increased attenuation, and a "D" by those that have decreased attenuation:
    __I__ Callus　　　__I__ Atrophy
    __I__ Acromegaly　__D__ Osteoporosis
    __D__ Ischemic necrosis　__D__ Osteolytic lesions
    __D__ Multiple myeloma　__I__ Osteosclerotic lesions

BIBLIOGRAPHY
Brower AC: *Arthritis in black and white,* Philadelphia, 1988, Saunders.
Greenfield GB: *Radiology of bone diseases,* ed 4, Philadelphia, 1990, Lippincott.
Greenspan A: *Orthopedic radiology: a practical approach,* Philadelphia, 1992, Lippincott.
Griffiths HJ: *Basic bone radiology,* Norwalk, 1987, Appleton & Lange.
Helms CA: *Fundamentals of skeletal radiology,* Philadelphia, 1989, Saunders.
Pressel DM: Evaluation of physical abuse in children, *Am Fam Physician,* May 15, 2000; aafp.org/aft/20000515/37.57.html
Resnick D, Niwayama G: *Diagnosis of bone and joint disorders,* Philadelphia, 1988, Saunders.
Rogers LF: *Radiology of skeletal trauma,* New York, 1992, Churchill Livingstone.

CHAPTER 4

Gastrointestinal System

■ **Prerequisite Knowledge**

The student should have a basic knowledge of the anatomy and physiology of the gastrointestinal system. In addition, proper learning and understanding of the material will be facilitated if the student has some clinical experience in gastrointestinal radiography and film evaluation, including a concept of the changes in technique required to compensate for density differences produced by a few of the underlying pathologic conditions.

■ **Goals**

To acquaint the student radiographer with the pathophysiology and radiographic manifestations of all of the common and some of the unusual disorders of the gastrointestinal system.

■ **Objectives**

1. To be able to classify the more common diseases in terms of their attenuation of x-rays
2. To be familiar with the changes in technical factors required for obtaining optimal quality radiographs in patients with various underlying pathologic conditions
3. To understand and be able to define or describe all bold-faced terms in this chapter
4. To be able to describe the physiology of the gastrointestinal system
5. To be able to identify anatomic structures on both diagrams and radiographs of the gastrointestinal system
6. To be able to describe the various pathologic conditions affecting the gastrointestinal system as well as their radiographic manifestations

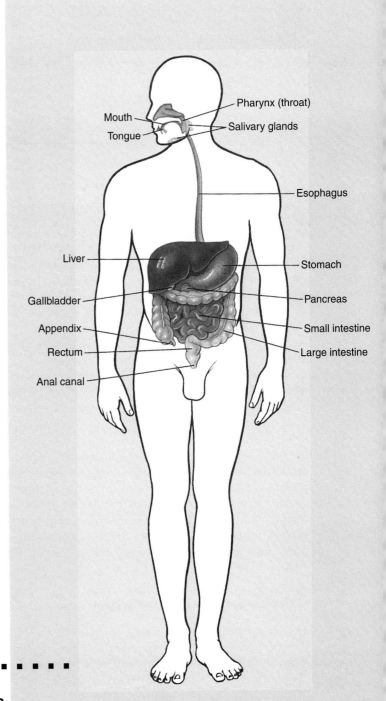

■ ■ ■ ■ ■ ■ ■ ■ ■ **Radiographer Notes**

Plain abdominal radiographs and contrast studies of the digestive tract remain the most common imaging examinations of the gastrointestinal system. Ultrasound and CT are the major imaging modalities for the pancreas and biliary tract, and MRI is now being used in some institutions to screen for hepatic metastases.

Plain abdominal radiographs must show an appropriate scale of contrast to demonstrate the many different densities in the abdominal cavity. Depending on the screen–film combination, this requires the use of a middle- to high-range kV range (70 to 80 kVp). Bony structures, such as the lumbar spine and its transverse processes, must be well demonstrated, as well as soft-tissue shadows of the liver, kidney, and psoas muscle. For barium studies of the gastrointestinal tract, adequate pen-

etration of the dense barium solution requires a high kV range (about 120 kVp). For double-contrast (air–barium) studies, a kVp range of 90 to 100 kVp is needed to allow penetration of the barium combined with excellent visualization of mucosal detail. Gallbladder studies require a shorter scale of contrast than other abdominal examinations and therefore are usually performed using a kVp in the low to middle range (about 70 kVp). Computed imaging systems tend to be more dependent on the kilovolts peak and require the use of slightly higher ranges (approximately 10 kVp higher) to produce the same images as obtained on film–screen systems. The technologist must select the proper algorithm (combination of procedure and position) to obtain an image with the proper contrast and density.

As in other body systems, certain pathologic conditions in the gastrointestinal system require alterations in the technical factors chosen for imaging. In patients with ascites, a common complication of advanced cirrhosis, an increased kVp is required to penetrate the additional fluid content of the abdomen. On the other hand, a decreased kVp is needed in patients with suspected large or small bowel obstruction because of the excessive amount of gas in the abdominal cavity.

The radiographer is usually called on to assist the radiologist during fluoroscopic examinations of the gastrointestinal tract. Indeed, it is generally the radiographer's task to coerce the patient into drinking (and not vomiting) the rather unpleasant-tasting contrast material and to urge the patient to turn around several times to provide adequate mucosal coating for the double-contrast upper gastrointestinal series. Similarly, the radiographer may have to convince the patient to retain barium and air during the often uncomfortable barium enema examinations. It is frequently time well spent for the radiographer to explain fully to the patient both the mechanics of the procedure and the extreme importance of patient cooperation.

■ **Physiology of the Digestive System**

The basic function of the digestive system is to alter the chemical and physical composition of food so that it can be absorbed and used by body cells. This process depends on secretions of the endocrine and exocrine

glands and on the controlled movement of ingested food through the tract so that absorption can occur.

Digestion begins in the mouth with chewing (**mastication**), the mechanical breakdown of food. The secretion of saliva moistens the food in preparation for swallowing. Swallowing (**deglutition**) is a complex process that requires coordination of many muscles in the head and neck and the precise opening and closing of esophageal sphincters. Digestion continues in the stomach with the churning movement of gastric contents that have become mixed with hydrochloric acid and the proteolytic enzyme pepsin. The resulting milky white **chyme** is propelled through the pyloric sphincter into the duodenum by rhythmic smooth muscle contractions called **peristalsis.**

The greatest amount of digestion occurs in the duodenum, the first part of the small bowel. In addition to intestinal secretions containing mucus and enzymes, secretions of the pancreas and liver enhance digestion in this region. The pancreas secretes enzymes for the digestion of proteins (trypsin and chymotrypsin), fat (lipase), and carbohydrates (amylase). It also secretes an alkaline solution to neutralize the acid carried into the small intestine from the stomach. Bile is secreted by the liver, is stored in the gallbladder, and enters the duodenum through the common bile duct. Bile is an **emulsifier,** a substance that acts like soap by dispersing the fat into very small droplets that permit it to mix with water.

When digestion is complete, the nutrients are absorbed through the intestinal mucosa into blood capillaries and lymph vessels of the wall of the small bowel. The inner surface area of the small bowel is increased by the formation of numerous fingerlike projections **(villi),** which provide the largest amount of surface area possible for digestion and absorption.

Material that has not been digested passes into the colon, where water and minerals are absorbed, and the remaining matter is excreted as feces. If the contents of the lower colon and rectum move at a rate that is slower than normal, extra water is absorbed from the fecal mass to produce a hardened stool and **constipation. Diarrhea** results from increased motility of the small bowel, which floods the colon with an excessive amount of water that cannot be completely absorbed.

The vermiform (worm-shaped) appendix arises from the inferomedial aspect of the cecum about 3 cm below the ileocecal valve. Although the appendix has no functional importance in digestion, it is often classified as an accessory digestive organ merely because of its location.

The liver is the largest gland in the body and is responsible for several vital functions. Liver cells detoxify (make harmless) a variety of poisonous substances that enter the blood from the intestines. Toxic chemicals that are changed to nontoxic compounds in the liver include ammonia (converted to urea and excreted by the kidneys), alcohol, and barbiturates. Liver cells secrete about 1 pint of bile each day. As mentioned, bile is an emulsifier; it is essential for the digestion and absorption of dietary fat and the fat-soluble vitamins A, D, E, and K. Bile is a greenish liquid consisting of water, bile salts, cholesterol, and bilirubin (a breakdown product of hemoglobin).

Liver cells play a vital role in the metabolism of proteins, fats, and carbohydrates. The liver is the major site of synthesis of the enzymes necessary for various cellular activities throughout the body. Liver cells also synthesize blood proteins, such as albumin, which maintains the correct amount of fluid within blood vessels, and the essential proteins required for blood clotting (fibrinogen and prothrombin). Therefore liver damage may result in edema (excess water in the soft tissues) and a serious bleeding tendency. The liver plays an important role in maintaining the proper level of glucose in the blood by taking up excess glucose absorbed by the small intestine and storing it as **glycogen.** When the level of circulating glucose falls below normal, the liver breaks down glycogen and releases glucose into the bloodstream. Liver cells also store iron and vitamins A, B_{12}, and D.

The gallbladder is a pear-shaped sac that lies on the undersurface of the liver. Its function is to store bile that enters by way of the hepatic and cystic ducts and to concentrate the bile by absorbing water. In response to the presence of dietary fat in the small bowel, the gallbladder contracts and ejects the concentrated bile into the duodenum.

The pancreas controls the level of circulating blood glucose by secreting insulin and glucagon in the islands of Langerhans. An increased concentration of glucose in the blood stimulates the beta cells to increase secretion of insulin, which decreases the blood glucose level probably by accelerating the transport of glucose into cells. A blood glucose concentration less than normal triggers the alpha cells to secrete glucagon, which accelerates the breakdown of glycogen into glucose by the liver.

As discussed, pancreatic secretions are vital for digestion. Pancreatic enzymes that pass through the pancreatic duct into the duodenum are necessary for the breakdown of proteins, carbohydrates, and fats.

▪ Esophagus

Tracheoesophageal fistula

CONGENITAL TYPE

Congenital tracheoesophageal (TE) fistulas result from the failure of a satisfactory esophageal lumen to develop completely separate from the trachea. Esophageal atresia and TE fistulas are often associated with other congenital malformations involving the skeleton, cardiovascular system, and gastrointestinal tract.

Radiographic appearance

In the second most common type of esophageal anomaly, type I, both the upper and lower segments of the esophagus are blind pouches. This anomaly can be differentiated from the type III lesion (the most common type) only by plain abdominal radiographs, which demonstrate the absence of air below the diaphragm in the type I lesion and air below the stomach in the type III lesion.

In the type II form of TE fistula, the upper esophageal segment communicates with the trachea, whereas the lower segment ends in a blind pouch. Because there is no connection between the trachea and the stomach, there is no radiographic evidence of gas within the abdomen. Oral administration of contrast material in this condition immediately outlines the tracheobronchial tree.

The type III TE fistula (seen in 85% to 90% of cases) consists of an upper segment that ends in a blind pouch at the level of the bifurcation of the trachea or slightly above it, and a lower segment attached to the trachea by a short fistulous tract. Radiographic demonstration of the looping of a small esophageal feeding tube indicates that the proximal esophagus ends in a blind pouch (Figure 4-1, *A*). Plain radiographs of the abdomen demonstrate the presence of air in the bowel that has freely entered the stomach

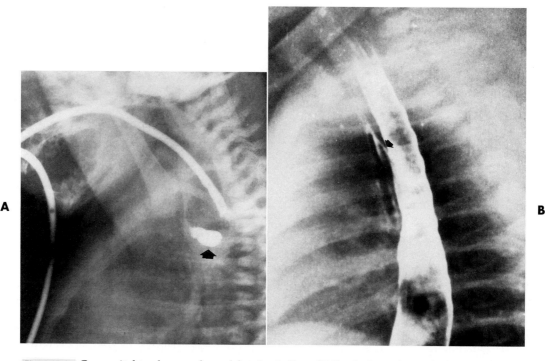

Figure 4-1 Congenital tracheoesophageal fistula. **A,** Type III fistula *(arrow)*, in which contrast material (injected through a feeding tube) demonstrates occlusion of proximal esophageal pouch. **B,** Type IV, or H, fistula *(arrow).*

through the fistulous connection between the trachea and the distal esophagus.

There are two forms of type IV TE fistula. In one, the upper and lower esophageal segments end in blind pouches, both of which are connected to the tracheobronchial tree. In this form, gas is seen in the stomach, and oral contrast material outlines both fistulas and the bronchial tree. In the other form of type IV fistula (called an H fistula), both the trachea and the esophagus are intact. These two structures are connected by a single fistulous tract that can be found at any level from the cricoid cartilage of the trachea to the tracheal bifurcation (see Figure 4-1, *B*). Unlike the other forms of TE fistula, the H fistula may not be identified in infancy and, if it is small and only occasionally causes emptying of material into the lungs, can permit survival into adulthood.

Treatment

Immediate surgical repair will prevent the infant from dying of starvation. If a fistula exists, delayed surgical repair may result in aspiration pneumonia.

ACQUIRED TYPE

About 50% of acquired fistulas between the trachea and esophagus are caused by malignancy in the mediastinum. Almost all the rest result from infectious processes or trauma.

Fistulization between the esophagus and the respiratory tract is a major late complication of esophageal carcinoma and is often a terminal event (Figure 4-2). A fistula can also be a complication of erosion into the esophagus by carcinoma of the lung arising near or metastasizing to the middle mediastinum, or by mediastinal metastases from other primary sites. Regardless of therapy, the overall prognosis of malignant TE fistulas is dismal, and more than 80% of patients with this complication die within 3 months from uncontrollable hemorrhage or from pulmonary infection caused by repeated episodes of aspiration pneumonia.

Fistulous communications between the esophagus and the tracheobronchial tree can be the result of esophageal instrumentation and perforation. This is most common after esophagoscopy but may also occur after instrumental dilatation of strictures by bougienage, pneumatic dilatation of the esophagus for the treatment of achalasia, or even the insertion of a nasogastric tube. Blunt or penetrating trauma to the chest, especially after crush injury, can result in esophageal perforation and fistulization.

Radiographic appearance

After traumatic perforation of the thoracic esophagus, chest radiographs may demonstrate air dissecting within the mediastinum and soft tissues, of-

Figure 4-2 Esophagorespiratory fistula between esophagus *(arrow)* and bronchial tree *(arrowheads),* seen as complication of esophageal carcinoma.

ten with pleural effusion or hydropneumothorax. The introduction of an oral contrast agent may demonstrate the site of perforation and the extent of fistulization.

Treatment

For patients with unresectable metastases or esophageal malignancies, using an interventional technique to place a stent to maintain the lumen may be the best palliative treatment available. Surgery may be performed if the benefit outweighs the risk.

Esophagitis

REFLUX (GASTROESOPHAGEAL REFLUX DISEASE)

Although the reflux of gastric acid contents is the most common cause of acute esophagitis, infectious and granulomatous disorders, physical injury (caustic agents, radiation injury), and medication may produce a similar inflammatory response. Gastroesophageal reflux disease (GERD) describes any symptomatic condition or structural changes due to reflux of the stomach contents into the esophagus. Alcohol, chocolate, caffeine, and fatty foods tend to decrease the pressure of the esophageal sphincter, allowing reflux to occur. Regardless of the cause,

acute esophagitis produces burning chest pain that may simulate the pain of heart disease. Superficial ulcerations are most typical of reflux. The esophagus is often dilated, with a loss of effective peristalsis. Nonpropulsive peristaltic waves, ranging from mild tertiary contractions to severe segmental spasms, are an early finding.

Reflux esophagitis develops when the lower esophageal sphincter fails to act as an effective barrier to the entry of gastric acid contents into the distal esophagus. Although there is a higher-than-normal likelihood of gastroesophageal reflux in patients with sliding hiatal hernias, reflux esophagitis can be endoscopically demonstrated in only about one fourth of these patients. On the other hand, esophagitis is often encountered in patients in whom no hiatal hernia can be demonstrated.

Several radiographic approaches have been suggested for the demonstration of gastroesophageal reflux. One procedure is to increase intraabdominal pressure by straight-leg raising or manual pressure on the abdomen, often with Valsalva's maneuver (forced expiration with the glottis closed). Turning the patient from prone to supine or vice versa may demonstrate reflux of barium from the stomach into the esophagus. It must be remembered, however, that the failure to demonstrate reflux radiographically does not exclude the possibility that a patient's esophagitis is related to reflux. As long as typical radiographic findings of reflux esophagitis are noted, there is little reason to persist in strenuous efforts to actually demonstrate retrograde flow of barium from the stomach into the esophagus.

Radiographic appearance

The earliest radiographic findings in reflux esophagitis are detectable on double-contrast studies. They consist of superficial ulcerations or erosions that appear as streaks or dots of barium superimposed on the flat mucosa of the distal esophagus. In single-contrast studies of patients with esophagitis, the outer borders of the barium-filled esophagus are not sharply seen but rather have a hazy, serrated appearance with shallow, irregular protrusions indicating erosions of varying length and depth. Widening and coarsening of edematous longitudinal folds can simulate filling defects. In addition to diffuse erosion, reflux esophagitis can result in large, discrete, penetrating ulcers in the distal esophagus (Figure 4-3) or in a hiatal hernia sac (Figure 4-4). Fibrotic healing of diffuse reflux esophagitis or a localized penetrating ulcer may cause narrowing of the distal esophagus. Strictures resulting from reflux esophagitis tend to be smooth and tapering with no demonstrable mucosal pattern (Figure 4-5).

Figure 4-3   Large, penetrating ulcer *(arrow)* in reflux esophagitis.

Figure 4-4   Ulcer *(arrows)* in large hiatal hernia sac.

BARRETT'S ESOPHAGUS

Barrett's esophagus is a condition related to severe reflux esophagitis in which the normal squamous lining of the lower esophagus is destroyed and replaced by columnar epithelium similar to that of the stomach. Ulceration in Barrett's esophagus typically occurs at the squamocolumnar junction (Z-line). In addition to exhibiting postinflammatory stricture, Barrett's esophagus has an unusually high propensity for developing malignancy in the columnar cell–lined portion. These tumors are almost always adenocarcinomas, which are otherwise very rare in the esophagus (comprising about 5% of esophageal cancers).

Radiographic appearance

Although a hiatal hernia with gastroesophageal reflux is commonly demonstrated, Barrett's ulcer is usually separated from the hiatal hernia by a variable length of normal-appearing esophagus (Figure 4-6), in contrast to reflux esophagitis, in which the distal esophagus is abnormal down to the level of the hernia. As in reflux esophagitis, fibrotic healing of the ulceration in Barrett's esophagus often leads to a smooth, tapered stricture (Figure 4-7).

Because the distal esophagus consists of a gastric type of mucosa in Barrett's esophagus, it actively takes up the intravenously injected radionuclide

Figure 4-5   Long esophageal stricture caused by reflux esophagitis. Note the associated hiatal hernia *(arrows).*

pertechnetate. The demonstration of a continuous concentration of the isotope from the stomach into the distal esophagus to a level that corresponds approximately to that of the ulcer or stricture is indicative of Barrett's esophagus.

Figure 4-6 Barrett's esophagus. Ulcerations *(arrow)* have developed at a distance from esophagogastric junction.

Figure 4-7 Barrett's esophagus. Note smooth, tapered stricture in upper thoracic esophagus.

CANDIDA AND HERPESVIRUS

Candida (fungal) and herpesvirus are the organisms most often responsible for infectious esophagitis, which usually occurs in patients with widespread malignancy who are receiving radiation therapy, chemotherapy, corticosteroids, or other immunosuppressive agents. It also can develop in patients with acquired immunodeficiency syndrome (AIDS) and even in otherwise healthy adults who have received antibiotics (especially tetracycline) for upper respiratory infection.

Radiographic appearance

The classic radiographic appearance is an irregular cobblestone pattern with a shaggy marginal contour of the esophagus caused by deep ulcerations and sloughing of the mucosa (Figure 4-8). *Candida* presents as plaques and nodules as a result of a superficial collection of fungi. Characteristics of herpetic esophagitis include small mucosal ulcers or plaques.

Treatments for esophagitis

Modifications to lifestyle including weight loss, changes in diet to prevent decreased esophageal sphincter control, and medications to reduce acidity are the first line of treatment. A new technique called proton pump inhibitor therapy (using esomeprazole) can help control progression in reflux and Barrett's esophagitis. If these therapies do not work, surgical fundoplication is an option. Infectious esophagitis caused by *Candida* or

Figure 4-8 *Candida* esophagitis. Multiple ulcers and nodular plaques produce the grossly irregular contour of shaggy esophagus. This manifestation of far-advanced candidiasis has become infrequent because of earlier and better treatment of the disease.

herpesvirus may require a regimen of antifungal or antiviral drugs to eradicate the cause.

Ingestion of corrosive agents

The ingestion of alkaline or acidic corrosive agents produces acute inflammatory changes in the esopha-gus. Superficial penetration of the toxic agent results in only minimal ulceration. Deeper penetration of the submucosa and muscular layers causes sloughing of destroyed tissue and deep ulceration. Ingesting strong alkaline agents causes deeper lesions than ingesting strong acids, and only half of those who ingest an acid suffer severe injury. Drug-induced esophagitis may occur in patients who have delayed esophageal transit time, which permits prolonged mucosal contact with the ingested substance. The most common drug causing esophageal ulceration is potassium chloride in tablet form. Other medications that can cause esophagitis are weak caustic agents that are harmless when they pass rapidly through the esophagus.

Radiographic appearance

Healing of the intense mucosal and intramural inflammation of acute esophagitis may lead to pronounced fibrosis and stricture formation. These benign strictures tend to be long lesions with tapered margins and relatively smooth mucosal surfaces (Figure 4-9), in contrast to the irregular narrowing, mucosal destruction, and overhanging margins that are generally associated with malignant processes.

Treatment

The type of agent ingested determines the therapy. Poison control is usually called for specific treatments if the situation is not drug induced. Vomiting is generally not induced because this would cause a repeated exposure to the esophagus. Dilution by administering milk or water is appropriate unless the corrosive agent is acidic (in this case, water should not be used as this would produce excessive heat).

Esophageal cancer

Progressive difficulty in swallowing (dysphagia) in a person older than 40 years must be assumed to be caused by cancer until proved otherwise. Because the symptoms of esophageal carcinoma tend to appear late in the course of the disease, and because the lack of a limiting outer layer (serosa) commonly permits direct extension of the tumor by the time of the initial diagnosis, carcinoma of the esophagus has a dismal prognosis. Most carcinomas of the esophagus are of the squamous cell type and they occur most often at the esophagogastric junction. The incidence of carcinoma of the esophagus is far higher in men than in women. There is a strong correlation between excessive alcohol intake, smoking, and esophageal carcinoma.

Radiographic appearance

The earliest radiographic evidence of infiltrating carcinoma of the esophagus appears on a double-contrast barium swallow film as a flat, plaquelike lesion, occasionally with central **ulceration,** that in-

Figure 4-9 Corrosive stricture resulting from ingestion of lye.

Figure 4-10 Early carcinoma of the esophagus. Flat, plaquelike lesion *(arrows)* involves the posterior wall of the esophagus.

Figure 4-11 Carcinoma of esophagus. Irregular narrowing with ulceration involves an extensive segment of the thoracic portion of the esophagus.

volves one wall of the esophagus (Figure 4-10). At this stage there may be minimal reduction in the caliber of the lumen. Unless the patient is carefully examined in various positions, this earliest form of esophageal carcinoma can be missed. As the **infiltrating** cancer progresses, irregularity of the wall is seen, indicating mucosal destruction. Advanced lesions encircle the lumen completely, causing annular constrictions with overhanging margins and often some degree of obstruction. The lumen through the stenotic area is irregular, and mucosal folds are absent or severely ulcerated (Figure 4-11). Less commonly, carcinoma of the esophagus can appear as a localized **polypoid** mass, often with deep ulceration and a fungating appearance.

Luminal obstruction as a result of carcinoma causes proximal dilatation of the esophagus and may result in aspiration pneumonia. Extension of the tumor to adjacent mediastinal structures may lead to fistula formation, especially between the esophagus and the respiratory tract (see Figure 4-15).

Computed tomography (CT) has become a major method of staging patients with esophageal

Figure 4-12 CT staging of esophageal carcinoma. **A,** Esophagram demonstrates infiltrating lesion causing irregular narrowing of the distal part of the esophagus. **B,** CT scan shows a mass of bulky carcinoma *(black arrows)* filling most of the lumen *(white arrow).* Obliteration of the fat plane adjacent to the aorta *(curved arrow)* indicates mediastinal invasion.

carcinoma (with 90% accuracy), providing information on tumor size, extension, and resectability that was previously available only at thoracotomy (Figure 4-12). Evidence of tumor spread includes the obliteration of fat planes between the esophagus and adjacent structures (left atrium, aorta), the formation of a fistula to the tracheobronchial tree, and recognition of metastatic disease (e.g., low-density masses in the liver; enlargement of draining lymph nodes).

Treatment

If the cancerous lesion has not extended into surrounding tissue, surgical resection may result in cure. When the cancerous lesion involves surrounding tissue, treatment becomes palliative surgery together with radiation therapy or chemotherapy. If the esophagus is severely narrowed, a technique known as bougienage can be employed; this is the introduction of a long instrument to dilate and help maintain an adequate lumen. Laser therapy aids in treating the dysphagia in patients with unresectable lesions. The prognosis of the patient who is diagnosed in the late stages is extremely poor.

Esophageal diverticula

Esophageal diverticula (outpouchings) are common lesions that either contain all layers of the wall (traction or true diverticula) or are composed of only mucosa and submucosa herniating through the muscular layer (pulsion or false diverticula). Small diverticula do not retain food or secretions and are asymptomatic. When the diverticulum fills with food or secretions, aspiration pneumonia may result.

Radiographic appearance

Zencker's diverticula arise from the posterior wall of the upper (cervical) esophagus (Figure 4-13). Occasionally, they can become so large that they almost occlude the esophageal lumen. Diverticula of the thoracic portion of the esophagus are primarily found opposite the bifurcation of the trachea in the region of the hilum of the lung (Figure 4-14). These **traction** diverticula reflect motor function disturbance and develop in response to the pull of fibrous adhesions after infection of the mediastinal lymph nodes. **Epiphrenic** diverticula arise in the distal 10 cm of the esophagus (Figure 4-15). They are associated with incoordination of esophageal peristalsis and sphincter

Figure 4-13 Small Zencker's diverticulum. Saccular outpouching *(arrow)* arising posteriorly just proximal to an impression produced by the cricopharyngeal muscle. (From Eisenberg RL: *Gastrointestinal radiology: a pattern approach,* Philadelphia, 1990, Lippincott.)

relaxation, which increases the intraluminal pressure in this segment.

Treatment

Diverticula do not require treatment unless they interfere with swallowing. In Zenker's diverticulum, surgery consists of excision of the diverticulum and correction of any motility issues.

Esophageal varices

Esophageal varices are dilated veins in the wall of the esophagus that are most commonly the result of increased pressure in the portal venous system (portal hypertension), which is in turn usually a result of cirrhosis of the liver. In patients with portal hypertension, much of the portal blood cannot flow along its normal pathway through the liver to the inferior vena cava and then on to the heart. Instead, it must go by a circuitous collateral route, and increased blood flow through these dilated veins causes the development of esophageal (and gastric) varices. Esophageal varices are infrequently demonstrated in the absence of portal hypertension. "Downhill" varices are produced when venous blood from the head and neck cannot reach the heart because of an obstruction of the superior vena cava caused by tumors or inflammatory disease in the mediastinum. In this situation blood flows "downhill" through the esophageal veins before eventually entering the portal vein, through

Figure 4-14 Traction diverticulum of the mid-thoracic portion of the esophagus. (From Eisenberg RL: *Gastrointestinal radiology: a pattern approach,* Philadelphia, 1990, Lippincott.)

which it flows to the inferior vena cava and the right atrium.

Radiographic appearance

The characteristic radiographic appearance of esophageal varices is serpiginous thickening of folds, which appear as round or oval filling defects resembling the beads of a rosary (Figure 4-16). Precise technique is required to demonstrate esophageal varices. A double-contrast barium swallow best demonstrates the serpiginous and wormlike filling defect. Complete filling of the esophagus with barium may obscure varices, and powerful contractions of the esophagus may squeeze blood out of the varices and make them impossible to detect. Upright and recumbent imaging may best demonstrate the varices dilated and empty, respectively.

The major complication of esophageal varices is bleeding. Their appearance in patients with cirrhotic liver disease implies significant portal venous hypertension and is an ominous sign, as up to 90% of the

Figure 4-15 Epiphrenic diverticulum. (From Eisenberg RL: *Gastrointestinal radiology: a pattern approach,* Philadelphia, 1990, Lippincott.)

Figure 4-16 Esophageal varices. Note diffuse round and oval filling defects, which resemble rosary beads.

deaths from liver disease in patients with cirrhosis occur within 2 years of the diagnosis of varices.

Treatment

Vasoconstrictor drugs to constrict the dilated vessels are commonly used to treat esophageal varices. Active bleeding can be controlled by a technique called balloon tamponade, which creates pressure to stop the bleeding. If bleeding cannot be controlled, surgery is performed to tie off collateral vessels.

Hiatal hernia

Hiatal hernia is the most frequent abnormality (occurring in 50% of the population) detected on upper gastrointestinal examination. Its broad radiographic spectrum ranges from large esophagogastric hernias, in which much of the stomach lies within the thoracic cavity and there is a predisposition to volvulus (twisting), to small hernias that emerge above the diaphragm only under certain circumstances (related to changes in intraabdominal or intrathoracic pressure) and easily slide back into the abdomen through the hiatus (sliding hiatal hernia). The symptoms associated with hiatal hernia, as well as its complications (esophagitis, esophageal ulcer, esophageal stenosis), are related to the presence of esophageal reflux rather than to the hiatal hernia itself. Most hiatal hernias do not produce symptoms and are clinically of no importance.

Radiographic appearance

Although the diagnosis of hiatal hernia generally requires a barium study (Figure 4-17), at times a large hi-

Figure 4-17 **A,** Large hiatal hernia *(arrows)*. **B,** This 65-year-old woman had right lower quadrant pain. Hiatal hernia was an incidental finding on CT scan of the abdomen with oral contrast agent. The stomach was shown to be in the retrocardiac area.

atal hernia may appear on plain chest radiographs as a soft-tissue mass in the posterior mediastinum, often containing a prominent air–fluid level (Figure 4-18). The esophagus and stomach are distinguished by their appearance; mucosal folds are linear and parallel in the esophagus, whereas in the stomach the folds appear numerous and thicker without a parallel orientation.

Treatment

In most cases, a hiatal hernia requires no treatment. If surgical intervention is necessary, the hiatus is tightened and the stomach secured below the diaphragm.

Achalasia

Achalasia is a functional obstruction of the distal section of the esophagus with proximal dilation caused by incomplete relaxation of the lower esophageal sphincter. It is related to a paucity or absence of ganglion cells in the myenteric neural plexuses of the distal esophageal wall.

Radiographic appearance

On plain chest radiographs, the dilated, tortuous esophagus may produce a widened mediastinum (often with an air–fluid level) on the right side adjacent to the cardiac shadow (Figure 4-19). The hallmark of achalasia, seen on barium studies, is a gradually tapered, smooth,

Figure 4-18 Air–fluid level *(arrow)* in a hiatal hernia seen on a lateral chest radiograph.

conical, 1- to 3-cm narrowing of the distal esophageal segment (rat-tail or beak appearance) (Figure 4-20). On sequential radiographs, especially with the patient upright, only small spurts of barium pass through the narrowed distal segment to enter the stomach.

Figure 4-19   Achalasia. Frontal chest radiograph demonstrates the margin of a dilated tortuous aorta *(arrows)* parallel with the right border of the heart producing a widened mediastinum. (From Eisenberg RL: *Gastrointestinal radiology: a pattern approach,* Philadelphia, 1990, Lippincott.)

Figure 4-20   Achalasia. **A,** "Rat-tail" narrowing of distal part of the esophagus *(arrow).* **B,** Small spurt of barium *(arrow)* enters stomach through narrowed distal segment (the jet effect). (From Eisenberg RL: *Gastrointestinal radiology: a pattern approach,* Philadelphia, 1990, Lippincott.)

Treatment

Medications are given before meals to assist in relaxing the esophageal sphincter. If these do not control the symptoms, endoscopic balloon dilation with a bougienage may be helpful. A last resort is surgery (Heller's myotomy) to open the sphincter.

Foreign bodies

A wide spectrum of foreign bodies can become impacted in the esophagus, usually in the cervical esophagus at or just above the level of the thoracic inlet (Figure 4-21). Symptomatically, the patient is unable to swallow without regurgitation. Most metallic

Figure 4-21 Fish bone *(arrow)* impacted in the lower cervical portion of the esophagus.

Figure 4-22 Meat impaction in the esophagus. Large bolus of hot dog *(arrow)* is trapped in the mid esophagus of a patient with quadriplegia. Note barium in the bronchial tree *(arrowheads)*, caused by aspiration.

objects, such as pins, coins, and small toys, are radiopaque and are easily visualized on radiographs or during fluoroscopy. Objects made of aluminum and some light alloys may be impossible to detect radiographically because the density of these metals is almost equal to that of soft tissue. It is essential that any suspected foreign body be evaluated on two projections to be certain that the object projected over the esophagus truly lies within it.

Radiographic appearance

Nonopaque foreign bodies in the esophagus, especially pieces of poorly chewed meat (masticated food bolus), can be demonstrated only after the ingestion of barium (Figure 4-22). Such foreign bodies usually become impacted in the distal esophagus just above the level of the diaphragm and are often associated with a distal stricture. These intraluminal filling defects usually have an irregular surface and may resemble a completely obstructing carcinoma.

Treatment

Medications are the first line of treatment to relax the esophagus and allow the foreign body to move naturally into the stomach. In some instances, especially for sharper-pointed objects, retrieval of the foreign body using endoscopy may be appropriate. Interventional approaches are attempted before taking the patient to surgery to remove the obstruction.

If the esophageal foreign body causes obstruction for more than 12 hours, there is an increased risk of perforation.

Perforation of the esophagus

Perforation of the esophagus may be a complication of esophagitis, peptic ulcer, neoplasm, external trauma, or instrumentation. At times, perforation of a previously healthy esophagus can result from severe vomiting (the most common cause) or coughing, often from dietary or alcoholic indiscretion. Complete rupture of the wall of the esophagus may cause the sudden development of severe upper gastric pain simulating myocardial infarction. In the **Mallory-Weiss syndrome,** an increase in intraluminal and intramural pressure associated with vomiting (severe retching) after an alcoholic bout causes superficial mucosal laceration or fissures near the esophagogastric junction that produce severe hemorrhage. Endoscopy is required to best demonstrate lacerations, especially those close to the sphincter.

Radiographic appearance

A perforation that extends throughout the entire esophageal wall can lead to free air in the mediastinum or periesophageal soft tissues. The administration of radiopaque contrast material may demonstrate extravasation through the perforation (Figure 4-23) or an intramural dissection channel separated by an intervening lucent line from the

Figure 4-23 A, Esophageal perforation. Extravasation of contrast material *(arrows)* is seen in previously healthy patient who experienced severe vomiting after excessive ingestion of alcohol. **B,** CT scan of the chest of a 41-year-old man illustrates perforation of the esophagus with drainage into the thoracic cavity.

Summary of Findings for the Esophagus

DISORDER	LOCATION	RADIOGRAPHIC APPEARANCE	TREATMENT
Tracheoesophageal atresia or fistula—congenital	Blind pouch superiorly Blind pouch distally or tracheal fistula	Blind pouch filled with contrast or NG tube Fistula track (if one exists), NG tube injection	Surgical repair—connect esophagus (anastomosis), fistula repair
Tracheoesophageal fistula—acquired	Usually at level of the carina or more proximal	Demonstration of connection between esophagus and tracheobronchial tree	Palliative—interventional stent placement Surgical—fistula repair
Reflux esophagitis	Distal esophagus	Streaks or dots superimposed on flat mucosa	Lifestyle modifications Weight-reduction diet Medication
Barrett's esophagitis	Mid to lower esophagus	Smooth tapered stricture(s)	Surgery—fundoplication
Candida (fungal) and herpesvirus esophagitis	Entire esophagus	Cobblestone pattern Shaggy marginal contour Possible plaques	Same treatment as for Barrett's, adding antifungal or antiviral medication
Ingestion of corrosive agents	Alkaline ingestion Acidic ingestion	Deeper ulceration Stricture formation Superficial minimal ulceration Stricture formation	Call poison control Water or milk dilution—alkaline

GI, Gastrointestinal; *NG,* nasogastric.

■ ■

Summary of Findings for the Esophagus—cont'd

DISORDER	LOCATION	RADIOGRAPHIC APPEARANCE	TREATMENT
Esophageal cancer	Distal esophagus, esophagogastric junction	Double-contrast barium swallow: • Flat plaquelike lesion • Infiltrating lesion (irregular wall) • Polypoid mass (deep ulceration)	Surgical resection—possible cure Palliative therapy—chemotherapy or radiation
Esophageal diverticula	Traction—all layers of wall Pulsion—mucosal and submucosal layers	Appears as an out-pouching or pocket filling with barium	Usually no treatment Surgery if diverticulum interferes with swallowing
Esophageal varices	Distal esophagus and stomach	Serpiginous thickening of folds—resembles rosary beads	Medication—vasoconstrictor drugs Active bleeding—interventional balloon tamponade or surgery to tie off collateral vessels
Hiatal hernia	Esophagogastric region	GI series—numerous thicker folds of the stomach above the diaphragm	No treatment in most instances Surgical intervention includes tightening the hiatus
Achalasia—functional obstruction	Distal esophagus with proximal dilation	Chest film—dilated esophagus GI series—narrowing of distal esophageal segment	Medication to relax sphincter Endoscopic balloon dilation Surgical myotomy
Foreign bodies—food bolus or nonopaque objects Foreign bodies—non–food-related (coin) or opaque	Any region of the esophagus	Barium swallow to demonstrate the level of impaction causing the obstruction	Medication to relax esophagus Endoscopy to retrieve foreign body Surgical retrieval if all interventional approaches fail
Esophageal perforation—inflammatory, neoplastic, or traumatic	Any region of the esophagus	Perforation through entire wall—air in the mediastinum Contrast material extravasaton through perforation	Interventional—expandable stent Treat complications Surgical band ligation

■ ■

normal esophageal lumen. CT is the preferred modality to define the extent of the process.

Treatment

Place an expandable stent and then treat the complications (chest tube for pneumothorax; antibiotics to prevent infection). A surgical procedure (band ligation) can be performed to close the perforation.

■ Stomach

Gastritis

Inflammation of the stomach can be the result of a variety of irritants including alcohol, corrosive agents, and infection. Gastritis changes the normal surface pattern of the gastric mucosa. *Helicobacter pylori* can cause chronic gastritis that may lead to peptic ulcer disease.

Radiographic appearance

Alcoholic gastritis may produce thickening of gastric folds (Figure 4-24), multiple superficial gastric erosions, or both. In **corrosive** gastritis, the acute inflammatory reaction heals by fibrosis and scarring, which results in severe narrowing of the antrum and may cause gastric outlet obstruction. In **bacterial** (phlegmonous) gastritis, inflammatory thickening of the gastric wall causes narrowing of the stomach that may mimic gastric cancer. The diagnosis of **infectious** gastritis can be made if there is evidence of gas bubbles (produced by the bacteria) in the stomach wall (Figure 4-25). These types of gastritis are known as erosive or acute gastritis.

Chronic atrophic gastritis (nonerosive) refers to severe mucosal atrophy (wasting) that causes thinning and a relative absence of mucosal folds, with the fundus or entire stomach having a bald appearance. This is a nonspecific radiographic pattern that can be related to such factors as age, malnutrition, medication, and complications of alcoholism. Chronic atrophic gastritis also occurs in patients with pernicious anemia, who cannot absorb vitamin B_{12} because of an inability of the stomach to secrete intrinsic factor (or hydrochloric acid).

Treatment

The causative agent in erosive gastritis determines treatment. Eliminating the causative agent, such as alcohol, reduces the changes in the mucosal lining as well as the symptoms. If overproduction of stomach acid produces the changes, acid-reduction medications are used to help maintain the mucous defense barrier. Antibiotics are the appropriate medication for bacterial or infectious gastritis. Patients with *H. pylori* gastritis receive a regimen of multiple antibiotics because this infection may be antibiotic resistant. Us-

Figure 4-24 Gastritis. Note pronounced thickening of rugal folds throughout the stomach.

Figure 4-25 Phlegmonous emphysematous gastritis. Note severe, irregular ulceration of the distal stomach, with air in the wall *(arrows)*.

ing a combination of antibiotics has resulted in an 80% to 90% cure rate.

Peptic ulcer disease

Peptic ulcer disease is an inflammatory process involving the stomach and duodenum. It is caused by the action of acid and the enzyme pepsin secreted by the stomach and occurs most frequently on the lesser curvature. The spectrum of peptic ulcer disease varies from small and shallow superficial erosions to huge ulcers that may perforate through the bowel wall.

The major complications of peptic ulcer disease are hemorrhage (20%), perforation (less than 5%), and gastric outlet obstruction (5% to 10%). Peptic ulcer disease is the most common cause of acute upper gastrointestinal bleeding. Free perforation of a peptic ulcer located in the anterior wall of the stomach or duodenum is the most frequent cause of pneumoperitoneum with peritonitis (see Pneumoperitoneum, later). Narrowing of the lumen of the distal stomach or duodenal bulb caused by peptic ulcer disease is by far the most common cause of gastric outlet obstruction.

DUODENAL ULCER

Duodenal ulcer is the most common manifestation of peptic ulcer disease. More than 95% of duodenal ulcers occur in the first portion of the duodenum (the duodenal bulb).

Radiographic appearance

An unequivocal diagnosis of active duodenal ulcer requires the demonstration of an ulcer crater, which appears in profile as a small collection of barium projecting from the lumen. When seen en face, the ulcer niche appears as a rounded or linear collection of contrast material surrounded by lucent folds that often radiate toward the crater (Figure 4-26). Secondary signs of duodenal ulcer disease include thickening of the mucosal folds and a deformity of the duodenal bulb. Acute ulcers incite muscular spasm, leading to deformity of the margins of the duodenal bulb that may be inconstant and varied during the examination. With chronic ulceration, fibrosis and scarring cause a fixed deformity that persists even though the ulcer heals. Symmetric narrowing of the duodenal bulb in its midportion may produce the typical cloverleaf deformity of chronic duodenal ulcer disease (Figure 4-27).

GASTRIC ULCER

Unlike duodenal ulcers, which are virtually always benign, up to 5% of gastric ulcers are malignant.

Radiographic appearance

Radiographic signs that indicate whether a gastric ulcer is more likely to be benign or malignant have been described. The classic sign of a benign gastric ulcer in profile is penetration, with clear projection of the ulcer outside the normal barium-filled gastric lumen because the ulcer represents an excavation in the wall of the stomach (Figure 4-28). A thin lucency at the

Figure 4-26 Duodenal ulcer. An ulcer niche appears as a rounded collection of barium *(white arrow)* surrounded by lucent edema. Multiple surgical clips are noted incidentally *(black arrow).*

Figure 4-27 Chronic duodenal ulcer disease. Typical cloverleaf deformity is visible *(arrows).*

Figure 4-28   Benign gastric ulcer. Penetration of contrast material outside normal, barium-filled gastric lumen associated with thin, sharply demarcated, lucent line with parallel straight margins *(arrows),* representing edema at the base of the ulcer crater.

Figure 4-29   Benign gastric ulcer. On en face projection, prominent radiating folds extend directly to the ulcer. Lucency around the ulcer *(arrows)* represents inflammatory mass effect. (From Margulis AR, Burhenne JH, editors: *Alimentary tract radiology,* ed 4, St Louis, 1989, Mosby.)

base of the ulcer, reflecting mucosal edema caused by inflammatory exudate, is another sign of benignancy. When viewed en face, a gastric ulcer appears as a persistent collection of barium surrounded by a halo of edema (the ulcer collar) (Figure 4-29).

A hallmark of benign gastric ulcer is radiation of mucosal folds to the edge of the crater. However, because radiating folds can be identified in both malignant and benign ulcers, the character of the folds must be carefully assessed. If the folds are smooth and slender and appear to extend into the edge of the crater, the ulcer is most likely benign (Figure 4-30, *A*). In contrast, irregular folds that merge into a mound of polypoid tissue around the crater are suggestive of malignancy (Figure 4-30, *B*).

Although the size, shape, number, and location of gastric ulcers have been suggested as criteria for distinguishing between benign and malignant lesions, these findings are of little practical value. One exception is ulcers in the gastric fundus above the level of the esophagogastric junction: essentially all of these are malignant.

An abrupt transition between the normal mucosa and the abnormal tissues surrounding a gastric ulcer is characteristic of a malignant lesion (Figure 4-31), in contrast to the diffuse and almost imperceptible transition between the normal gastric mucosa and the mound of edema surrounding a benign ulcer. Neo-

plastic tissue surrounding a malignant ulcer is usually nodular, unlike the smooth contour of the edematous mound around a benign ulcer. A malignant ulcer does not penetrate beyond the normal gastric lumen but remains within it, because the ulcer merely represents a necrotic area within an intramural or intraluminal mass.

Most benign gastric ulcers heal completely with medical therapy (Figure 4-32). Complete healing does not necessarily mean that the stomach returns to an absolutely normal radiographic appearance; bizarre deformities can result because of fibrotic retraction and stiffening of the stomach wall. Although many malignant ulcers show significant healing, there is almost never complete disappearance of the ulcer crater.

The role of endoscopy in evaluating patients with gastric ulcers is controversial. At present, endoscopy is indicated whenever the radiographic findings are not typical for a benign ulcer, if healing of the ulcer does not progress at the expected rate, or if the mucosa surrounding a healed ulcer crater has a nodular surface or any other feature suggestive of an underlying early gastric cancer.

SUPERFICIAL GASTRIC EROSIONS
Superficial gastric erosions are ulcerations that are so small and shallow that they are rarely demonstrated

Figure 4-30 Radiating folds in gastric ulcers. **A,** Small, slender folds extending to edge of crater *(arrow)* indicate the benign nature of this ulcer. **B,** In this malignant gastric ulcer, thick folds radiate to an irregular mound of tissue around the ulcer *(arrow)*.

Figure 4-31 Malignant gastric ulcer. An abrupt transition occurs between normal mucosa and abnormal tissue surrounding an irregular gastric ulcer *(arrows)*.

Figure 4-32 A healing gastric ulcer. Folds converge to a residual central depression *(arrow)*.

on conventional single-contrast upper gastrointestinal examinations. With the increasing use of double-contrast techniques, a superficial gastric erosion typically appears radiographically as a tiny fleck of barium, which represents the erosion, surrounded by a radiolucent halo, which represents a mound of edematous mucosa (Figure 4-33). Possible factors implicated in the production of superficial gastric erosions include alcohol, antiinflammatory drugs (aspirin, steroids), Crohn's disease (see Crohn's Disease [Regional Enteritis], later), and candidiasis (see *Candida* and Herpesvirus, earlier).

Figure 4-33 Superficial gastric erosions in patient with gastritis. Collection of barium represents shallow erosion surrounded by a radiolucent halo *(arrow)*.

Figure 4-34 Gastric carcinoma producing linitis plastica pattern.

Treatment of ulcers

Lifestyle modifications are the first line of treatment for ulcers. First, the patient should avoid foods that cause an increase in the acid secretions (i.e., alcohol, caffeine). Antacids aid in neutralizing stomach acid. If stress is the cause of the increase in acidic secretions, stress management is appropriate. When the ulceration is caused by an infection *(H. pylori),* antibiotics are given to kill the bacteria. If the acidic secretions cannot be controlled by these methods, histamine H$_2$ antagonists help in reducing stomach acids and protecting the stomach lining. Surgical treatment for management of complications may be necessary when patients do not respond to other treatments.

Cancer of the stomach

Because pain is infrequently an early symptom, carcinoma of the stomach is rarely noted until the disease is far advanced and thus has a dismal prognosis (survival rate, 10%). The incidence of gastric cancer varies widely throughout the world. It is very high in Japan, Chile, and parts of Eastern Europe. It is low in the United States, where for reasons unknown it has been decreasing.

Several conditions appear to predispose persons to the development of carcinoma of the stomach. There is an increased risk of gastric cancer in patients with atrophic gastric mucosa, as in pernicious anemia, and in persons 10 to 20 years after a partial gastrectomy for peptic ulcer disease. A suggestive laboratory sign is achlorhydria, the absence of hydrochloric acid in gastric secretions obtained by means of a stomach

tube. Most carcinomas occur in the distal stomach and are adenomatous in nature.

Radiographic appearance

Gastric carcinoma can present a broad spectrum of radiographic appearances. Tumor infiltration of the gastric wall may stimulate intense fibrosis, which produces diffuse thickening, narrowing, and fixation of the stomach wall (a linitis plastica pattern) (Figure 4-34). The stomach is contracted into a tubular structure without normal pliability. This fibrotic process usually begins near the pylorus and progresses slowly upward; the fundus is the area least involved.

Another major form of gastric carcinoma is a large irregular polypoid mass (about one third of cancers). Irregularity and ulceration within the mass are suggestive of malignancy, whereas the presence of a stalk or normal-appearing gastric folds extending to the tumor are signs of benignancy. Ulceration can develop in any gastric carcinoma and occurs in approximately one third. This varies from shallow erosions in relatively superficial mucosal lesions to huge excavations within fungating polypoid masses (Figure 4-35).

CT is of major value in the staging of gastric carcinoma, in planning its treatment, in assessing the response to therapy, and in detecting tumor recurrence (Figure 4-36). Carcinoma of the stomach may appear as thickening of the gastric wall or as an intraluminal mass. Obliteration of the fat planes (the covering layers of fat) around the stomach is a reliable indicator of the extragastric spread of tumor. CT can demon-

Figure 4-35   Gastric carcinoma producing a large polypoid mass with associated ulceration *(arrow)*.

Figure 4-36   CT staging of gastric carcinoma. **A,** Double-contrast study demonstrates large lesser-curvature mass *(arrows)*. **B,** CT image shows a thickened gastric wall; the contrast agent demonstrates the lumen of the stomach.

Summary of Findings for the Stomach

DISORDER	LOCATION	RADIOGRAPHIC APPEARANCE	TREATMENT
Gastritis	Alcohol—gastric folds	Thickened gastric folds	Depends on cause:
	Corrosive—narrowing of antrum	Gastric outlet obstruction	Avoid long term irritants Acid-reduction
	Bacterial or infectious— gastric wall	Thickened gastric wall causing narrowing of stomach	medications Antibiotics for infections
	Chronic atrophic	Thinning and absence of mucosal folds ("bald")	Treat cause
Peptic ulcer	Inflammatory	Small shallow erosions to perforations—bleeding ulcer	Avoid foods causing increased acid secretion
	Duodenal ulcer	Rounded or linear collection of contrast material surrounded by lucent folds that often radiate toward the crater	(alcohol, caffeine) Antibiotics for infectious process
	Gastric ulcer	Benign—mucosal folds are smooth and slender and appear to extend into the edge of the crater	Histamine H_2 antagonist to reduce acidic secretions
		Malignant—irregular folds merge into a mound of polypoid tissue around the crater	
	Superficial gastric erosions	Fleck of barium with radiolucent halo	
Cancer	Gastric wall infiltration	Diffuse thickening, narrowing, and fixation of stomach wall	Surgical resection of all or part of stomach
	Polypoid mass	Irregularity and ulceration suggest malignancy	

strate direct tumor extension to intraabdominal organs, and distant metastases, especially to the liver.

Treatment

In most cases, treatment consists of surgical resection of all or part of the stomach.

Lymphoma of the stomach

(See Lymphoma in Chapter 8.)

■ Small Bowel

Crohn's disease (regional enteritis)

Crohn's disease is a chronic inflammatory disorder of unknown cause that most often involves the terminal area of the ileum but can affect any part of the gastrointestinal tract. Although it can occur at any age, Crohn's disease is most common in young adults. The underlying cause is unknown, although there appears to be some psychogenic element; stress or emotional

upsets are frequently related to the onset or relapse of the disease.

The granulomatous inflammatory process in Crohn's disease is frequently discontinuous, with diseased segments of bowel separated by apparently healthy portions (skip areas). Diffuse inflammation with edema involves all layers of the intestinal wall. Ulceration is common, and fistulas running in the bowel wall or extending to other organs are not infrequent.

The clinical spectrum of Crohn's disease is broad, ranging from a relatively benign course with unpredictable acute attacks and remissions to severe diarrhea and an acute condition in the abdomen. Although acute Crohn's disease may produce right lower quadrant pain simulating appendicitis, there is often blood in the stools that has come from the intensely congested mucous membranes. Small bowel obstruction and fistula formation occur in up to half of patients. Rectal fissures and perirectal abscesses occur in about one third.

Figure 4-37 Crohn's disease. Cobblestone appearance is produced by transverse and longitudinal ulcerations separating islands of thickened mucosa and submucosa.

Figure 4-38 Crohn's disease. Arrows point to widely separated areas of disease (skip lesions). The lesions are greatly narrowed segments of small bowel (string sign).

Radiographic appearance

In the small bowel, the earliest radiographic changes of Crohn's disease include irregular thickening and distortion of mucosal folds caused by submucosal inflammation and edema. Transverse and longitudinal ulcerations can separate islands of thickened mucosa and submucosa, leading to a characteristic rough cobblestone appearance (Figure 4-37). Rigid thickening of the entire bowel wall produces pipelike narrowing. Continued inflammation and fibrosis can result in a severely narrowed, rigid segment of small bowel in which the mucosal pattern is lost (string sign) (Figure 4-38). When several areas of small bowel are diseased, involved segments of varying length are often sharply separated from radiographically normal segments (skip lesions).

Fistula formation, a hallmark of chronic Crohn's disease, is found in at least half of all patients with this condition (Figure 4-39). The diffuse inflammation of the serosa and mesentery in Crohn's disease causes involved loops of bowel to be firmly matted together by fibrous peritoneal and mesenteric bands. Fistulas apparently begin as ulcerations that burrow through the bowel wall into adjacent loops of small bowel and colon. In addition to fistulas between loops of bowel, a characteristic finding in Crohn's disease is the appearance of fistulous tracts ending blindly in abscess cavities surrounded by dense inflammatory tissue. These abscess cavities can produce palpable masses, persistent fever, or pain. Although less common than bowel-to-bowel fistulas, internal fistulas extending

Figure 4-39 Crohn's disease. Note fistulization between the terminal ileum and the sigmoid colon (*solid arrow*) as well as along the cecum (*open arrow*).

from the bowel to the bladder or vagina can occur. A common complication is the development of external gastrointestinal fistulas, which usually extend to the perianal area and may be associated with fissures and perirectal abscesses.

Figure 4-40 Small bowel obstruction. Supine **(A)** and upright **(B)** projections demonstrate large amounts of gas in dilated loops of small bowel with multiple prominent air–fluid levels. Single, small collection of gas *(arrow)* remains in colon.

Treatment

Whenever possible, Crohn's disease is treated with medications, and surgery is performed only if complications require it. Surgical resection of an involved segment of small bowel is associated with a high incidence of recurrence of Crohn's disease adjacent to the anastomosis.

Small bowel obstruction

Fibrous adhesions caused by previous surgery or peritonitis account for almost 75% of all small bowel obstructions. External hernias (inguinal, femoral, umbilical, incisional) are the second most frequent cause. Other general causes of mechanical small bowel obstruction include luminal occlusion (gallstone, intussusception) and intrinsic lesions of the bowel wall (neoplastic or inflammatory strictures, vascular insufficiency).

Radiographic appearance

Distended loops of small bowel containing gas and fluid can usually be recognized within 3 to 5 hours of the onset of complete obstruction. Almost all gas proximal to a small bowel obstruction represents swallowed air. On upright or lateral decubitus projections, the interface between gas and fluid forms a straight horizontal margin (Figure 4-40). Although the presence of gas–fluid levels at different heights in the same loop has traditionally been considered evidence for mechanical obstruction, an identical pattern can also be demonstrated in some patients with adynamic ileus (see next section). The caliber of the air-filled bowel appears as a dilated proximal bowel and a collapsed distal bowel. On upright films, a string-of-beads sign appears. In adynamic ileus, the bowel has no caliber change.

As time passes, the small bowel may become so distended as to be almost indistinguishable from the colon. To make the critical differentiation between small and large bowel obstruction, it is essential to determine which loops of bowel contain abnormally large amounts of air. Small bowel loops generally occupy the more central portion of the abdomen, whereas colonic loops are positioned laterally around the periphery of the abdomen or inferiorly in the pelvis (Figure 4-41). Gas within the lumen of the small bowel outlines the thin valvulae conniventes, which completely encircle the bowel. In contrast, colonic haustral markings are thicker and farther apart and occupy only a portion of the transverse diameter of the bowel.

The site of obstruction can usually be predicted with considerable accuracy if the number and position of dilated bowel loops are analyzed. The presence of a few dilated loops of small bowel located high in the abdomen (in the center or slightly to the left) indicates an obstruction in the distal duodenum or jejunum. The involvement of additional small bowel loops is suggestive of a lower obstruction. As more loops are affected, they appear to be placed one above the other upward and to the left, producing a characteristic stepladder appearance (Figure 4-42). The point of obstruction is always distal to the lowest loop of dilated bowel.

Patients with complete mechanical small bowel obstruction demonstrate little or no gas in the colon.

Figure 4-41 Small bowel obstruction. Dilated loops of small bowel occupy the central portion of the abdomen, with the nondilated cecum and ascending colon positioned laterally around the periphery of the abdomen *(arrows)*.

Figure 4-42 Low small bowel obstruction. Dilated loops of gas-filled bowel appear to be placed one above the other, upward and to the left, producing the characteristic stepladder appearance.

This is a valuable point in the differentiation between mechanical obstruction and adynamic ileus, in which gas is seen within distended loops throughout the bowel. Although a small amount of gas or fecal accumulation may be present at an early stage of a small bowel obstruction (see Figure 4-41), the detection of a large amount of gas in the colon effectively eliminates this diagnosis.

The bowel proximal to an obstruction can contain no gas but be completely filled with fluid. This may produce a confusing picture of a normal-appearing abdomen or a large soft-tissue abdominal mass.

Plain abdominal radiographs are occasionally insufficient for a distinction to be made between small and large bowel obstruction. In these instances a carefully performed barium enema examination will document or eliminate the possibility of large bowel obstruction. If it is necessary to determine the precise site of small bowel obstruction, barium can be administered in either a retrograde (by means of an enema) or an antegrade (by way of the mouth) manner. Orally administered barium (*not* water-soluble agents) is the most effective contrast material for demonstrating the site of small bowel obstruction (Figure 4-43). The large amount of fluid proximal to a small bowel obstruction prevents any trapped

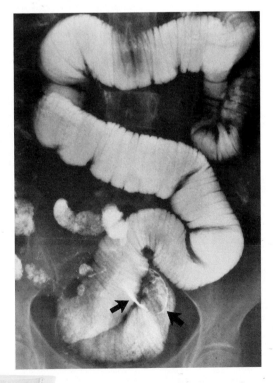

Figure 4-43 Barium upper gastrointestinal series demonstrates an impacted bezoar *(arrows)* to be the cause of a small bowel obstruction.

barium from hardening or increasing the degree of obstruction. The density of barium permits excellent visualization far into the intestine; water-soluble agents, however, are lost to sight because of dilution and absorption. It must be emphasized that if plain radiographs clearly demonstrate a mechanical small bowel obstruction, *any* contrast examination is unnecessary.

Strangulation of bowel caused by interference with the blood supply is a serious complication of small bowel obstruction. In a closed-loop obstruction (e.g., volvulus, incarcerated hernia) (Figure 4-44), the loops going both toward (afferent) and away from (efferent) the area of narrowing become obstructed. The involved segments usually fill with fluid and appear radiographically as a tumorlike soft-tissue mass. A closed loop is a clinically dangerous form of obstruction, since the continuing outpouring of fluid into the enclosed space can raise intraluminal pressure and rapidly lead to occlusion of the blood supply to that segment of bowel. Because venous pressure is normally lower than arterial pressure, blockage of venous outflow from the strangulated segment occurs before obstruction of the mesenteric arterial supply. Ischemia can rapidly cause necrosis of the bowel with sepsis, peritonitis, and a potentially fatal outcome.

CT may aid in demonstrating small bowel obstruction when the plain abdominal radiographs are normal or nonspecific. In addition to showing the site, level, and cause of the obstruction, this modality may indicate whether there is strangulation of the involved loops of bowel. CT appears to be the most valuable modality for patients with a history of abdominal malignancy and for those who have signs of infection, bowel infarction, or a palpable abdominal mass (Figure 4-45).

Treatment

Surgery is usually required to decompress the bowel as soon as possible to prevent necrosis or bowel perforation from occurring.

Adynamic ileus

Adynamic ileus is a common disorder of intestinal motor activity in which fluid and gas do not

Figure 4-44 CT scan of bowel obstructions. **A,** Herniation of small bowel and stomach through anterior abdominal wall. **B,** Scrotal herniation of large bowel causing bowel obstruction. **C,** Dilated sigmoid colon caused by obstruction.

progress normally through a nonobstructed small and large bowel. A variety of neural, hormonal, and metabolic factors can precipitate reflexes that inhibit intestinal motility. Adynamic ileus occurs to some extent in almost every patient who undergoes abdominal surgery. Other causes of adynamic ileus include peritonitis, medications that decrease intestinal peristalsis (those with an atropine-like effect),

electrolyte and metabolic disorders, and trauma. Adynamic ileus (or paralytic ileus) occurs more often than mechanical bowel obstruction. The clinical findings in patients with adynamic ileus vary from minimal symptoms to generalized abdominal distention with a sharp decrease in the frequency and intensity of bowel sounds.

Radiographic appearance

The radiographic hallmark of adynamic ileus is the retention of large amounts of gas and fluid in dilated small and large bowel. The entire small and large bowel in adynamic ileus, unlike in mechanical small bowel obstruction, appears almost uniformly dilated with no demonstrable point of obstruction (Figure 4-46).

There are two major variants of adynamic ileus. **Localized ileus** refers to an isolated distended loop of small or large bowel (the sentinel loop), which is often associated with an adjacent acute inflammatory process. The portion of the involved bowel can offer a clue to the underlying disease. Localized segments of the jejunum or transverse colon are frequently dilated in patients with acute pancreatitis. Similarly, the hepatic flexure of the colon can be distended in acute cholecystitis, the terminal ileum can be dilated in acute appendicitis, the descending colon can be distended in acute diverticulitis and dilated loops can be seen along the course of the ureter in acute ureteral colic (Figure 4-47). Unfortunately,

Figure 4-45 CT diagnosis of clinically unsuspected small bowel obstruction caused by adhesions. Note transition point between the dilated loops of small bowel *(B)* and the collapsed ileum *(black arrow)*. Note also the collapsed terminal ileum *(open arrow)*. (From Jeffrey RB: *CT and sonography of the acute abdomen*, New York, 1989, Raven Press.)

Figure 4-46 Adynamic ileus. Large amounts of gas and fluid are retained in loops of dilated small and large bowel. The entire bowel, small and large, appears almost uniformly dilated with no demonstrable point of obstruction.

Figure 4-47 Localized ileus in patient with acute ureteral colic. Arrow points to impacted ureteral stone.

Figure 4-48 Colonic ileus. Massive distention of large bowel without obstruction in a patient with severe diabetes and electrolyte abnormalities.

isolated segments of distended small bowel are commonly seen in patients with abdominal pain and thus the sentinel loop may be found "guarding" the wrong area.

Colonic ileus refers to selective or disproportionate gaseous distention of the large bowel without an obstruction (Figure 4-48). Massive distention of the cecum, which is often horizontally oriented, characteristically dominates the radiographic appearance. Colonic ileus usually accompanies or follows an acute abdominal inflammatory process or abdominal surgery. The clinical presentation and the findings on plain abdominal radiographs simulate those of mechanical obstruction of the colon. A barium enema examination is usually necessary to exclude an obstructing lesion.

Treatment

Adynamic ileus caused by surgery usually resolves itself spontaneously in 36 to 48 hours if no complications are involved. Treatment includes insertion of a nasogastric tube to aspirate the stomach, decompress the bowel, and allow the intestine to rest. Electrolyte and fluid imbalances are corrected by IV injection.

Intussusception

Intussusception is a major cause of bowel obstruction in children; it is much less common in adults. Intussusception is the telescoping of one part of the intestinal tract into another because of peristalsis, which forces the proximal segment of bowel to move distally within the ensheathing outer portion. Once such a lead point has been established, it gradually progresses forward and causes increased obstruction. This can compromise the vascular supply and produce ischemic necrosis of the intussuscepted bowel.

In children, intussusception is most common in the region of the ileocecal valve. The clinical onset tends to be abrupt, with severe abdominal pain, blood in the stool ("currant jelly"), and often a palpable right-sided mass. If the diagnosis is made early and therapy instituted promptly, the mortality of intussusception in children is less than 1%. However, if treatment is delayed more than 48 hours after the onset of symptoms, the mortality increases dramatically. In adults, intussusception is often chronic or subacute and is characterized by irregular recurrent episodes of colicky pain, nausea, and vomiting. A specific cause of intussusception often cannot be detected in children. In adults, however, the leading edge is frequently a polypoid tumor with a stalk (pedunculated) or an inflammatory mass.

Radiographic appearance

Radiographically, an intussusception produces the classic coiled-spring appearance of barium trapped between the intussusceptum and the surrounding portions of bowel (Figure 4-49, *A*). Reduction of a colonic intussusception can sometimes be accomplished by a barium enema examination (Figure 4-49, *B* and *C*), although great care must be exercised to prevent excessive intraluminal pressure, which may lead to perforation of the colon.

Ultrasound, used especially in children, demonstrates the obstructive mass as a doughnut-shaped lesion on the transverse scan and as a "pseudokidney" on longitudinal scan (Figure 4-50).

Treatment

Reduction of intussusceptions by rectal insufflation of air (instead of barium) has been reported to be an effective technique in children. In older children and adults, a repeat barium enema after reduction is necessary to determine whether an underlying polyp or a tumor caused the intussusception.

Malabsorption disorders

The term **malabsorption disorder** refers to a multitude of conditions in which there is defective absorption of carbohydrates, proteins, and fats from the small bowel. Regardless of the cause, malabsorption results in steatorrhea—the passage of bulky, foul-smelling, high-fat-content stools that float.

Radiographic appearance

Many of the diseases that cause malabsorption produce radiographic abnormalities in the small bowel, although malabsorption can exist without any de-

Figure 4-49　Intussusception. Obstruction of the colon at the hepatic flexure produces the characteristic coiled-spring appearance of intussuscepted bowel **(A)**. Partial **(B)** and complete **(C)** reduction of intussusception by careful barium enema examination.

Figure 4-50　Intussusception. Ultrasound image illustrates doughnut-shaped lesion marked for measurement.

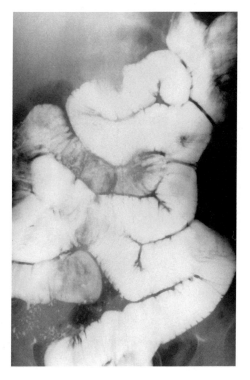

Figure 4-51 Diffuse dilatation of entire small bowel with excessive intraluminal fluid in a patient with malabsorption caused by sprue.

Figure 4-52 Diffuse, irregular thickening of small bowel folds in a patient with malabsorption secondary to Whipple's disease.

Summary of Findings for the Small Bowel

DISORDER	LOCATION	RADIOGRAPHIC APPEARANCE	TREATMENT
Crohn's disease (regional enteritis)	Most often in terminal ileum	Irregular thickened mucosal folds Cobblestone appearance String and skip signs Ulcerations—fistula formation	Medications Surgery if complications occur
Small bowel obstruction	Mechanical	Caliber of the air-filled bowel appears as a dilated proximal bowel and a collapsed distal bowel Stepladder appearance	Decompression as soon as possible Usually surgery
Adynamic ileus	Motility loss in small bowel	Large amounts of gas and fluid in small and large bowel	Usually resolves itself in 36-48 hr Place NG tube and balance fluids
Intussusception	Children—ileocecal valve	Radiograph—coiled spring appearance on contrast enema US—doughnut-shaped lesion	Reduction of telescoping bowel (rectal insufflation) Therapeutic enema of air or barium
Malabsorption disorders	Throughout small bowel	• Dilation with normal folds • Irregular distorted folds	Medications to increase nutrient absorption

NG, Nasogastric; *US,* ultrasound.

tectable small bowel changes. The two major radiographic appearances are (1) small bowel dilatation with normal folds (Figure 4-51) and (2) a pattern of generalized, irregular, distorted small bowel folds (Figure 4-52).

Treatment

Patients afflicted with malabsorption disorders take medications to assist in absorbing key nutrients to keep the body's systems in good health. Probiotics are live microbial food supplements that aid in improving the intestinal microbial balance. These supplements enhance the bioavailability of nutrients to the body.

■ Colon

Appendicitis

Acute appendicitis develops when the neck of the appendix becomes blocked by a fecalith or by postinflammatory scarring that creates a closed-loop obstruction within the organ. Because of inadequate drainage, fluid accumulates in the obstructed portion and serves as a breeding ground for bacteria. High intraluminal pressure causes distention and thinning of the appendix distal to the obstruction, which interferes with the circulation and may lead to gangrene and perforation. If the process evolves slowly, adjacent organs (terminal ileum, cecum, omentum) may wall off the appendiceal area so that a localized abscess develops; rapid vascular compromise may permit free perforation with the spilling of fecal material into the peritoneal cavity and the development of generalized peritonitis. Appendicitis occurs in all age-groups but is more common in children and adolescents.

The clinical symptoms of acute appendicitis are usually so characteristic that there is no need for routine radiographs to make the correct diagnosis. The presence of severe right lower quadrant pain, low-grade fever, and slight leukocytosis, especially in younger adults, is presumed to be evidence of appendicitis. However, in some patients, especially the elderly, the clinical findings may be obscure or minimal. In addition, because the appendix is mobile and may be in an unusual location, the pain of acute appendicitis may mimic cholecystitis, diverticulitis, or pelvic inflammatory disease. When the symptoms are confusing, radiographic examination may be necessary for prompt diagnosis and surgical intervention before perforation occurs.

Radiographic appearance

Plain abdominal radiographs may demonstrate a round or oval, laminated calcified fecalith in the appendix (appendicolith) (Figure 4-53) in about one

Figure 4-53   Laminated calcification in appendicolith.

third of patients. Surgical experience indicates that the presence of an appendicolith in combination with symptoms of acute appendicitis usually implies that the appendix is gangrenous (necrotic) and likely to perforate. Most appendicoliths are located in the right lower quadrant overlying the iliac fossa. Depending on the length and position of the appendix, however, an appendicolith can also be seen in the pelvis or in the right upper quadrant (retrocecal appendix), where it can simulate a gallstone.

Because of the danger of perforation, barium enema examination is usually avoided in acute appendicitis. If it is performed, an irregular impression of the base of the cecum (caused by inflammatory edema), in association with failure of barium to enter the appendix, is a characteristic finding. Nevertheless, failure of barium to fill the appendix is not a reliable sign of appendicitis, because the appendix does not fill in about 20% of normal patients. Partial filling of the appendix with distortion of its shape or caliber strongly suggests acute appendicitis (Figure 4-54), especially if there is a cecal impression. In contrast, a

Figure 4-54   Acute appendicitis. Spot radiograph from barium enema examination shows incomplete filling of appendix. (From Rice RP et al: *Radiographics* 4:393-409, 1984.)

Figure 4-55   Ultrasound images of appendicitis. **A,** Sagittal sonogram shows inflamed appendix *(A),* which is elongated and hypoechoic. **B,** Transverse scan shows appendiceal lumen surrounded by hypoechoic inflamed tissue *(arrows).* (Courtesy Carol Krebs, R.T., Shreveport, La.)

patent (open) appendiceal lumen effectively excludes the diagnosis of acute appendicitis, especially when barium extends to fill the rounded appendiceal tip.

When the clinical presentation is unclear, high-resolution ultrasound with graded compression is the imaging modality of choice for diagnosing acute appendicitis, especially when ionizing radiation is contraindicated in the patient. A noncompressible appendix measuring 7 mm or more in maximal outer diameter is considered virtually pathognomonic of acute appendicitis (Figure 4-55).

CT, the gold standard, shows an appendiceal abscess as a round or oval mass of soft-tissue density that may contain gas. After administration of IV con-

Figure 4-56   CT scan of the abdomen shows an appendix with an enlarged thickened wall indicating inflammation. An appendicolith can be seen in the appendix *(arrows)*.

Figure 4-57   Diverticulosis. The typical saw-toothed configuration is produced by thickened circular muscle and is associated with multiple diverticula.

trast material, the appendix appears as a dilated structure with a thickened, circumferentially enhancing wall (Figure 4-56). This modality provides a more precise evaluation of the nature, extent, and location of the pathologic process and can detect intraabdominal disease unrelated to appendicitis, which may explain the patient's clinical presentation.

Treatment

When diagnosed with appendicitis, an immediate appendectomy should be performed before perforation occurs to prevent complications (e.g., peritonitis, gangrene, abscess formation). If perforation occurs, a regimen of antibiotics helps to reduce the risk of peritonitis and sepsis.

Diverticulosis

Colonic diverticula are outpouchings that represent acquired herniations of mucosa and submucosa through the muscular layers at points of weakness in the bowel wall. The incidence of colonic diverticulosis increases with age. Rare in persons less than 30 years of age, diverticula can be demonstrated in up to half of persons over 60 years of age. Diverticular disease is presumed to occur in individuals who frequently exert high pressures in the lumen while straining to pass a large bulk of stool. Those consuming low-fiber and low-bulk meals are more susceptible. Diverticula occur most commonly in the sigmoid colon and decrease in frequency in the proximal colon. Although most patients with diverticulosis have no symptoms, a substantial number have chronic or intermittent lower abdominal pain, frequently related to meals or emotional stress,

and alternating bouts of diarrhea and constipation. Bleeding may be caused by inflammatory erosion of penetrating blood vessels at the base of the diverticulum. The leading cause of massive lower gastrointestinal bleeding in adults and guaiac-positive (indicating occult blood) stools in the elderly is diverticular disease.

Radiographic appearance

Colonic diverticula appear radiographically as round or oval outpouchings of barium projecting beyond the confines of the lumen. They vary in size from barely visible dimples to saclike structures 2 cm or more in diameter. Giant sigmoid diverticula up to 25 cm in diameter, which probably represent slowly progressing chronic diverticular abscesses, may appear as large, well-circumscribed, lucent cystic structures in the lower abdomen.

Diverticula are usually multiple and tend to occur in clusters, although a solitary diverticulum is occasionally found. When diverticula are multiple, deep criss-crossing ridges of thickened circular muscle (saw-toothed configuration) can produce a characteristic series of sacculations (Figure 4-57).

Diverticula also commonly occur in the esophagus and duodenum and infrequently may develop in the jejunum and ileum.

Diverticulitis

Diverticulitis is a complication of diverticular disease of the colon (necrosing inflammation in the diverticula), especially in the sigmoid region, in which perforation of a diverticulum leads to the development of a peridiverticular abscess. It is estimated that up to 20% of patients with diverticulosis eventually develop acute diverticulitis. Retained fecal material trapped in a diverticulum by the narrow opening of the diverticular neck causes inflammation of the mucosal lining, which then leads to perforation of the diverticulum. This usually results in a localized peridiverticular abscess that is walled off by fibrous adhesions. The inflammatory process may localize within the wall of the colon and produce an intramural mass, or it may dissect around the colon, causing segmental narrowing of the lumen. Extension of the inflammatory process along the colon wall can involve adjacent diverticula, resulting in a longitudinal sinus tract along the bowel wall. A common complication of diverticulitis is the development of fistulas to adjacent organs (bladder, vagina, ureter, small bowel).

Radiographic appearance

The radiographic diagnosis of diverticulitis requires direct or indirect evidence of diverticular perforation. The most specific sign is extravasation, which can appear either as a tiny projection of contrast material from the tip of a diverticulum (Figure 4-58, *A*) or as an obvious filling of a pericolic abscess (Figure 4-58, *B*). A more common, although somewhat less specific, sign of diverticulitis is the demonstration of a pericolic soft-tissue mass that is attributable to a localized abscess and represents a walled-off perforation. This extraluminal mass appears as a filling defect causing eccentric narrowing of the bowel lumen. The adjacent diverticula are spastic, irritable, and attenuated and frequently seem to drape over the mass. It is important to remember, however, that a peridiverticular abscess caused by diverticulitis can occur without radiographically detectable diverticula (Figure 4-59).

Severe spasm or fibrotic healing of diverticulitis can cause a rigidity and progressive narrowing of the colon that simulates annular carcinoma. Although radiographic distinction from carcinoma may be impossible, findings favoring the diagnosis of diverticulitis include the involvement of a relatively long segment, a gradual transition from diseased to normal colon, a relative preservation of mucosal detail, and fistulous tracts and intramural abscesses. At times, colonoscopy or surgery may be required to make a definitive diagnosis.

CT demonstrates pericolic fluids or gas collections, usually with nonspecific colonic wall thickening that produces narrowing of the bowel lumen (Figure 4-60). Inflammatory stranding may appear in the adjacent fat.

Treatment of diverticulosis and diverticulitis

Noninvasive treatment is the first choice, using dietary modifications and exercise (to increase peristalsis). If diverticulitis has developed, antibiotics and

Figure 4-58   Diverticulitis. **A,** Thin projection of contrast material *(arrow)* implies extravasation from colonic lumen. Note severe spasm of the sigmoid colon caused by intense adjacent inflammation. **B,** The pericolic abscess is clearly filled with contrast material *(arrows).*

diet adjustments (liquids) are given until the bowel heals. Perforation requires surgical repair and a regimen of antibiotics.

Ulcerative colitis

Ulcerative colitis is one of the two major inflammatory bowel diseases (the other is Crohn's colitis; see later). It primarily affects young adults and is highly variable in severity, clinical course, and ultimate prognosis. The cause is unknown, although an autoimmune cause has been suggested and a psychogenic factor may be involved because the condition is often aggravated by stress. The onset of the disease, as well as subsequent exacerbations, can be insidious or abrupt. The main symptoms include

Figure 4-59 Sigmoid diverticulitis. Severe narrowing of the long involved portion of the sigmoid colon *(arrows)* in a patient with no radiographically detectable diverticula.

Figure 4-61 Toxic megacolon in ulcerative colitis. Note dilatation of the transverse colon with multiple pseudo-polypoid projections extending into the lumen *(arrows)*.

Figure 4-60 Diverticulitis. CT scan illustrates thickened small bowel wall. The tissue has a "dirty" appearance *(arrow)*.

bloody diarrhea, abdominal pain, fever, and weight loss. A characteristic feature of ulcerative colitis is alternating periods of remission and relapse. Most patients have intermittent episodes of symptoms, with complete remission between attacks. In fewer than 15% of patients, ulcerative colitis is an acute severe process with a far higher incidence of serious complications such as toxic megacolon (extreme dilatation of a segment of colon with systemic toxicity) and free perforation into the peritoneal cavity. Usually, ulcerative colitis involves only the mucosal layer of the colon.

Radiographic appearance

In the radiographic evaluation of a patient with known or suspected ulcerative colitis, plain abdominal radiographs are essential. Large nodular protrusions of hyperplastic mucosa, deep ulcers outlined by intraluminal gas, or polypoid changes along with a loss of haustral markings (normal indentations in the wall of the colon) may indicate the diagnosis. Plain abdominal radiographs can also demonstrate evidence of toxic megacolon, a dramatic and ominous complication of ulcerative colitis that is characterized by extreme dilatation of a segment of colon (Figure 4-61), or evidence of an entire diseased colon, combined with systemic toxicity (abdominal pain and tenderness, tachycardia, fever, and leukocytosis). Toxic megacolon can lead to spontaneous perforation of the colon, which can be dramatic and sudden and can cause irreversible shock. Because there is such a high danger of spontaneous perforation, barium enema examination is absolutely contraindicated during a recognized attack of toxic megacolon.

Ulcerative colitis has a strong tendency to begin in the rectosigmoid area. Although by radiographic criteria alone the rectum appears normal in about 20% of patients with ulcerative colitis, true rectal sparing is infrequent, and there is usually evidence of disease on sigmoidoscopy or rectal biopsy. Isolated right colon disease with a normal left colon does not occur, and ulcerative colitis may spread to involve the entire colon (pancolitis). The disease is almost always continuous, without evidence of the skip areas seen

Figure 4-62 Ulcerative colitis involving primarily the rectosigmoid. Distal rectosigmoid mucosa *(white arrow)* is finely granular compared with the normal-appearing mucosa *(black arrow)* in the more proximal colon.

Figure 4-64 Chronic ulcerative colitis (lead-pipe colon). Muscular hypertrophy and spasm cause shortening and rigidity of the colon with loss of haustral markings.

Figure 4-63 Ulcerative colitis. Progression of disease results in deep ulcerations (collar-button ulcers) extending into the submucosal layer.

in Crohn's disease. Except for "backwash ileitis" (minimal inflammatory changes involving a short segment of terminal ileum), ulcerative colitis does not involve the small bowel, a feature distinguishing it from Crohn's disease, which may involve both the large and the small intestines.

On double-contrast studies, the earliest detectable radiographic abnormality in ulcerative colitis is fine granularity of the mucosa corresponding to the hyperemia and edema seen endoscopically (Figure 4-62). Once superficial ulcers develop, small flecks of adherent barium produce a stippled mucosal pattern. As the disease progresses, the ulcerations become deeper. Extension into the submucosa may produce broad-based ulcers with a collar-button appearance (Figure 4-63). Perirectal inflammation can cause widening of the soft-tissue space between the anterior sacrum and the posterior rectum (retrorectal space).

When the disease is chronic, fibrosis and muscular spasm cause progressive shortening and rigidity of the colon (Figure 4-64). The haustral pattern is absent, and the bowel contour is relatively smooth because of ulcer healing and subsequent reepithelization. Eventually, the colon may appear as a symmetric, rigid, tubular structure (lead-pipe colon).

Carcinoma of the colon is about 10 times more frequent in patients with ulcerative colitis than in the general population. During the first 10 years of disease, there is only a small risk of malignancy. Thereafter, it is estimated that there is a 20% chance per decade that a patient with ulcerative colitis will

Figure 4-65   Carcinoma of the colon developing in a patient with long-standing chronic ulcerative colitis. A long, irregular lesion with a bizarre pattern is visible in the transverse colon *(arrows)*.

develop carcinoma. Malignant lesions in ulcerative colitis generally occur at a much younger age than they occur in the general population, and they tend to be extremely virulent. Carcinoma of the colon in patients with chronic ulcerative colitis often appears as a bizarre stricture rather than with the more characteristic polypoid or apple-core appearance of a primary colonic malignancy (Figure 4-65). The tumor typically produces a narrowed segment with an eccentric lumen, irregular contours, and margins that are rigid and tapered. Because it is frequently difficult to distinguish carcinoma from benign stricture in patients with ulcerative colitis, colonoscopy or surgery is often required for an unequivocal diagnosis.

Crohn's colitis

Crohn's disease of the colon, the second major cause of inflammatory bowel disease, is identical to Crohn's disease in the small bowel and must be distinguished from ulcerative colitis. The proximal portion of the colon is most frequently involved in Crohn's disease; associated disease of the terminal ileum is seen in up to 80% of these patients. Unlike in ulcerative colitis, in Crohn's colitis the rectum is often spared, and isolated rectal disease very rarely occurs. Crohn's disease usually has a patchy distribution, with involvement of multiple noncontiguous segments of colon (skip lesions), unlike the continuous colonic involvement in ulcerative colitis. Perirectal abnormalities (fissures, abscesses, fistulas) occur at some point during the course of disease in half of patients with Crohn's co-

litis but are rare in ulcerative colitis. Crohn's disease involves all layers of the gastrointestinal tract.

Radiographic appearance

The earliest radiographic findings of Crohn's disease of the colon are seen on double-contrast examinations. Isolated tiny, discrete erosions (aphthous ulcers) appear as punctate collections of barium with a thin halo of edema around them (Figure 4-66). Aphthous ulcers in Crohn's disease have a patchy distribution against a background of normal mucosa, unlike the blanket of abnormal granular mucosa seen in ulcerative colitis.

As Crohn's colitis progresses, the ulcers become deeper and more irregular, with a great variation in size, shape, and overall appearance. Deep linear, transverse, and longitudinal ulcers often separate intervening mounds of edematous but nonulcerating mucosa, producing a characteristic cobblestone appearance (see Figure 4-37). If the penetrating ulcers extend beyond the contour of the bowel, they can coalesce to form long tracts running parallel to the long axis of the colon (Figure 4-67). The penetration of ulcers into adjacent loops of bowel or into the bladder, vagina, or abdominal wall causes fistulas, which can often be demonstrated radiographically. Inflammatory and fibrotic thickening of the bowel wall leads to narrowing of the lumen and stricture formation. Occasionally, an eccentric stricture with a suggestion of overhanging edges can be difficult to distinguish from annular carcinoma (Figure 4-68). In most instances, however, characteristic features of Crohn's disease elsewhere in the colon (deep ulcerations, pseudo-

Figure 4-66   Diffuse aphthous ulcers (*arrowheads*) in early Crohn's colitis. (From Caroline DF, Evers K: Colitis: radiographic features and differentiation of idiopathic inflammatory bowel disease, *Radiol Clin North Am* 25:47-66, 1987.)

polyps, skip lesions, sinus tracts, fistulas) clearly indicate the correct diagnosis.

CT demonstrates the mesenteric and extraintestinal extent of the disease, and any abscess formation or colonic wall thickening. Magnetic resonance (MR) spectroscopy is currently under investigation to help distinguish ulcerative colitis from Crohn's. Preliminary results indicate that this technique is able to differentiate between the two inflammatory bowel diseases in more than 90% of the cases.

Patients with Crohn's colitis appear to have a higher incidence of developing colon cancer than the general population, although this association is less striking than that between colon cancer and ulcerative colitis. Carcinoma complicating Crohn's colitis is most common in the proximal portion of the colon and usually appears radiographically as a fungating mass with typical malignant features, unlike the mildly irregular stricture characteristic of colon cancer in patients with ulcerative colitis. A small bowel examination may be necessary to demonstrate the terminal ileum.

Treatment of ulcerative colitis and Crohn's colitis

The initial treatments for ulcerative colitis and Crohn's disease are identical, as both are inflammatory bowel diseases. First, nutritional supplements and dietary modifications (decrease bulk to reduce stool frequency)

begin to decrease the inflammatory process. A regimen of antiinflammatory drugs interrupts the inflammatory cycle. Stress-related conditions require psychological support to control episodes. For ulcerative colitis, surgical resection may be necessary to prevent the spread of the condition. With proper treatment or spontaneous remission, many of the radiographic changes in this disease are reversible. In Crohn's, surgery is usually ineffective because the area adjacent to the anastomosis becomes involved as a result of the resection. For severe cases of Crohn's, parenteral (IV) nutrition allows the intestine time to heal.

Ischemic colitis

Ischemic colitis is characterized by the abrupt onset of lower abdominal pain and rectal bleeding. Diarrhea is common, as is abdominal tenderness on physical examination. Most patients are older than 50 years, and many have a history of prior cardiovascular disease.

Radiographic appearance

The initial radiographic appearance of ischemic colitis is fine superficial ulceration caused by inflammatory edema of the mucosa. As the disease progresses, deep penetrating ulcers, pseudopolyps, and characteristic "thumbprinting" can be demonstrated. Thumbprinting refers to sharply defined, fingerlike indentations along the margins of the colon wall (Figure 4-69). In most cases the radiographic appearance of the colon returns to normal within 1 month if good collateral circulation is established. Extensive fibrosis during the healing phase can cause tubular narrowing and a smooth stricture. If blood flow is insufficient, acute bowel necrosis and perforation may result.

Treatment

In some cases no intervention is needed as the bowel heals itself. Patients taking vasoconstriction drugs are most susceptible, and when the diagnosis is ischemic colitis these medications are discontinued and supportive is care given. Immediate surgical intervention is required for bowel infarctions and other complications.

Irritable bowel syndrome

The term **irritable bowel syndrome** refers to several conditions that have an alteration in intestinal motility as the underlying pathophysiologic abnormality. Most consider these conditions to be functional disorders, as there is a disruption of the food sequence breakdown in the stomach and intestines. Patients with irritable bowel syndrome may complain primarily of chronic abdominal pain and constipation (spastic colitis), chronic intermittent watery diarrhea, often without pain, or alternating bouts of constipation and diarrhea.

Figure 4-67 Crohn's colitis. Note long intramural fistula *(arrowheads)* in transverse colon. (From Lichtenstein JE: Radiologic-pathologic correlation of inflammatory bowel disease, *Radiol Clin North Am* 25:3-23, 1987.)

Figure 4-68 Chronic Crohn's colitis. Benign stricture with overhanging edges in transverse colon simulates carcinoma *(arrow)*.

Figure 4-69 Ischemic colitis. Soft-tissue polypoid densities *(arrow)* protrude into lumen of descending colon in a patient with acute abdominal pain and rectal bleeding.

Radiographic appearance

Although there are no specific radiographic findings in irritable bowel syndrome, patients with this condition usually undergo a barium enema examination to exclude another chronic disorder as the cause of the symptoms. When the patient is symptomatic, a barium enema may demonstrate areas of irritability and spasticity and accentuated haustration, although similar radiographic findings may be observed in normal asymptomatic persons, especially those who have received laxatives and enemas.

Treatment

No cure exists for irritable bowel syndrome. As the precise cause of this functional disorder has not been determined, symptomatic relief is provided. It is necessary to identify trigger foods so that they can be avoided, thus decreasing the spasms and pain. Alternative therapies, relaxation, meditation, and physical exercise have value if the patient can use them to help ease some of the spasms and pain.

Cancer of the colon

Carcinoma of the colon and rectum is the leading cause of death from cancer in the United States, even though it can be more easily diagnosed than most other malignant neoplasms. About half of colon carcinomas occur in the rectum and sigmoid, where they can be felt by rectal examination or seen with a sigmoidoscope. Carcinoma of the colon and rectum is primarily a disease of older persons, with a peak incidence in the 50- to 70-year range, and twice as common in men. Two diseases predispose to the development of cancer of the colon: long-standing ulcerative colitis and familial polyposis, a hereditary disease in which innumerable polyps develop in the colon and elsewhere in the intestinal tract.

Radiographic appearance

Because cancer of the colon is curable if discovered early in the course, delay in diagnosis is the most significant factor in the poor prognosis. There is considerable evidence to indicate that many, if not most, carcinomas of the colon arise in preexisting polyps. Therefore the early diagnosis of colonic cancer depends on polyp detection. Malignant polyps (Figure 4-70) tend to be sessile lesions (without stalks) with an irregular or lobulated surface, unlike benign polyps that are usually smooth and often have a stalk (are pedunculated). Other radiographic criteria suggestive that a polyp is malignant include large size (especially if greater than 2 cm in diameter), retraction or indentation (puckering) of the colon wall seen on profile view at the site of origin of a sessile polyp, and evidence of interval growth of a polyp on sequential examinations.

Figure 4-70   Carcinoma of rectum. Bulky lesion *(arrows)* could be felt on rectal examination.

Figure 4-71   Annular carcinoma of sigmoid colon. Note sharply defined proximal and distal margins of this relatively short, apple-core lesion *(arrow)*.

Annular carcinoma (described as apple-core or napkin-ring carcinoma) is one of the most typical forms of primary colonic malignancy (Figure 4-71). Annular carcinomas appear to arise from flat plaques of tumor (saddle lesions) that involve only a portion of the circumference of the colon wall. Unless meticulous care is taken to search for an area of minimal straightening or slight contour defects, the small and subtle, but lethal, saddle carcinomas can be easily overlooked. As the tumor grows, it characteristically infiltrates the bowel wall rather than forming a bulky intraluminal mass. This produces a classic bilateral contour defect with ulcerated mucosa, eccentric and irregular lumen, and overhanging margins. Progressive constriction of the bowel can cause complete colonic obstruction, most commonly in the sigmoid region.

Ulceration is common in carcinoma of the colon. It can vary from an excavation within a large fungating mass to mucosal destruction within an annular apple-core tumor.

A patient with carcinoma of the colon has a 1% risk of having multiple synchronous (occurring simultaneously) colon cancers. Therefore it is essential to examine carefully the rest of the colon once an obviously malignant lesion has been detected. In addition, such a patient has a 3% risk of developing additional metachronous cancers later.

CT is a major modality for staging carcinoma of the colon and for assessing tumor recurrence (Figure 4-72). Carcinoma causes asymmetric or circumferential thickening of the bowel wall with narrowing and deformity of the lumen. CT can demonstrate local extension of tumor to the pelvic organs as well as lymphadenopathy and metastases to the adrenal glands or liver (Figure 4-73).

Transrectal ultrasound produces the most accurate images for staging local rectal cancer by demonstrating the depth of invasion within the bowel wall. Ultrasound also may determine the presence of a tumor in adjacent, normal-size lymph nodes.

Positron emission tomography with 18-fluorodeoxyglucose (FDG-PET), although less specific than CT and ultrasound, has a higher accuracy for detecting distant nodular metastases.

Treatment

Surgical resection is required to remove a solitary carcinoma. Postoperative treatment may include chemotherapy or radiation therapy. Following resection, FDG-PET in combination with a CT scan helps rule out recurrence. FDG-PET images can differentiate recurrence of the tumor from adhesions or scar tissue resulting from the resection. The presence of multiple lesions requires radiation and chemotherapy.

Large bowel obstruction

About 70% of large bowel obstructions result from primary colonic carcinoma. Diverticulitis and volvulus account for most other cases. Colonic obstructions tend to be less acute than small bowel obstructions; the symptoms develop more slowly, and fewer fluid and electrolyte disturbances are produced.

Figure 4-72 CT scan of a patient with rectal carcinoma shows a soft-tissue mass on the lateral wall of the rectum containing a central ulceration *(straight arrows)*. Thickening of the perirectal fascia *(curved arrow)*, the presence of multiple lymph nodes (on the more cephalic images), and increased soft-tissue density of perirectal fat were suggestive of tumor extension beyond the bowel wall, which was confirmed at surgery. (From Butch RJ: In Taveras JM, Ferruci JT, editors: *Radiology: diagnosis, imaging, intervention*, Philadelphia, 1987, Lippincott.)

Figure 4-73 CT scan. Retroperitoneal and periaortic lymphadenopathy *(arrows)* in a 51-year-old woman with colon cancer.

Radiographic appearance

The radiographic appearance of colonic obstruction depends on the competency of the ileocecal valve. If the ileocecal valve is competent, obstruction causes a large, dilated colon with a greatly distended, thin-

Figure 4-74 Large bowel obstruction. Huge dilatation of cecum (up to 13 cm in diameter) without perforation.

walled cecum and little small bowel gas (Figure 4-74). The colon distal to the obstruction is usually collapsed and free of gas. If the ileocecal valve is incompetent, there is distention of gas-filled loops of both colon and small bowel, which may simulate an adynamic ileus.

The major danger in colonic obstruction is perforation. If the ileocecal valve is competent, the colon behaves like a closed loop, and the increased pressure caused by the obstruction cannot be relieved. Because the cecum is spherical and has a large diameter, it is the most likely site for perforation. In acute colonic obstruction, perforation is very likely if the cecum distends to more than 10 cm; in intermittent or chronic obstruction, however, the cecal wall can become hypertrophied, and the diameter of the cecum can greatly exceed 10 cm without perforation (see Figure 4-74). In the patient with suspected large bowel obstruction, a low-pressure barium enema can be safely performed and will demonstrate the site and often the cause of the obstruction (Figure 4-75).

Some professionals recommend an abdominal/pelvic CT scan as an initial examination, especially for patients without a surgical history who have symptomatic signs suggesting infection, bowel infarction, or palpable mass. CT can demonstrate causes of an obstruction such as diverticulitis or appendicitis.

Volvulus of the colon

Volvulus refers to a twisting of the bowel on itself that may lead to intestinal obstruction. Because twisting of the bowel usually requires a long, movable mesentery, volvulus of the large bowel most frequently involves the cecum and sigmoid colon. The transverse colon, which has a short mesentery, is rarely affected by volvulus. A sigmoid volvulus, more commonly found in the elderly, results from a bulky high-residue diet causing constipation.

CECAL VOLVULUS

The ascending colon and the cecum may have a long mesentery as a fault of rotation and fixation during the embryonic development of the gut. This situation predisposes to volvulus, with the cecum twisting on its long axis. It should be stressed, however, that only a few patients with an extremely mobile cecum ever develop cecal volvulus.

Radiographic appearance

In cecal volvulus, the distended cecum tends to be displaced upward and to the left, although it can be found anywhere within the abdomen. A pathognomonic sign of cecal volvulus is a kidney-shaped mass (representing the twisted cecum) with the twisted and thickening mesentery mimicking the renal pelvis (Figure 4-76, *A*). A barium enema examination is usually required for definite confirmation of the diagnosis. This study demonstrates obstruction of the contrast column at the level of the stenosis, with the tapered edge of the column pointing toward the site of the twist (Figure 4-76, *B*).

SIGMOID VOLVULUS

A long, redundant loop of sigmoid colon can undergo a twist on its mesenteric axis and form a closed-loop obstruction. In sigmoid volvulus, the greatly inflated sigmoid loop appears as an inverted U-shaped shadow that rises out of the pelvis in a vertical or oblique direction and can even reach the level of the diaphragm. The affected loop appears devoid of haustral markings and has a sausage or balloon shape.

Radiographic appearance

A barium enema examination demonstrates an obstruction to the flow of contrast material at the site of volvulus and considerable distention of the rectum. The lumen of the sigmoid tapers toward the site of stenosis, and a pathognomonic bird's-beak appearance is produced (Figure 4-77).

Figure 4-75 Large bowel obstruction caused by annular carcinoma of the sigmoid. **A,** Plain abdominal radiograph demonstrates pronounced dilatation of gas-filled transverse and ascending colon. **B,** Barium enema demonstrates typical apple-core lesion *(arrow)* producing the colonic obstruction.

Figure 4-76 Cecal volvulus. **A,** Dilated, gas-filled cecum appears as a kidney-shaped mass with twisted and thickening mesentery *(arrow)* mimicking the renal pelvis. **B,** Barium enema examination demonstrates obstruction of the contrast column at the level of stenosis *(arrow);* tapered edge of column points toward the torsion site.

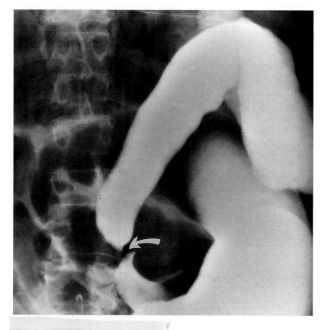

Figure 4-77 Sigmoid volvulus. Luminal tapering at site of stenosis produces characteristic bird's-beak configuration.

Figure 4-78 Hemorrhoids. Multiple rectal filling defects *(arrows)* simulate polyps.

Treatment for large bowel obstruction or volvulus

Surgical detorsion is usually required, although a water-soluble enema may be therapeutic and resolve the obstruction.

Hemorrhoids

Hemorrhoids are varicose veins of the lower end of the rectum that cause pain, itching, and bleeding. Like varicose veins in the leg, hemorrhoids are caused by increased venous pressure. The most common cause of increased pressure is chronic constipation with resulting excessive muscular straining needed to empty the bowel. Increased venous pressure can also be produced by a pelvic tumor or a pregnant uterus.

Radiographic appearance

On barium enema examinations, hemorrhoids occasionally can produce single or multiple rectal filling defects that simulate polyps (Figure 4-78). The proper diagnosis can easily be made by inspection, digital examination, or direct vision through the anoscope.

Treatment

Hemorrhoids may be treated nonsurgically and surgically. The nonsurgical approach consists of rubber band ligation. The surgical intervention consists of cir-cumferential mucosectomy, which is a stapled hemorrhoidectomy, a safe and effective procedure for advanced stages (third- and fourth-degree hemorrhoidal prolapse).

■ Gallbladder

Gallstones (cholelithiasis)

Gallstones consist of two major types: cholesterol stones and pigment stones. Cholesterol stones are predominant (75%) in the United States, whereas pigment stones occur more frequently in the tropics and the Orient. Genetic predispositions associated with higher incidence include family history of the disorder, age over 40 years, excess weight, and female sex. Gallstones can develop whenever bile contains insufficient bile salts and lecithin in proportion to cholesterol to maintain the cholesterol in solution. This situation can result from a decrease in the amount of bile salts present (because of decreased reabsorption in the terminal ileum as a result of inflammatory disease or surgical resection), or it can be caused by increased hepatic synthesis of cholesterol.

Radiographic appearance

Because cholesterol is not radiopaque, most gallstones are radiolucent and visible only on contrast examinations or ultrasound. In up to 20% of patients, however, gallstones contain sufficient calcium to be detectable

- -

Summary of Findings for the Colon

DISORDER	LOCATION	RADIOGRAPHIC APPEARANCE	TREATMENT
Appendicitis	Appendix	KUB—appendicolith US—7 mm or more outer diameter CT—round or oval mass, possibly containing gas Dilated lumen with thickened circumferentially enhancing wall	Appendectomy should be performed before perforation
Diverticulosis	Most common in sigmoid	Round or oval out-pouching projecting beyond lumen; usually multiple	Noninvasive: —Dietary modifications and exercise —Antibiotics for diverticulitis Invasive: —Surgery for perforated diverticula
Diverticulitis	Inflammation of diverticula	Diverticular perforation with possible abscess	
Ulcerative colitis	Superficial and acute; beginning in rectosigmoid area with continuous involvement throughout colon	KUB—deep ulcers with intraluminal gas or polypoid changes, loss of haustral markings BE (double contrast)—fine granularity of mucosa collar-button appearance	Nutritional supplements Dietary modifications (to decrease bulk) Antiinflammatory drugs Surgical resection for severe ulcerative colitis
Crohn's disease	Terminal ileum and proximal colon most often	BE (double contrast)—patchy distribution, noncontiguous segments (skip lesions)	Nutritional supplements Dietary modifications (to decrease bulk) Antiinflammatory drugs
Ischemic colitis	Entire colon	Fine superficial ulceration Characteristic "thumbprinting" Tubular narrowing and a smooth stricture	Many cases resolve spontaneously Restrict vasoconstrictor drugs and give supportive care Immediate surgery for infarctions and complications
Irritable bowel syndrome	Alteration of intestinal motility	No specific findings Rule out other disorders	No cure exists; treatments aid in alleviating the symptoms Identify and avoid trigger foods to reduce pain Alternative therapies: relaxation, meditation to reduce stress

- -

BE, Barium enema; *KUB,* kidney–ureter–bladder radiograph; *PET,* positron emission tomography; *US,* ultrasound.   *Continued*

■ ■

Summary of Findings for the Colon—cont'd

DISORDER	LOCATION	RADIOGRAPHIC APPEARANCE	TREATMENT
Cancer	50% in rectum and sigmoid region	Sessile lesion: irregular, lobulated surface Larger than 2 cm: "apple core" or "napkin ring" appearance CT—circumferential bowel wall thickening, metastasis, lymphadenopathy US—transrectal; depth of tumor invasion into bowel wall PET—detection of distant nodular metastasis	Solitary lesion: surgical resection, with or without chemotherapy Multiple or distant lesions: chemotherapy and/or radiation therapy
Large bowel obstruction	Large bowel	Ileocecal valve competent: large dilated colon, thin-walled cecum, little small-bowel gas Ileocecal valve incompetent: gas-filled loops of colon and of small bowel	Surgical detorsion Water-soluble enema may be therapeutic
Volvulus	Cecal or sigmoid colon	Distended cecum, displaced upward and to the left Distended rectum, devoid of haustral markings and a sausage or balloon shape Bird's-beak appearance	
Hemorrhoids	Distal rectum	Single or multiple rectal filling defects simulating polyps	Nonsurgical—rubber-band ligations Surgical—circumferential mucosectomy

■ ■

BE, Barium enema; *KUB*, kidney–ureter–bladder radiograph; *PET*, positron emission tomography; *US*, ultrasound.

on plain abdominal radiographs (Figure 4-79). Gallstones can have a central nidus (or focus) of calcification, a laminated appearance (with alternating opaque and lucent rings), or calcification around the periphery. Occasionally, a nonopaque stone may contain gas-filled fissures that produce the "Mercedes-Benz" sign, a characteristic triradiate pattern similar to the German automobile trademark (Figure 4-80).

Oral cholecystography (OCG) is the traditional technique for the diagnosis of gallstones, although it has been replaced in most institutions by ultrasound (see later). Gallstones appear as freely movable filling defects in the opacified gallbladder. They fall by gravity to the dependent portion of the gallbladder and frequently layer out at a level that depends on the relationship of the specific gravity of the stone to that of

the surrounding bile (Figure 4-81). Solitary gallstones are usually rounded; multiple stones are generally faceted. Large numbers of stones can have a sandlike or gravel-like consistency and be visible only when they layer out on radiographs obtained using a horizontal beam and with the patient in an erect or lateral decubitus position. Infrequently, a gallstone is coated with tenacious mucus and adheres to the gallbladder wall.

Malabsorption of the radiopaque contrast material, hepatocellular dysfunction (serum bilirubin ≥2 mg/dl), and intrinsic disease of the gallbladder (cystic duct obstruction, chronic cholecystitis) can lead to nonvisualization of the gallbladder on OCG. If these causes can be excluded, failure of the gallbladder to opacify after the administration of two doses of orally

Figure 4-80   Mercedes-Benz sign of fissuring in gallstone *(arrow)*. Note adjacent gallstone with radiopaque rim.

Figure 4-79   Calculi in gallbladder *(solid arrows)* and bile ducts *(open arrow)*. Calculi *(arrowheads)* lie in common bile duct, some of which overlie spine and are difficult to detect. (Courtesy Stephen R. Baker, New York, N.Y.)

administered cholecystographic contrast material is highly reliable evidence of gallbladder disease.

Ultrasound is now the major imaging modality for demonstrating gallstones. This noninvasive technique is as accurate as OCG, is independent of hepatic function, and does not rely on patient compliance in taking oral contrast agents. In addition to imaging the gallbladder, ultrasound can provide important additional information by effectively demonstrating the biliary tree and hepatic parenchyma. Gallstones appear on ultrasound as foci of high-amplitude echoes associated with posterior acoustic shadowing (Figure 4-82). The mobility of free-floating gallstones may be demonstrated by performing the examination with the patient in various positions.

Acute cholecystitis

Acute cholecystitis (inflammation of the gallbladder) usually (in 95% of cases) occurs after obstruction of the cystic duct by an impacted gallstone. Gallstones may injure the mucosal wall, allowing bacteria to enter.

Radiographic appearance

Either ultrasound or radionuclide scanning can be used. The sonographic diagnosis of acute cholecysti-

A   **B**

Figure 4-81   Oral cholecystogram showing multiple gallstones. **A,** With the patient supine, the stones are poorly defined and have a gravel-like consistency. **B,** On an erect film taken with a horizontal beam, the innumerable gallstones layer out and are easily seen.

tis requires the demonstration of a distended gallbladder containing gallstones. Important additional findings include edema of the gallbladder wall and focal tenderness elicited directly over the gallbladder. A normal gallbladder ultrasound image virtually excludes the diagnosis of acute cholecystitis. Because many disorders may mimic acute cholecystitis, ultrasound can also be used to evaluate the remainder of

Figure 4-82 Ultrasound scan of gallstones. Echogenic focus *(white arrow)* in otherwise sonolucent gallbladder *(G)* represents large gallstone. Notice acoustic shadowing immediately inferior to the stone *(black arrows).*

the right upper quadrant to detect any other acute abnormality.

When the results of a radionuclide cholescintigram are normal, they demonstrate the bile ducts, the gallbladder, and early excretion of radionuclide into the duodenum and proximal jejunum within 30 minutes after the IV injection of the radionuclide (technetium-99m) (Figure 4-83). Failure to accumulate radioactivity (after 4 hours) in the gallbladder is highly sensitive (98%) and specific for cystic duct obstruction. If associated with appropriate symptoms, this finding is virtually diagnostic of acute cholecystitis.

When ultrasound is inconclusive, MR cholangiopancreatography can demonstrate the cystic duct and any obstructing calculi located in the gallbladder neck. MR does not, however, evaluate the gallbladder wall thickness as well as ultrasound.

Emphysematous cholecystitis

Emphysematous cholecystitis is a rare condition in which the growth of gas-forming organisms in the gallbladder is facilitated by stasis and ischemia caused by cystic duct obstruction (most often by stones). Emphysematous cholecystitis occurs most frequently in elderly men and in patients with poorly controlled diabetes mellitus.

Radiographic appearance

Plain abdominal radiographs demonstrate gas in the gallbladder lumen that dissects into the wall or peri-

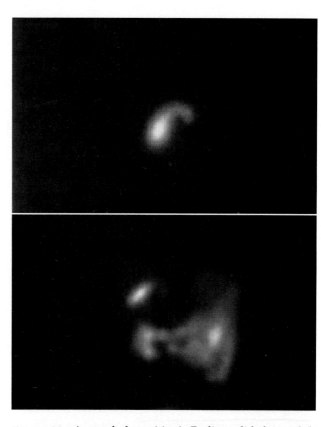

Figure 4-83 Acute cholecystitis. **A,** Radionuclide hepatobiliary study using technetium-99m Hepatolite in a 51-year-old woman with right upper quadrant pain demonstrates an engorged gallbladder at 1 hour after injection. **B,** At 28 minutes after injection of cholecystokinin (CCK), the gallbladder empties into the small bowel with an ejection fraction of 83%, which is normal.

cholecystic tissues. This produces the pathognomonic appearance of a rim of lucent bubbles or streaks of gas outside of and roughly parallel to the gallbladder lumen (Figure 4-84).

Treatment for cholecystitis

No treatment is necessary for asymptomatic patients. For acute impaction and biliary colic, prompt treatment using an antispasmodic and an analgesic helps alleviate symptoms. Interventional treatments available today include extracorporeal shockwave therapy (lithotripsy), stone removal by endoscopic retrograde cholangiopancreatography (ERCP), and chemical dissolution. The most common surgical approach used currently is the laparoscopic cholecystectomy.

Porcelain gallbladder

Porcelain gallbladder refers to extensive calcification in the wall of the gallbladder, which forms an oval den-

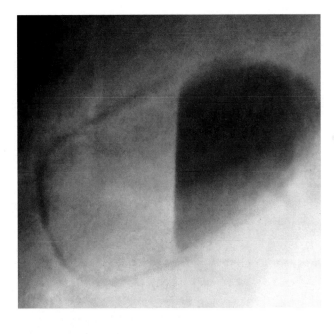

Figure 4-84 Emphysematous cholecystitis. Gas is found in both lumen and wall of gallbladder. (From Eisenberg RL: *Gastrointestinal radiology: a pattern approach*, Philadelphia, 1990, Lippincott.)

Figure 4-85 Porcelain gallbladder. Note extensive mural calcification around perimeter of gallbladder.

sity that corresponds to the size and shape of the organ (Figure 4-85). Because chronic cholecystitis produces a loss of wall function, the gallbladder becomes fibrotic and calcified. The term reflects the blue discoloration and brittle consistency of the gallbladder wall.

Radiographic appearance

The calcification in a porcelain gallbladder can appear as a broad continuous band in the muscular layers, or it may be multiple and punctate and occur in the glandular spaces of the mucosa.

- -

Summary of Findings for the Gallbladder

DISORDER	LOCATION	RADIOGRAPHIC APPEARANCE	TREATMENT
Gallstones	Gallbladder and biliary tree	KUB—cholelithiasis evident if calcified US—foci of high-amplitude echoes associated with acoustic shadowing	Asymptomatic—no treatment Noninvasive: lithotripsy; chemical dissolution Invasive: ERCP for stone retrieval; laparoscopic cholecystectomy
Acute cholecystitis	Gallbladder and biliary tree	US—demonstrates distended gallbladder containing gall-stones and possibly edema of the gallbladder wall NM cholescintigram—failure to accumulate radioactivity after 4 hr MR cholangiopancreatography—demonstrates the cystic duct and obstructing calculi located in gallbladder neck	
Emphysematous cholecystitis	Gallbladder	KUB—demonstrates gas in the gallbladder lumen that dis-sects into the wall to produce appearance of a rim of lucent bubbles or streaks of gas out-side of and roughly parallel to the gallbladder lumen	
Porcelain gallbladder	Extensive calcification in the wall	Broad continuous band of calci-fication in the muscular layers, or multiple and punctate calci-fications in the glandular spaces of mucosa	Prophylactic cholecystectomy

- -

ERCP, Endoscopic retrograde cholangiopancreatography; *KUB*, kidney–ureter–bladder radiograph; *NM*, nuclear medicine; *US*, ultrasound.

The detection of extensive calcification in the wall of the gallbladder should indicate the possibility of carcinoma. Although a porcelain gallbladder is un-common in cases of carcinoma of the gallbladder, there is a striking incidence of carcinoma in patients with porcelain gallbladder (up to 60% of the cases).

Treatment

Because of this high incidence, patients with porcelain gallbladder are usually subjected to prophylactic cholecystectomy even if they are asymptomatic.

■ Liver

Cirrhosis of the liver

Cirrhosis refers to the chronic destruction of liver cells and structure, with nodular regeneration of liver parenchyma and fibrosis; it is an end-stage liver dis-ease. The major cause of cirrhosis is chronic alcoholism (i.e., 10 to 20 years of alcohol abuse), in which damage to the liver is related either to the toxic effect of alco-hol or to the malnutrition that frequently accompanies chronic alcoholism. Other causes of liver destruction leading to cirrhosis include postnecrotic viral hepati-tis, hepatotoxic drugs and chemicals that destroy liver cells, disease of the bile ducts (primary and secondary biliary cirrhosis), and excessive deposition of iron pig-ment within the liver (hemochromatosis).

Regardless of the cause, fibrous connective tissue replaces the destroyed liver cells with cells that have no liver cell function. Initially, the liver enlarges be-cause of regeneration, but it eventually becomes smaller as the fibrous connective tissue contracts, and the surface becomes bumpy and nodular.

Figure 4-86 Fatty infiltration of the liver in cirrhosis. CT scan shows generalized decrease in attenuation value of liver *(L),* which is far less than that of spleen *(S).* Portal veins appear as high-density structures *(arrows)* surrounded by a background of low-density hepatic fat.

Radiographic appearance

Cirrhosis causes many physiologic changes that can be detected clinically or radiographically. In alcoholic cirrhosis a large amount of fat accumulates within the liver. This fatty infiltration is beautifully demonstrated on CT. In normal individuals the liver always appears brighter than the spleen, whereas in patients with cirrhosis the liver is much darker because of the large amount of fat (Figure 4-86). The portal veins appear as high-density structures surrounded by a background of low density caused by hepatic fat; this is the opposite of the normal pattern of portal veins, which as low-density channels on noncontrast scans.

Nodular regeneration of the liver combined with fibrosis causes obstruction of the portal vein, which drains blood from the gastrointestinal tract through the liver before emptying into the inferior vena cava near the heart. Increased pressure within this vessel causes pronounced enlargement of the spleen (splenomegaly). Because blood cannot flow through the obstructed portal vein, it must find an alternative route to bypass the liver. This leads to the development of collateral circulation, with large dilated veins becoming prominent on the abdominal wall in the area of the umbilicus. Another alternative route for blood to take in its return to the heart is the periesophageal veins, which dilate to become esophageal varices, which then can rupture and result in fatal hemorrhage (see Figure 4-16).

Destruction of liver cells substantially decreases the ability of the organ to synthesize proteins, such as albumin and several of the factors required for blood clotting. A deficiency of albumin (hypoalbuminemia) results in fluid leaking out of the circulation and the development of generalized edema, which is evidenced by swelling of the lower extremities. When edema in-

volves the wall of the intestinal tract, it can produce regular, uniform thickening of small bowel folds.

One of the most characteristic symptoms of cirrhosis is the accumulation of fluid in the peritoneal cavity (ascites), which causes characteristic abdominal distention. The abdomen is tight and quite hard, and an increase in exposure factors is required if a large amount of fluid has accumulated. Ascites develops because of a combination of albumin deficiency and increased pressure within obstructed veins, which permits fluid to leak into the abdominal cavity. Large amounts of ascitic fluid are easily detectable on plain abdominal radiographs as a general abdominal haziness (ground-glass appearance) (Figure 4-87, *A*). With the patient in a supine position, the peritoneal fluid tends to gravitate to dependent portions of the pelvis and accumulate within the pelvic peritoneal reflections, thus filling the recesses on both sides of the bladder and producing a symmetric density resembling dog's ears. Smaller amounts of fluid (300 to 1000 ml) may widen the flank stripe and obliterate the right lateral inferior margin of the liver (the hepatic angle). Ascites is exquisitely shown on ultrasound as a mobile, echo-free fluid region shaped by adjacent structures (Figure 4-87, *B*), or on CT as an extravisceral collection of fluid with a low attenuation value (Figure 4-87, *C*).

Cirrhosis may lead to the development of jaundice, either from destruction of liver cells or obstruction of bile ducts. Because the liver cannot perform its usual task of inactivating the small amounts of female sex hormones secreted by the adrenal glands in both men and women, men with cirrhosis often develop breast enlargement (gynecomastia). The inability of necrotic liver cells to detoxify harmful substances leads to an accumulation of ammonia and other poisonous material in the circulation. The patient becomes confused and disoriented, develops a typical flapping tremor or shaking, becomes abnormally sleepy (exhibits somnolence), and may lapse into a potentially fatal hepatic coma. Ascites occurs in advance stages of cirrhosis; of those afflicted, only 20% survive 5 years.

Treatment

The damage caused by cirrhosis is irreversible and incurable except by liver transplant. Most patients without a liver transplant die within 15 years of diagnosis. The patient may control the process by choosing a nutritional diet that decreases the metabolic load on the liver, stopping alcohol consumption, resting, and managing the complications liver failure.

Hepatocellular carcinoma

In the United States, primary liver cell carcinoma most commonly occurs in patients with underlying diffuse hepatocellular disease, especially alcoholic or postnecrotic cirrhosis. The clinical presentation varies

Figure 4-87 Ascites. **A,** Plain radiograph shows general abdominal haziness (ground-glass appearance). **B,** On an ultrasound image, a large amount of sonolucent ascitic fluid (*a*) separates liver (*L*) and other soft-tissue structures from the anterior abdominal wall. Note the relative thickness of the gallbladder wall (*arrow*). **C,** CT scan through the lower abdomen shows a huge amount of low-density ascitic fluid (*a*) with medial displacement of ascending and descending colon (*c*).

from mild right upper quadrant discomfort and weight loss, to hemorrhagic shock from massive intraperitoneal bleeding, which reflects rupture of the tumor into the peritoneal cavity. Invasion of the biliary tree may produce obstructive jaundice.

Radiographic appearance

CT is the modality of choice in the diagnosis of hepatocellular carcinoma. The tumor appears as a large mass, with an attenuation value close to that of normal parenchyma, that tends to alter the contour of the liver by projecting beyond its outer margin (Figure 4-88). Af-

ter the rapid administration of IV contrast material, there is usually dense, diffuse, and nonuniform enhancement of the tumor. Unlike metastases, hepatocellular carcinoma tends to be a solitary mass or to produce a small number of lesions (thus appearing multinodular). Hepatocellular carcinoma tends to invade the hepatic and portal venous systems, and tumor thrombi within these veins are well demonstrated on CT.

Currently a three-phase contrast helical study is performed to image the arterial phase, the portal circulation, and the contrast-staining tumor in the venous or excretory phase (Figure 4-89). Sonography is used to screen

Figure 4-88 Hepatocellular carcinoma. CT scan shows huge mass *(H)* with attenuation value slightly less than that of normal liver. Black arrows point to interface between tumor and normal liver. Incidentally noted is a pancreatic pseudocyst *(white arrow)* in the lesser sac between stomach *(S)* and pancreas *(p)*.

Figure 4-89 Three-phase CT imaging of the normal liver. **A,** Hepatic arteries. The bolus of contrast material is in the abdominal aorta. **B,** The inferior vena cava and the portal system are visible. **C,** The liver parenchyma is homogeneous, which indicates a normal study.

chronic hepatitis B virus carriers. MRI may permit a specific diagnosis by demonstrating (during the arterial phase, after gadolinium injection) a characteristic capsule of compressed liver tissue, an accumulation of fat within the tumor, and the propensity of the tumor to spread into the hepatic and portal venous system.

Treatment

Although the overall prognosis for patients with hepatocellular carcinoma remains bleak, radiographic studies can determine whether the tumor can be successfully removed surgically. If the tumor is confined to one lobe of the liver and there is no evidence of metastases, arteriography is usually indicated to demonstrate the precise surgical anatomy and to detect small, staining tumor nodules that cannot be identified with noninvasive imaging techniques. Surgery and chemotherapy are the treatments of choice. Metastases occur late and are usually not the cause of death. A common cause of death is catastrophic bleeding into the peritoneal cavity from hepatic failure or esophageal varices.

Hepatic metastases

Metastases are by far the most common malignant tumors involving the liver. Although some types of metastases (especially mucinous carcinoma of the colon or rectum) may produce diffuse, finely granular calcifications that can be seen on plain radiographs, the diagnosis of hepatic metastases usually requires CT, ultrasound, MRI, or radionuclide studies.

Radiographic appearance

CT and MRI are probably the most sensitive techniques for detecting hepatic metastases. On CT, most metastases are relatively well marginated and appear less dense than normal liver parenchyma (Figure 4-90). Although frequently detectable on non-contrast scans, most metastatic lesions are best seen as areas of increased density adjacent to normally enhancing hepatic parenchyma after the administration of IV contrast material. CT-guided fine-needle aspiration biopsy can be used to obtain cells that can be studied for a definitive diagnosis. MRI demonstrates liver metastases as areas of low signal intensity on T1-weighted sequences and bright lesions on T2-weighted sequences. This modality is especially important for patients who cannot receive IV iodinated contrast agents.

Ultrasound and radionuclide scans can demonstrate hepatic metastases, but these modalities are slightly less sensitive than CT. CT has the additional advantage of being able to detect extrahepatic metastases, such as those to abdominal lymph nodes.

Figure 4-90 Hepatic metastases. **A,** CT scan shows multiple low-density metastases with high-density centers *(arrows)*. **B,** Ultrasound image of the liver demonstrates a diffuse, patchy, nodular appearance *(arrows)*.

Treatment

Once diagnosed with hepatic metastases, most patients face imminent death (within months).

■ Pancreas

Acute pancreatitis

Acute pancreatitis is an inflammatory process in which protein- and lipid-digesting enzymes become activated within the pancreas and begin to digest the organ itself. Occasionally this necrotic process extends into blood vessels, causing bleeding (acute hemorrhagic pancreatitis), which may be life-threatening.

The most common cause of acute pancreatitis is excessive alcohol consumption. Less frequently, acute pancreatitis is related to gallstones, which may enter the common bile duct and obstruct the ampulla of

▪ ▪

Summary of Findings for the Liver

DISORDER	LOCATION	RADIOGRAPHIC APPEARANCE	TREATMENT
Cirrhosis	Liver cells and structure	KUB—haziness in ascites CT—fatty infiltration in liver, portal vein involvement/ obstruction, ascites, extravisceral fluid collection	Dietary modifications Stop alcohol consumption Irreversible—curable only by liver transplant
Hepatocellular carcinoma	Previously injured liver cells are most susceptible	CT—diffuse infiltrate, solitary multinodular mass	Poor prognosis Surgery and chemotherapy are treatments of choice
Hepatic metastases	Liver	CT—increased density adjacent to normal parenchyma when IV contrast administered MRI—low signal intensity on T_1-weighted, high signal intensity on T_2-weighted images	Terminal Treatment palliative only

▪ ▪

KUB, Kidney–ureter–bladder radiograph.

Vater, forcing bile to reflux into the pancreas and causing an inflammatory reaction.

The first symptoms of acute pancreatitis usually include the sudden onset of severe, steady abdominal pain that radiates to the back; this may indicate a perforated ulcer. Nausea and vomiting are common, and jaundice may develop if inflammatory edema of the head of the pancreas sufficiently obstructs the common bile duct. If a large area of the pancreas is affected, the absence of lipid enzymes from the pancreas prevents the proper absorption of fat, leading to the malabsorption syndrome. Blood tests and urinalysis typically show a high level of the pancreatic enzyme amylase, which confirms the diagnosis of acute pancreatitis.

Radiographic appearance

The findings on plain abdominal radiographs are often normal in the patient with acute pancreatitis; even when abnormal, they are usually nonspecific and consistent with any intraabdominal inflammatory disease. The most frequent abnormalities include a localized adynamic ileus, usually involving the jejunum (the "sentinel loop"); generalized ileus with diffuse gas–fluid levels; isolated distention of the duodenal sweep (C-loop); and localized distention of the transverse colon to the level of the splenic flexure (the colon cutoff sign). Pancreatic calcifications indicate that the patient has chronic pancreatitis, and moreover they may indicate an exacerbation of the inflammatory disease.

Ultrasound and CT are the imaging modalities that most precisely define the degree of pancreatic inflammation and the pathways of its spread throughout the abdomen. They are also of great clinical importance in the early diagnosis of complications of acute pancreatitis, such as abscess, hemorrhage, and pseudocyst formation.

CT in acute pancreatitis demonstrates diffuse or focal enlargement of the gland. The margins of a normal pancreas are sharply delineated by surrounding peripancreatic fat. Spread of inflammation and edema beyond the confines of the pancreas obscures the peripancreatic soft tissues and often thickens the surrounding fascial planes (Figure 4-91), which makes CT superior to ultrasound.

Acute pancreatitis may alter both the size and the parenchymal echogenicity of the gland on ultrasound examination. Although the pancreas usually enlarges symmetrically and retains its initial shape, nonspecific enlargement of the pancreatic head or tail can simulate focal pancreatic carcinoma. Gallstones causing pancreatitis can be demonstrated. The accompanying interstitial inflammatory edema causes the pancreas to appear relatively sonolucent when compared with the adjacent liver (Figure 4-92). One limitation of ultrasound in patients with acute pancreatitis is the frequent occurrence of adynamic ileus with excessive

Figure 4-91   Acute pancreatitis. CT scan demonstrates diffuse enlargement of the pancreas *(P)* with obliteration of peripancreatic fat planes by an inflammatory process. Extension of the inflammatory reaction into the transverse mesocolon *(arrows)* is shown. (From Jeffrey RB, Federle MP, Laing FC: Computed tomography of mesenteric involvement in fulminant pancreatitis, *Radiology* 147:185-192, 1983.)

Figure 4-92   Acute pancreatitis. Transverse sonogram illustrates multiple hypoechoic areas in the head of the pancreas *(arrows),* causing biliary tree dilation.

intestinal gas, which may prevent adequate visualization of the gland.

Chronic pancreatitis

Chronic pancreatitis results when frequent intermittent injury to the pancreas causes increasing damage that produce scar tissue. Recurring episodes usually result

from chronic alcohol abuse, which may cause the gland to lose its ability to produce digestive enzymes, insulin, and glucagon. Three symptoms that help identify chronic pancreatitis are pain, malabsorption causing weight loss (exocrine failure—digestive enzymes), and diabetes (endocrine failure—insulin and glucagon).

Radiographic appearance

Pancreatic calcifications are a pathognomonic finding in chronic pancreatitis, developing in about one third of patients with this disease (Figure 4-93). The small, irregular calcifications are seen most frequently in the head of the pancreas and can extend upward and to the left to involve the body and tail of the organ.

On ultrasound examination, the major feature of chronic pancreatitis is an alteration of the intrinsic echo pattern caused by calcification and fibrosis (Figure 4-94). The pancreas may be atrophic as a result of fibrous scarring or appear significantly enlarged during recurrences of acute inflammation. Dilatation of the pancreatic duct as a result of gland atrophy and obstruction can be seen, although a similar pattern can be produced by the ductal obstruction in pancreatic cancer. CT can also demonstrate ductal dilatation, calcification, and atrophy of the gland in patients with chronic pancreatitis. However, since similar information can be obtained less expensively and without ionizing radiation by ultrasound, CT is usually reserved for patients with chronic pancreatitis in whom technical factors make ultrasound suboptimal.

Enlargement of the pancreatic head can cause widening and pressure changes on the inner aspect of the duodenal sweep on barium studies. This produces narrowing of the lumen (the double-contour effect) and spiny protrusions of mucosal folds (spiculation) that can be indistinguishable from those of pancreatic carcinoma.

Treatment of acute and chronic pancreatitis

Most cases of acute pancreatitis require supportive treatment only (e.g., IV fluids, pain and nausea medications), because the pancreas will self-heal. If acute pancreatitis is caused by stone blockage, procedures to remove the stone (e.g., ERCP) or possibly surgery to remove the gallbladder should be done. In some cases, IV antibiotics are given to help reduce the inflammatory process and prevent infection.

In chronic pancreatitis, treatment is directed toward controlling pain and managing nutritional and metabolic problems. Consumption of alcohol must cease. Dietary changes reduce fat and protein intake; supplements containing pancreatic enzymes are taken to aid in digestion. If the blood sugar becomes uncontrolled, insulin is prescribed. Most patients who follow their prescribed treatment do well.

Figure 4-93 Chronic pancreatitis. Diffuse pancreatic calcifications.

Figure 4-94 Chronic pancreatitis in a 40-year-old man with abdominal pain; he has a history of chronic alcoholism. **A,** In April, an ultrasound image shows the pancreas to be inhomogeneous with a patchy appearance. **B,** On the follow-up scan in May, the pancreatic ducts are considerably dilated *(cursors).*

Pancreatic pseudocyst

Pancreatic pseudocysts are loculated (walled-off) fluid collections arising from inflammation, necrosis, or hemorrhage associated with acute pancreatitis or trauma (Figure 4-95). When the infected or traumatized pancreas continues to release enzymes, pseudocysts are commonly formed. The pseudocyst has a shaggy lining surrounded by dense white scar tissue and may or may not connect with the pancreatic duct.

Radiographic appearance

On ultrasound examination, a pseudocyst typically appears as an echo-free cystic structure with a sharp posterior wall (Figure 4-96). Hemorrhage

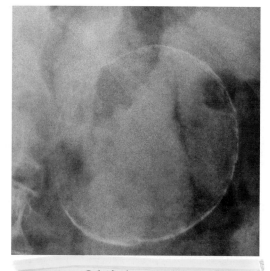

Figure 4-95   Calcified pancreatic pseudocyst.

Figure 4-97   Multiple pancreatic pseudocysts. CT scan after IV administration of contrast material demonstrates four sharply marginated, fluid-filled collections.

Figure 4-96   Ultrasound image of pancreatic pseudocyst. Longitudinal sonogram of right upper quadrant demonstrates irregularly marginated pseudocyst *(PC)* with acoustic shadowing *(arrow)*. *L,* Liver.

into the pseudocyst produces a complex fluid collection containing septations of echogenic areas. CT demonstrates pseudocysts as sharply marginated, fluid-filled collections that are often best delineated after the administration of IV contrast material (Figure 4-97).

Large pseudocysts are visible on plain radiographs of the abdomen when they displace the gas-filled stomach and bowel. Similarly, pseudocysts in the head of the pancreas can cause pressure defects and widening of the duodenal sweep, whereas those arising from the body or tail of the pancreas can displace and deform the stomach, proximal jejunum, or colon. However, because ultrasound is highly accurate in diagnosing pancreatic pseudocysts, it has completely replaced plain abdominal radiographs and barium studies, which display only indirect signs.

Treatment

Pseudocysts may undergo spontaneous resolution or persist as chronic collections that may require surgical intervention. Because ultrasound is relatively inexpensive and does not involve ionizing radiation, serial sonograms are usually used to monitor the progression of a pancreatic pseudocyst. Percutaneous drainage of a pseudocyst and endoscopic drainage for cysts extending into the stomach are interventional therapies used today.

Cancer of the pancreas

The most common pancreatic malignancy is adenocarcinoma (90%), which often is far advanced and has metastasized before it is detected and thus has an extremely poor survival rate. Of these malignancies, 60% occur in the head of the pancreas. Less common pancreatic tumors include hormone-secreting neoplasms of the islet cells of the islands of Langerhans. Production of insulin by an **insulinoma** can lower blood glucose, leading to attacks of weakness, unconsciousness, and insulin shock. This tumor occurs most frequently in the tail and is usually benign. **Ulcerogenic islet cell**

Figure 4-98   Pancreatic adenocarcinoma in a 66-year-old man with a 10-day history of painless jaundice and weight loss. Ultrasound image demonstrates a heterogeneous hypoechoic mass (dark area with measurements) in the pancreatic head and uncinate process; the mass is producing an obstruction of the pancreatic and common bile ducts.

Figure 4-99   Carcinoma of the pancreas. **A,** Noncontrast CT scan demonstrates homogeneous mass *(M)* in the body of the pancreas. **B,** After IV injection of a bolus of contrast material, there is enhancement of the normal pancreatic parenchyma and the surrounding vascular structures. The pancreatic carcinoma remains unchanged and thus appears as a low-density mass. (From Federle MP, Goldberg HL: In Moss AA, Gamsu G, Genant HK, editors: *Computed tomography of the body,* Philadelphia, 1992, Saunders.)

tumors (**gastrinomas**—usually malignant) produce the Zollinger-Ellison syndrome, which is characterized by intractable ulcer symptoms, hypersecretion of gastric acid, and diarrhea. **Diarrheogenic islet cell tumors** produce the WDHA syndrome; this acronym stands for watery diarrhea, hypokalemia (low serum potassium), and achlorhydria (low serum chloride), which are major features of the clinical picture. Adrenocorticotropic hormone (ACTH) production by pancreatic islet cell tumors causes Cushing's syndrome; the release of serotonin by pancreatic tumors may cause the carcinoid syndrome. Because these functional islet cell tumors usually become apparent by their hormonal effects rather than by the consequences of tumor bulk, they are often small and difficult to detect.

Radiographic appearance

Because it is noninvasive and relatively inexpensive, ultrasound is often the initial screening modality for a patient with suspected pancreatic carcinoma. Ultrasound can demonstrate most tumors greater than 2 cm in diameter that lie in the head of the pancreas, but lesions in the body and tail of the pancreas are more difficult to detect. Pancreatic carcinoma typically causes the gland to have an irregular contour and a semisolid pattern of intrinsic echoes (Figure 4-98).

CT is the most effective modality for detecting pancreatic cancer in any portion of the gland and for defining its extent. CT can demonstrate the mass of the tumor, ductal dilatation, and invasion of neighboring structures. After the administration of IV contrast material, the relatively avascular tumor appears as an area of decreased attenuation when compared with the normal pancreas (Figure 4-99). CT is the best procedure for staging pancreatic carcinoma and may prevent needless surgery in patients with nonresectable lesions. This technique may permit detection of hepatic metastases or involvement of regional vessels and adjacent retroperitoneal lymph nodes.

Cytologic examination of tissue obtained by percutaneous fine-needle aspiration under ultrasound or CT guidance can often provide the precise histologic diagnosis of a neoplastic mass, thus making surgical intervention unnecessary.

Carcinoma of the head of the pancreas often causes obstructive jaundice and the appearance of narrowing of the distal common bile duct on transhepatic cholangiography (Figure 4-100) or ERCP. Percuta-

Figure 4-100 Carcinoma of the head of the pancreas. Transhepatic cholangiogram shows irregular narrowing of the common bile duct *(arrows)*. Calcifications reflect underlying chronic pancreatitis.

Summary of Findings for the Pancreas

DISORDER	LOCATION	RADIOGRAPHIC APPEARANCE	TREATMENT
Pancreatitis	Acute—pancreatic ducts	US—altered echogenicity CT—diffuse or focal enlargement	Supportive treatment IV antibiotics
	Chronic—pancreatic parenchyma	US—intrinsic echo pattern, alteration by calcification and fibrosis CT—ductal dilatation, calcification, atrophy, and pseudocyst formation	Reduce fat/protein intake Pancreatic enzyme supplements Insulin for uncontrolled blood sugar levels
Pseudocyst	Cyst walled off from ductal system	US—echo-free cyst with sharp posterior wall CT—sharply marginated fluid-filled collection(s) best seen with IV contrast	Spontaneous resolution Drainage (percutaneous or endoscopic) Surgical correction
Cancer	Adenocarcinoma Head of pancreas in 60%	US—tumor 2 cm or greater, irregular contour and semi-solid pattern of intrinsic echoes CT (most effective)—tumor mass, ductal dilation, and invasiveness	Survival, 2% Surgery Radiation therapy Chemotherapy Biological therapy

US, Ultrasound

neous biliary drainage may represent an alternative to surgical intervention for relieving biliary obstruction in patients with pancreatic carcinoma who cannot be cured. Although the transhepatic insertion of biliary drainage tubes does not alter the dismal prognosis, it can reduce patient morbidity and the need for hospitalization.

Barium upper gastrointestinal series demonstrate distortion of the mucosal pattern and configuration of the duodenal sweep in about half of patients with carcinoma of the head of the pancreas. Early or small lesions, however, rarely produce detectable radiographic abnormalities; tumors of the body or tail of the pancreas must be quite large to be visible on barium examinations.

Treatment

Finding pancreatic cancer in the earliest stages can result in a cure (2% 5-year survival rate). In most cases, the diagnosis of the disease occurs after metastasis and most patients die within 12 to 24 months of diagnosis. Nevertheless, treatment can improve the quality of life. Surgical resection, radiation therapy, chemotherapy, and biological therapy help alleviate the patient's symptoms.

Surgical resection (total pancreatectomy) includes the removal of the entire pancreas, duodenum, common bile duct, gallbladder, spleen, and surrounding lymph nodes. The Whipple procedure consists of removing only the head of the pancreas, the duodenum, a portion of the stomach, and other nearby tissue. If a distal pancreatectomy is performed, only the body and tail of the pancreas are removed. In most cases the purpose of the surgery is to alleviate biliary and small bowel obstruction. Surgery and chemotherapy are most effective for islet cell cancers.

■ Pneumoperitoneum

Free air in the peritoneal cavity associated with significant abdominal pain and tenderness is often caused by perforation of a gas-containing viscus and indicates a surgical emergency. Less frequently, pneumoperitoneum results from abdominal, gynecologic, intrathoracic, or iatrogenic causes and does not require operative intervention.

Radiographic appearance

The radiographic demonstration of free air in the peritoneal cavity is a valuable sign in the diagnosis of perforation of the gastrointestinal tract. As little as 1 cc of free intraperitoneal gas can be identified. Free air is best demonstrated by examination of the patient in the upright position with a horizontal beam (Figure 4-101). Because the gas rises to the highest point in the

Figure 4-101 Pneumoperitoneum. Gas accumulating beneath dome of right hemidiaphragm *(arrow)* appears as a sickle-shaped lucency on this erect chest film obtained with a horizontal beam.

peritoneal cavity, it accumulates beneath the domes of the diaphragm. Free intraperitoneal gas appears as a sickle-shaped lucency that is easiest to recognize on the right side between the diaphragm and the homogeneous density of the liver. On the left side, the normal gas and fluid shadows present in the fundus of the stomach can be confusing. The free air is shown to best advantage if the patient remains in an upright (or lateral decubitus) position for 10 minutes before a radiograph is obtained.

If the patient is too ill to sit or stand, a lateral decubitus view (preferably with the patient on the left side) can be used. In this position, free air moves to the right side and collects between the lateral margin of the liver and the abdominal wall (Figure 4-102). Some gas also collects in the right iliac fossa and, when large amounts are involved, can be seen along the flank down to the pelvis.

When the patient is in the supine position, free intraperitoneal gas accumulates between the intestinal loops and is much more difficult to demonstrate. However, a large quantity of gas can be diagnosed indirectly because the outer margins of the intestinal wall can be visualized (Figure 4-103). The demonstration of distinct inner and outer contours of the bowel wall is often the only sign of pneumoperitoneum in patients who are in such poor condition that they cannot be turned on their side or be examined upright.

In children, pneumoperitoneum can be manifest as a generalized greater-than-normal lucency of the

A

B

Figure 4-102   Pneumoperitoneum. **A,** Semierect projection obtained without a horizontal beam shows no evidence of free intraperitoneal gas beneath the domes of the diaphragm. **B,** On a lateral decubitus projection obtained with a horizontal beam on the same patient, free intraperitoneal gas is clearly seen collecting under the right side of the abdominal wall *(arrows).* Gas can even be seen extending down the flank to the region of pelvis.

Figure 4-103   Double-wall sign of pneumoperitoneum demonstrated on supine projection. Large quantities of free intraperitoneal gas may be diagnosed indirectly because gas permits visualization of both inner and outer margins of the intestinal wall *(arrows).*

Figure 4-104   Falciform ligament sign of pneumoperitoneum. On supine projection, falciform ligament appears as a curvilinear water-density shadow *(arrows)* in the upper abdomen to the right of the spine. This finding implies that pneumoperitoneum with gas is on both sides of the ligament.

- -

Summary of Findings for Pneumoperitoneum

DISORDER	LOCATION	RADIOGRAPHIC APPEARANCE	TREATMENT
Pneumoperitoneum	Abdominal cavity	Upright abdominal film (1st choice) shows 1 cc free intraperitoneal gas (air) under diaphragm Left lateral decubitus (2nd choice) shows air collection between lateral margin of liver and outer abdominal wall	Immediate surgery for visceral perforation, IV antibiotics

- -

entire abdomen. An important sign of pneumoperitoneum on the supine radiograph is demonstration of the falciform ligament. This almost vertical, curvilinear, water-density shadow in the upper abdomen to the right of the spine is outlined only when there is gas on both sides of it, as in pneumoperitoneum (Figure 4-104).

The most frequent cause of pneumoperitoneum with associated inflammation is perforation of a peptic ulcer, either gastric or duodenal. Colonic perforations, especially those involving the cecum, give the most abundant quantities of free intraperitoneal gas. Septic infection of the peritoneal cavity by gas-forming organisms can result in the production of a substantial amount of gas and the radiographic appearance of pneumoperitoneum. Pneumoperitoneum can also develop after penetrating injuries of the abdominal wall and after blunt trauma causing rupture of a hollow viscus.

Iatrogenic pneumoperitoneum is generally asymptomatic and usually follows abdominal surgery. Postoperative pneumoperitoneum can be radiographically detectable for up to 3 weeks after surgery, but usually it can no longer be demonstrated after the first postoperative week. Rarely, free air in the peritoneal cavity may be the result of perforation during an endoscopic procedure.

Treatment

Immediate surgical repair of a perforation is required to reduce the risk of peritonitis and sepsis. IV antibiotics help control infection.

■ Spleen

Enlargement

Enlargement of the spleen (splenomegaly) is associated with numerous conditions, including infections (subacute bacterial endocarditis, tuberculosis, infectious mononucleosis, malaria), connective tissue disorders, neoplastic hematologic disorders (lymphoma, leukemia), hemolytic anemia and hemoglobinopathies, and portal hypertension (cirrhosis).

Radiographic appearance

Plain abdominal radiographs can demonstrate the inferior border of the enlarged spleen well below the costal margin. An enlarged spleen can elevate the left hemidiaphragm, impress the greater curvature of the barium-filled stomach, and displace the entire stomach toward the midline. Splenomegaly can also cause downward displacement of the left kidney and the splenic flexure of the colon.

CT is of value when it is unclear whether a mass palpated in the left upper quadrant represents an enlarged spleen or a separate abdominal mass. When splenomegaly is present (Figure 4-105), CT findings may indicate the cause of the splenic enlargement by demonstrating a tumor (Figure 4-106), abscess, or cyst. Associated abdominal lymph node enlargement is suggestive of lymphoma; characteristic alterations in the size and shape of the liver and prominence of collateral venous structures in the splenic hilum indicate that splenomegaly may be a result of cirrhosis and portal hypertension.

Rupture

Rupture of the spleen is usually caused by trauma. Infrequently, it may be a complication of the palpation of a spleen enlarged by infection (especially infectious mononucleosis) or leukemia. In many patients suffering traumatic rupture of the spleen, the severity of clinical symptoms and the rapid loss of blood into the abdominal cavity require immediate surgery without radiographic investigation. However, in patients in whom bleeding stops temporarily or in whom there is slow bleeding over several

Figure 4-105   Splenomegaly. CT demonstrates a homogeneous and extremely enlarged spleen.

Figure 4-106   Lymphoma of spleen. CT scan shows focal low-attenuation lesion *(arrowheads)* posteriorly in this greatly enlarged spleen. (From Koehler RE: Spleen. In Lee JKT, Sagel SS, Stanley RJ, editors: *Computed body tomography*, New York, 1983, Raven Press.)

days, radiographic studies may be of diagnostic value.

Radiographic appearance

CT is the best imaging procedure for screening patients with blunt abdominal trauma for the presence of splenic injury. Indeed, its almost 100% sensitivity in detecting splenic injury has substantially decreased the need for abdominal arteriography and exploratory surgery. Subcapsular hematomas appear on CT as crescentic collections of fluid that flatten or indent the lateral margin of the spleen (Figure 4-107). Splenic lacerations, which may occur with or without an accompanying subcapsular hematoma, produce a CT appearance of splenic enlargement, an irregular cleft or defect in the splenic border, and free blood in the peritoneal cavity.

Before the advent of CT, splenic arteriography was the procedure of choice for demonstrating splenic rupture. Major positive findings include extravasation of contrast material into the splenic parenchyma, obstruction of a major splenic artery, and, in an enlarged spleen, vascular defects that indicate sites of rupture and hematoma.

Treatment of splenic disorders

Treatment depends on the causative factors. Very enlarged spleens have a higher incidence of rupture and thus the patient should limit physical activity to avoid trauma. In most cases, splenomegaly does well with

Figure 4-107   CT image from a patient who was ejected from a motor vehicle. Traumatic splenic rupture and hematoma are illustrated by decreased attenuation surrounding spleen.

conservative treatment. Aggressive treatment would include possible embolization of the splenic artery to stop the bleeding in a splenic rupture. Surgical procedures include laparoscopic splenectomy and distal pancreatectomy, if necessary.

■ ■

Splenic Disorders

DISORDER	LOCATION	RADIOGRAPHIC APPEARANCE	TREATMENT
Splenomegaly	Enlarged spleen	Abdominal film—elevated left diaphragm, stomach displacement CT—demonstrates tumor, abscess, or cyst causing splenomegaly	Treat cause Limited physical activity to prevent traumatic rupture
Splenic rupture	Fracture by trauma	CT—subcapsular hematoma with splenic laceration	Embolization of splenic artery Laparoscopic splenectomy

■ ■

QUESTIONS

1. Visualization of which of the following structures indicates that the correct contrast scale has been used for a plain abdominal radiograph?
   I. Liver, kidneys, and psoas muscle shadows
   II. Lumbar spine and transverse processes
   III. Kidneys and psoas muscle shadows
   IV. Lumbar spine and psoas shadows
   A. Both I and IV C. I only
   B. Both I and II D. IV only

2. The rhythmic smooth muscle contractions found in the upper gastrointestinal system are called
   A. Chyme C. Peristalsis
   B. Digestion D. Mastication

3. The greatest amount of digestion occurs in which portion of the intestines?
   A. Duodenum C. Ileum
   B. Jejunum D. Colon

4. Detoxification of poisonous substances takes place in which organ?
   A. Kidneys C. Pancreas
   B. Liver D. Spleen

5. Which organ controls the level of glucose in the circulating blood?
   A. Kidneys C. Pancreas
   B. Liver D. Spleen

6. The telescoping of one part of the intestinal tract into another is termed _____.
   A. Intussusception C. Crohn's disease
   B. Volvulus D. Ileus

7. Twisting of the bowel upon itself is termed _____.
   A. Intussusception C. Crohn's disease
   B. Volvulus D. Ileus

8. What is now considered to be the major imaging modality for the demonstration of gallstones?
   A. OCG C. CT
   B. MRI D. Ultrasound

9. What is the major cause of cirrhosis in the United States and Europe?
   A. Hepatitis C. Alcoholism
   B. Elevated cholesterol D. Cholecystitis

10. Rupture of the spleen as a result of blunt abdominal trauma can be best demonstrated by what imaging procedure?
    A. OCG C. CT
    B. MRI D. Ultrasound

11. If a patient is too ill to stand, what projection can be used to demonstrate pneumoperitoneum?
    A. Right lateral decubitus, patient on left side
    B. Right lateral decubitus, patient on right side
    C. Left lateral decubitus, patient on left side
    D. Left lateral decubitus, patient on right side

12. Extensive calcification in the wall of the gallbladder is termed _____.
    A. Cholelithiasis C. Cholecystitis
    B. Porcelain gallbladder D. A or B

13. Varicose veins of the rectum are termed _____.
    A. Polyps C. Ulcerations
    B. Hemorrhoids D. Carcinomas

14. *Apple-core* and *napkin-ring* are common descriptive terms for annular carcinoma of the _____.
    A. Small intestine C. Jejunum
    B. Stomach D. Colon

15. Crohn's disease occurs in what organ(s)?
    A. Colon
    B. Small bowel
    C. Stomach
    D. All of the above

16. The presence of large amounts of gas and fluid in uniformly dilated loops of small and large bowel, often seen after abdominal surgery, is termed _____.
    A. Adynamic ileus
    B. Localized ileus
    C. Colonic ileus
    D. Ileus

17. What medical term is used to denote difficulty in swallowing?
    A. Mastication
    B. Dysphagia
    C. Deglutition
    D. B and C

18. Gastric contents that are mixed with hydrochloric acid and pepsin are called _____.
    A. Chyme
    B. Digest
    C. Enzyme
    D. Emulsifier

19. To demonstrate esophageal reflux, the patient is often asked to perform _____.
    A. Trendelenburg's maneuver
    B. Sims' maneuver
    C. Fowler's maneuver
    D. The Valsalva maneuver

20. An abnormal connection between the esophagus and trachea is termed _____.

21. An abnormal accumulation of fluid in the peritoneal cavity is termed _____.
    A. Pneumoperitoneum
    B. Ascites
    C. Volvulus
    D. Hydroperitoneum

22. Herniations, or outpouchings, of the walls of a hollow organ are termed _____.
    A. Ulcers
    B. Diverticula
    C. Hemorrhoids
    D. Polyps

23. A colonic intussusception can sometimes be reduced by what radiographic procedure?
    A. Upper GI series
    B. Small bowel series
    C. Enteroclysis
    D. Barium enema

24. Patients older than 40 years with a history of difficulty in swallowing are usually assumed, until proven otherwise, to have what pathologic condition?
    A. Esophageal varices
    B. Esophageal carcinoma
    C. Esophageal fistula
    D. Esophageal hernia

25. What is the most common manifestation of peptic ulcer disease?
    A. Gastric ulcer
    B. Esophageal ulcer
    C. Duodenal ulcer
    D. Peritoneal ulcer

26. If loops of bowel are distended by abnormally large amounts of air and are occupying the central portion of the abdomen, the patient most likely has a _____.
    A. Small bowel obstruction
    B. Large bowel obstruction
    C. Gastric obstruction
    D. A and B

BIBLIOGRAPHY

Eisenberg RL: *Gastrointestinal radiology: a pattern approach,* Philadelphia, 1990, Lippincott.

Farman J: *Gastrointestinal radiology,* New York, 1989, Gower Medical.

Gore RM, Levine MS, Laufer I: *Textbook of gastrointestinal radiology,* Philadelphia, 1993, Saunders.

Jones B, Braver JM: *Essentials of gastrointestinal radiology,* Philadelphia, 1982, Saunders.

Margulis AR, Burhenne HJ: *Alimentary tract radiology,* ed 4, St Louis, 1989, Mosby.

Meyers MA: *Dynamic radiology of the abdomen,* New York, 1994, Springer-Verlag.

CHAPTER 5

Urinary System

■ **Prerequisite Knowledge**

The student should have a basic knowledge of the anatomy and physiology of the urinary system. In addition, proper learning and understanding of the material will be facilitated if the student has some clinical experience in urinary radiography and film evaluation.

■ **Goals**

To acquaint the student radiographer with the pathophysiology and radiographic manifestations of all of the common and some of the unusual disorders of the urinary system

■ **Objectives**

1. To be able to classify the more common diseases in terms of their attenuation of x-rays
2. To be familiar with the changes in technical factors required for obtaining optimal-quality radiographs in patients with various underlying pathologic conditions
3. To understand and be able to define or describe all bold-faced terms in this chapter
4. To be able to describe the physiology of the urinary system
5. To be able to identify anatomic structures on both diagrams and radiographs of the urinary system
6. To be able to describe the various pathologic conditions affecting the urinary system as well as their radiographic manifestations

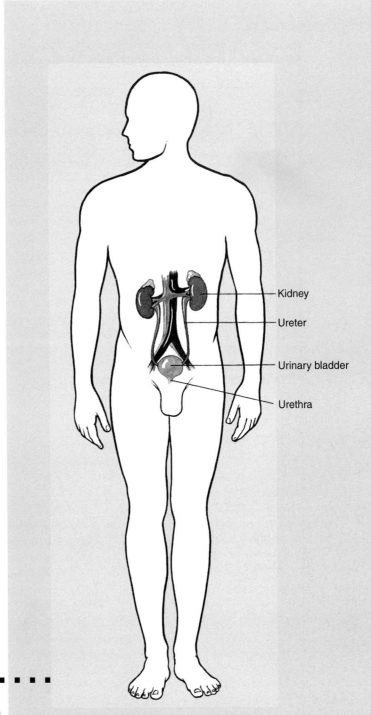

Kidney

Ureter

Urinary bladder

Urethra

■ ■ ■ ■ ■ ■ ■ ■ ■ **Radiographer Notes**

Although ultrasound and CT are being used with increasing frequency, plain radiography with contrast material introduced intravenously or by means of a catheter remains a major technique for imaging the urinary system. For excretory urography, the radiographer is responsible for preparing sterile injections of contrast material as well as for operating the equipment properly and positioning the patient. In some instances the radiographer may have to perform these functions in an operating room using sterile technique.

All radiographic studies begin with a "scout" film that is obtained before the injection of any contrast material. The radiographer should evaluate this film for proper technique and positioning so that any required alterations can be made on subsequent radiographs during the procedure. A film with correct density and contrast should demonstrate the kidney and psoas muscle shadows and the lumbar vertebrae and their transverse processes. A correctly positioned film should show all of both kidneys down to the superior portion of the pubic bones (to ensure that all of the bladder is included). The radiograph must be in a true anteroposterior position with the pelvis appearing symmetric and the spinous processes of the lumbar vertebrae projected over the central portions of the vertebral bodies. The radiologist evaluates the scout radiograph to make certain that the technique and positioning are appropriate for the clinical problem and to evaluate proper patient preparation. The radiograph is also checked for any radiopaque calculi or other abnormality that might be obscured after the injection of contrast material.

The radiographer must be alert to the possibility of an allergic reaction whenever contrast agents are used. It is essential that the radiographer be aware of the proper procedures to follow in the event of an allergic reaction and be able to initiate and maintain basic life support until advanced life-support personnel have arrived. Depending on departmental policy, it is usually the radiographer's responsibility to assist during resuscitation procedures. Therefore it is essential that the radiographer be familiar with the contents of the emergency cart and take responsibility for ensuring that the cart is completely stocked with appropriate medications.

All radiographs of the urinary system must be made with the patient in full exhalation so that the diaphragm assumes its highest position and does not compress the abdominal contents. Depending on the specific area being evaluated, the radiographer may have to perform oblique or erect projections, coned-down views of the kidneys or bladder, tomograms, or films made with abdominal compression. In certain pathologic conditions, radiographs must be obtained at precisely timed intervals, and delayed films may be necessary.

■ Physiology of the Urinary System

The urinary system consists of the kidneys, ureters, and bladder. The functional unit of the kidney is the nephron. Each kidney contains more than a million nephrons, which filter waste products from the blood, reabsorb water and nutrients (e.g., glucose, amino acids) from the tubular fluid, and secrete excess substances in the form of urine. In an average person, the nephron filters about 190 L of water out of glomerular blood each day. This enormous amount is many times the total volume of blood in the body. However, only a small proportion of this water (1 to 2 L) is excreted in the urine. Therefore more than 99% of water is reabsorbed into tubular blood.

The formation of urine begins in the **glomerulus,** a tuft of capillaries with very thin walls and a large surface area. The blood pressure within the glomerulus is higher than that in **Bowman's capsule,** which surrounds it. This causes the filtration of fluid into Bowman's capsule that is equivalent to plasma containing neither protein nor red blood cells (if the nephron is healthy). The initial urine proceeds into the **proximal convoluted tubule,** where a large amount of water and virtually all nutrients are reabsorbed into the blood capillaries surrounding the tubules. The amount of sodium and chloride reabsorbed is determined by the concentration of these substances in the body, and it occurs at a variable rate designed to keep the osmotic pressure of the body constant. This process is greatly influenced by two hormones, antidiuretic hormone (ADH), secreted by the posterior pituitary gland, and aldosterone, secreted by the adrenal glands.

After passing through the proximal tubule, the fluid flows through the **loop of Henle,** a complex structure consisting of a descending limb, a loop, and an ascending limb. In addition to reabsorbing salt and water, the loop of Henle permits the excretion of a concentrated urine by actively secreting substances such as potassium (K^+) and hydrogen (H^+) ions, and

Figure 5-20   **A,** Spiral CT image done at 5-mm intervals on an 11-year-old boy, demonstrating bilateral renal calculi with caliectasis (dilated calyces) and kidney enlargement. **B,** Staghorn calculi fill renal pelves bilaterally. Of incidental note is residual contrast material *(arrow)* from prior myelogram. **C,** Nephrostomy tube placement in the left renal pelvis to drain the kidney.

hydronephrosis; however, stones smaller than 3 mm may not produce a detectable acoustic shadow. This modality is used when ionizing radiation is contraindicated.

When CT is unavailable, excretory urography is used to detect these otherwise invisible, nonopaque stones that appear as filling defects in the contrast-filled collecting system. In patients with acute renal colic caused by an obstructing stone in the ureter, excretory urography may demonstrate the point of cut-off and dilatation of the proximal ureter and pelvicalyceal system. With acute obstruction, the intrapelvic pressure may increase to such an extent that there is little or no glomerular filtration, resulting in a delayed and prolonged nephrogram and a lack of calyceal filling on the affected side.

Small renal stones (3 mm or less) may pass spontaneously in the urine. At times, a stone may completely fill the renal pelvis (**staghorn** calculus) (see Figure 5-20, *B*), blocking the flow of urine. Figure 5-20, *C*, shows nephrostomy placement to drain the kidney.

Calcium can also deposit within the renal parenchyma (**nephrocalcinosis**) (Figure 5-21). This calcification varies from a few scattered punctate densities to very dense and extensive calcifications throughout both kidneys. The most common causes of nephrocalcinosis include hyperparathyroidism, increased intestinal absorption of calcium (sarcoidosis, hypervitaminosis D, milk-alkali syndrome), and renal tubular acidosis, a disorder in which the kidney is unable to excrete an acid urine (below pH 5.4).

Figure 5-21   Nephrolithiasis. Multiple deposits are scattered throughout parenchyma of left kidney.

Figure 5-22   Obstructing ureteral calculus. Excretory urogram demonstrates prolonged nephrogram and pronounced dilatation of collecting system and pelvis proximal to obstructing stone *(arrow)*.

Stones can also form in other portions of the genitourinary tract. Ureteral calculi almost invariably result from the downward movement of kidney stones (Figure 5-22). They are usually small, irregular, and poorly calcified and are therefore easily missed on abdominal radiographs that are not of good quality. Calculi most commonly lodge in the lower portion of the ureter, especially at the ureterovesical junction and at the pelvic brim (Figure 5-23). They are often oval, with their long axes paralleling the course of the ureter. Ureteral calculi must be differentiated from the far more common phleboliths, which are spherical and located in the lateral portion of the pelvis below a line joining the ischial spines. In contrast, ureteral stones are situated medially above the interspinous line.

Stone formation in the bladder is a disorder primarily of elderly men with obstruction or infection of the lower urinary tract (Figure 5-24, *A*). Frequently associated lesions include bladder-outlet obstruction, urethral strictures, neurogenic bladder, and bladder diverticula (Figure 5-24, *B*). At times, upper urinary tract stones migrate down the ureter and are retained in the bladder. Bladder calculi can be single or multiple. They vary in size from tiny concretions, each the size of a grain of sand, to an enormous single calculus occupying the entire bladder lumen. Most bladder calculi are circular or oval; however, almost any shape can be encountered. They can be amorphous, laminated (layered), or even spiculated. One unusual type with a characteristic radiographic appearance is the hard burr, or jackstone, variety, which gets its name from the many irregular prongs that project from its surface and simulate the child's toy.

Treatment

Preventive measures include increasing fluid intake and decreasing the intake of the stone-forming substances. In the past, surgery was frequently necessary to remove large kidney stones. More recently, medication introduced into the upper urinary tract by means of a percutaneous catheter has been used to dissolve large kidney stones into smaller pieces that pass easily (chemolysis). Lithotripsy is a technique to break up the stone using an external source of shock waves that shatter the hard stones into sand-sized particles, which are then excreted in the urine. This technique works well for stones in the kidney or the upper ureter (above the pelvic brim). For stones in the lower ureter (in the pelvis), cystoscopic retrieval (ureteroscopy basket) or laser destruction is an option. The last resort is performing surgery, as this traumatizes the patient and requites a longer recovery period.

■ Urinary Tract Obstruction

Urinary tract obstruction produces anatomic and functional changes that vary with regard to rapidity of onset, degree of occlusion, and distance between the kidney and the obstructing lesion. In adults, urinary calculi, pelvic tumors, urethral strictures, and enlargement of the prostate gland are the major causes. In children, congenital malformations (ureteropelvic junction narrowing, ureterocele, retrocaval ureter, posterior urethral valve) are usually responsible for

Figure 5-23 Ureteral calculus. **A,** Stone appears as nonopaque filling defect *(arrows)* in distal portion of ureter. **B,** CT image done at 5-mm intervals without contrast material demonstrates a stone in the right kidney. **C,** A scan of the lower pelvis demonstrates a second stone in the distal portion of the ureter.

Figure 5-24 Bladder calculi. **A,** Plain radiograph of pelvis shows large laminated stone on the left and multiple smaller calculi on the right. **B,** Excretory urogram demonstrates large stone *(arrows)* in the bladder diverticulum on the left side. Multiple smaller calculi on the right have been obscured by overlying contrast material.

mechanical obstruction. Normal points of narrowing, such as the ureteropelvic and ureterovesical junctions, the bladder neck, and the urethral meatus, are common sites of obstruction. Blockage above the level of the bladder causes unilateral dilatation of the ureter **(hydroureter)** and renal pelvicalyceal system **(hydronephrosis);** if the lesion is at or below the level of the bladder, as in prostatic hypertrophy or tumor, bilateral involvement is the rule.

Radiographic appearance

Noncontrast helical CT scanning detects mass effects, stones, or other causes of obstruction better than excretory urography. A contrast agent may be used to demonstrate renal function and the renal vascular structures if needed. In acute urinary tract obstruction, diminished filtration of urographic contrast material results in parenchymal opacification that is delayed compared with that of the nonobstructed kidney. The nephrogram eventually becomes more dense than normal because of a decreased rate of flow of fluid through the tubules, which results in enhanced water reabsorption by the nephrons and greater concentration of the contrast material (Figure 5-25). There is delayed and decreased pelvicalyceal filling because of dilatation and elevated pressure in the collecting system. The radiographic study may have to be prolonged for up to 48 hours after the administration of contrast material to determine the precise site of obstruction.

Figure 5-25   Urinary tract obstruction. **A,** Excretory urogram demonstrates prolonged nephrogram on the left and no calyceal filling. Arrow points to obstructing stone in the proximal left ureter. **B,** In another patient, there is a prolonged and intensified obstructive nephrogram of right kidney. On the left, there is pronounced dilatation of the pelvicalyceal system but no persistent nephrogram, reflecting intermittent chronic obstruction on this side. **C,** CT scan on a different patient shows large renal calyces, hydronephrosis, and a hydroureter on the left.

In the patient with acute urinary tract obstruction, the kidney is generally enlarged, and the calyces are moderately dilated. An uncommon but pathognomonic urographic finding in acute unilateral obstruction (usually caused by a ureteral stone) is opacification of the gallbladder 8 to 24 hours after the injection of contrast material. This "vicarious excretion" is related to increased liver excretion of contrast material that cannot be promptly excreted by the kidneys.

As an obstruction becomes more chronic, the predominant urographic finding is a greatly dilated

Figure 5-26 Hydronephrosis. Dilatation of the entire pelvicalyceal system proximal to an obstructing *Cryptococcus* fungus ball *(arrow)* at the ureteropelvic junction.

pelvicalyceal system and ureter proximal to the obstruction (Figure 5-26). Prolonged increased pressure causes progressive papillary atrophy, leading to calyceal clubbing. Gradual enlargement of the calyces and renal pelvis with progressive destruction of renal parenchyma may continue until the kidney becomes a nonfunctioning hydronephrotic sac in which its normal anatomy is obliterated.

Whenever possible, the site of obstruction should be demonstrated. Although excretory urography with delayed films may accomplish this purpose, antegrade pyelography is often required. In this procedure, a catheter or needle is placed percutaneously into the dilated collecting system under ultrasound or fluoroscopic guidance, and contrast material is then introduced. This approach has the added advantage of providing immediate and certain decompression of a unilateral obstructing lesion.

Ultrasound is of particular value in detecting hydronephrosis in patients with such severe urinary tract obstruction and renal dysfunction that there is no opacification of the kidneys and collecting systems on excretory urograms. The dilated calyces and pelvis become large, hydronephrotic, echo-free sacs separated by septa of compressed tissue and vessels (Figure 5-27, *A*). With increased duration and severity of hydronephrosis, the intervening septa may disappear, leaving a large fluid-filled sac with no evidence of internal structure and no normal parenchyma apparent at its margins (Figure 5-27, *B*).

A physiologic form of hydronephrosis often develops during pregnancy. The enlarging uterine mass and physiologic hormonal changes cause extrinsic pressure on the ureter, leading to progressive dilatation of the proximal collecting systems (Figure 5-28). Often bilateral, the dilatation usually is more prominent and

A   **B**

Figure 5-27 Hydronephrosis. Longitudinal ultrasound images demonstrating dilatation of renal collecting system appearing as echo-free sacs *(dark areas)* in this 73-year-old patient. **A,** Left kidney with perirenal fluid *(arrow)*. **B,** Right kidney demonstrates more severe dilatation.

Figure 5-28 Hydronephrosis of pregnancy. Excretory urogram performed 3 days postpartum demonstrates bilateral large kidneys with dilatation of ureters and pelvicalyceal systems, especially on the right. The large pelvic mass (*arrows*) indenting the superior surface of the bladder represents the uterus, which is still causing extrinsic pressure on the ureters.

Summary of Findings for Urinary Obstructions

DISORDER	LOCATION	RADIOGRAPHIC APPEARANCE	TREATMENT
Calculi	Most commonly form in the kidney	KUB—radiopaque calcium renal stones CT—demonstrates location of stone IVU—noncalcium stones cause filling defects US—demonstrates an echogenic region with acoustic shadowing	Medications administered into upper urinary tract Lithotripsy to break up the stone Cystoscopy for retrieval or laser destruction Surgery
Obstruction	Internal or external pressure prevents normal urine flow	CT—demonstrates mass effects, stones, or other causes of obstruction IVU—dense nephrogram, delayed or decreased pelvicalyceal filling Chronic shows dilated pelvicalyces Percutaneous nephrostomy to demonstrate obstruction and provide drainage US—chronic hydronephrosis with echo-free sacs	Decompress urinary tract to prevent damage Treat cause of obstruction

IVU, Intravenous urography; *KUB,* kidney–ureter–bladder radiograph; *US,* ultrasound.

develops earlier on the right side. After delivery, the urinary tract returns to normal within several weeks. In some women, however, persistent dilatation of the ovarian vein can compress the ureter and result in prolonged postpartum hydronephrosis.

Treatment

Appropriate treatment requires decompressing the urinary tract to prevent parenchymal damage and possible ureteral rupture due to the blockage. Percutaneous nephrostomy provides drainage and may help demonstrate the site of obstruction (see Figure 5-20, C). Once the cause of the obstruction is determined, therapy for that specific cause can be initiated.

■ Cysts and Tumors

Renal cyst

Simple renal cysts are the most common unifocal masses of the kidney. They are fluid filled and usually unilocular, although septa sometimes divide the cyst into chambers, which may or may not communicate with each other. Cysts vary in size, and they may occur at single or multiple sites in one or both kidneys. Thin curvilinear calcifications can be demonstrated in the wall of about 3% of simple cysts. However, this peripheral type of calcification is not pathognomonic of a benign process, as malignant kidney lesions can produce a similar pattern.

Radiographic appearance

As a simple renal cyst slowly increases in size, its protruding portion elevates the adjacent edges of the cortex. The cortical margin appears on nephrotomography as a very thin, smooth, radiopaque rim about the bulging lucent cyst (beak sign) (Figure 5-29). Although the beak sign is generally considered characteristic of benign renal cysts, it merely reflects a slow expansion of a mass and thus may occasionally be seen in slow-growing solid lesions, including carcinoma. Thickening of the rim about a lucent mass is suggestive of bleeding into a cyst, cyst infection, or a malignant lesion. Renal cysts cause focal displacement of adjacent portions of the pelvicalyceal system. The displaced, attenuated collecting structures remain smooth, unlike the shagginess and obliteration that often occur when focal displacement is caused by a malignant neoplasm.

Ultrasound is the modality of choice for distinguishing fluid-filled simple cysts from solid mass lesions. Fluid-filled cysts classically appear as echo-free structures with strongly enhanced posterior walls (Figure 5-30), in contrast to solid or complex lesions, such as tumors, that appear as echo-filled masses without posterior wall enhancement. CT is also highly accurate in detecting and characterizing

Figure 5-29 Renal cyst. Nephrotomogram shows smooth-walled, fluid-filled mass *(arrows)*.

Figure 5-30 Huge renal cyst. Anechoic lesion *(dark round area)* with a well-defined posterior wall.

simple renal cysts. On unenhanced scans, the cyst has a uniform attenuation value near that of water. After the injection of contrast material, a simple cyst becomes more apparent as the contrast material is concentrated by the normal surrounding parenchyma (Figure 5-31). The cyst itself shows no change in attenuation value, unlike a solid renal neoplasm, which always shows a small but definite increase in density. Because of the accuracy of CT and ultrasound, percutaneous cyst puncture is rarely necessary if these modalities provide unequivocal evidence of a simple cyst.

Figure 5-31   Renal cyst appears as a nonenhancing left renal mass *(C)* with sharply marginated border and thin wall.

However, because abscesses, cystic or necrotic tumors, and inflammatory or hemorrhagic cysts can mimic simple cysts, cyst puncture should be performed if there is an atypical appearance or a strong clinical suspicion of abscess, or if the patient has hematuria or hypertension. Fluid aspirated from a renal cyst can be clearly differentiated from that obtained from an abscess or a renal tumor. The introduction of contrast material or air after the cyst fluid has been removed demonstrates the smooth inner wall of the cyst and further decreases the possibility of missing a malignant neoplasm (Figure 5-32).

Treatment

Following needle puncture, a catheter can be placed for drainage if needed. An injection of iodine or alcohol may obliterate the cyst.

Polycystic kidney disease

Polycystic kidney disease is an inherited disorder in which multiple cysts of varying size cause lobulated enlargement of the kidneys and progressive renal impairment, which presumably results from cystic compression of nephrons, which in turn causes localized intrarenal obstruction. One third of patients with this condition have associated cysts of the liver, which do not interfere with hepatic function. About 10% have one or more saccular (berry) aneurysms of cerebral arteries, which may rupture and produce a fatal subarachnoid hemorrhage. Many patients with polycystic disease are hypertensive, a condition that may cause further deterioration of renal function and increase the likelihood that a cerebral aneurysm will rupture. Because patients tend to be asymptomatic during the first three decades of life, early diagnosis

A

B

Figure 5-32   Renal cyst puncture. **A,** Instillation of contrast material shows a smooth inner wall characteristic of a benign cyst. **B,** In another patient, injection of contrast material reveals a highly irregular inner border of a necrotic renal cell carcinoma.

is made either by chance or as a result of a specific search prompted by the discovery of findings in the family history.

Radiographic appearance

Excretory urography demonstrates enlarged kidneys with a multilobulated contour. The pelvic and infundibular structures are elongated, effaced, and often displaced around larger cysts, producing a crescentic outline. The nephrogram typically has a distinctive mottled or Swiss cheese pattern caused

Figure 5-34 Polycystic kidney disease. Right kidney longitudinal ultrasound scan demonstrating multiple cysts *(dark areas).*

Figure 5-33 Polycystic kidney disease. Nephrogram phase from selective arteriography of left kidney demonstrates innumerable cysts ranging from pinhead size to 2 cm. The opposite kidney had an identical appearance. (From Bosniak MA, Ambos MA: Polycystic kidney disease, *Semin Roentgenol* 10:133-143, 1975.)

Figure 5-35 Polycystic kidney disease. **A,** CT scan shows contrast-enhancing rims *(arrowheads)* in severely thinned renal parenchyma about innumerable large renal cysts. **B,** CT scan at higher level also shows diffuse cystic involvement of liver.

by the presence of innumerable lucent cysts of varying size throughout the kidneys (Figure 5-33). Plaques of calcification occasionally occur in cyst walls.

Ultrasound demonstrates grossly enlarged kidneys containing multiple cysts that vary considerably in size and are randomly distributed throughout the kidney (Figure 5-34). The renal parenchyma becomes hyperechoic because of small cysts that do not appear as fluid filled but are large enough to cause echoes. The demonstration of similar hepatic cysts further strengthens the diagnosis. Ultrasound is also of value in screening family members of a patient known to have this hereditary disorder. In patients with bilateral kidney enlargement and poor renal function, ultrasound permits the differentiation of polycystic kidney disease from multiple solid masses.

The multiple cysts in polycystic kidney disease can also be detected on CT scans (Figure 5-35) and magnetic resonance imaging (MRI). Although most individual cysts are histologically identical to simple cysts, intracystic hemorrhage is common. Unlike simple renal cysts, which demonstrate low attenuation on CT scan, hemorrhagic cysts have high attenuation values. On MRI a hemorrhagic cyst has high signal intensity on both T1- and T2-weighted images, unlike simple renal cysts, which have low signal intensity on T1-weighted images.

A rare, usually fatal form of polycystic disease can present at birth; it involves diffusely enlarged kidneys, renal failure, and maldevelopment of intrahepatic bile ducts. The margins of the kidneys are smooth in infantile polycystic disease, unlike the irregular renal contours in the adult form of polycystic disease that are attributable to the protrusion of innumerable cysts from the kidney surface. When renal function is sufficient, excretory urography results in a striking nephrogram in which a streaky pattern of alternating dense and lucent bands reflects contrast material puddling in elongated cystic spaces that radiate perpendicularly to the cortical surface (Figure 5-36). Ultrasound shows distortion of the intraparenchymal architecture, although the individual cysts are too small to be visualized.

Treatment

No cure is available. Medications are prescribed to control pain, high blood pressure, and infection related to the disease. Renal failure due to the loss of functioning kidney tissue requires dialysis, and renal transplantation may be considered.

Renal carcinoma

Renal cell carcinoma (**hypernephroma**) is the most common renal neoplasm, occurring predominantly in patients older than 40 years and often presenting with painless hematuria. About 10% of hypernephromas involve calcification, usually located in reactive fibrous zones about areas of tumor necrosis. In the differentiation of solid tumor from fluid-filled benign cysts, the location of calcium within the mass is more important than the pattern of calcification. Of all masses containing calcium in a nonperipheral location, almost 90% are malignant. The classic triad of symptoms (seen in about 10% of cases) includes hematuria, flank pain, and possibly a palpable abdominal mass. Although peripheral curvilinear calcification is much more suggestive of a benign cyst, hypernephromas can have a calcified fibrous pseudocapsule that results in an identical radiographic appearance.

Radiographic appearance

Hypernephromas typically produce urographic evidence of localized bulging or generalized renal en-

Figure 5-36 Infantile polycystic kidney disease. Excretory urogram in a young boy with large, palpable abdominal masses demonstrates renal enlargement with characteristic streaky densities leading to calyceal tips. There is only minimal distortion of the calyces.

largement. The tumor initially causes elongation of adjacent calyces; progressive enlargement and infiltration lead to distortion, narrowing, or obliteration of part or all of the collecting system (Figure 5-37). Large tumors may partially obstruct the pelvis or upper ureter and cause proximal dilatation. Complete loss of function on excretory urography usually indicates tumor invasion of the renal vein.

On nephrotomography, a hypernephroma generally appears as a mass with indistinct outlines and a density similar to that of normal parenchyma, unlike the classic radiolucent mass with sharp margins and a thin wall that represents a benign cyst. Necrotic neoplasms can also appear cystic, although they are usually surrounded by thick, irregular walls (Figure 5-38).

Ultrasound shows a renal carcinoma as a solid mass with numerous internal echoes and no evidence of the acoustic enhancement seen with renal cysts (Figure 5-39). On unenhanced CT scans, a hypernephroma appears as a solid neoplasm that is often not homogeneous and has an attenuation value near that of normal renal parenchyma, unlike a simple cyst, which has a uniform attenuation value near that of water. After the injection of contrast material, a simple cyst shows no change in attenuation value, whereas a solid renal neoplasm demonstrates a small but definite increase in density that is probably attributable primarily to vascular perfusion. However,

Figure 5-37   Renal cell carcinoma. Upward displacement of right kidney and distortion of collecting system by a large lower pole mass.

Figure 5-38   Renal cell carcinoma. Nephrotomogram demonstrates lucent, well-demarcated renal mass with thick wall *(arrows)*. (From Bosniak MA, Faegenburg D: *Radiology* 84:692-698, 1965.)

this increased density is much less than that of surrounding normal parenchyma, which also tends to concentrate the contrast material, and thus renal neoplasms become more apparent on contrast-enhanced scans (Figure 5-40).

CT is also an accurate method for detecting local and regional spread of hypernephroma. It can usually distinguish between neoplasms confined to the renal capsule and those that have extended beyond it. CT is also the most accurate method for detecting enlargement of paraaortic, paracaval, and retrocrural lymph nodes and spread to the ipsilateral renal vein and inferior vena cava (Figure 5-41).

MRI allows detailed demonstration of the renal anatomy and approaches the accuracy of CT in staging the abdominal extent of tumor in the patient with renal cell carcinoma (Figure 5-42, *A*). Advantages of MRI include its ability to determine the origin of the mass, to detect perihilar and perivascular lymph node metastases, and to demonstrate tumor invasion of adjacent organs. The superb delineation of blood vessels with MRI permits evaluation of tumor thrombus extension into the renal veins (a common occurrence) and into the inferior vena cava without the need for intravenous contrast material (Figure 5-42, *B*).

The most common sites of metastasis from renal cell carcinoma include the lungs, liver, bones, and brain.

Treatment

Nephrectomy, the most common treatment, is associated with a 40% survival rate.

Wilms' tumor (nephroblastoma)

Wilms' tumor is the most common abdominal neoplasm of infancy and childhood. The lesion arises from embryonic renal tissue, it may be bilateral, and it tends to become very large and appear as a palpable mass.

Wilms' tumor (highly malignant) must be differentiated from neuroblastoma, a tumor of adrenal medullary origin that is the second most common malignancy in children. Peripheral cystic calcification occurs in about 10% of Wilms' tumors, in contrast to the fine, granular, or stippled calcification seen in about half of the cases of neuroblastoma.

Radiographic appearance

At excretory urography, the intrarenal Wilms' tumor causes pronounced distortion and displacement of the pelvicalyceal system (Figure 5-43). The major effect of

Figure 5-39 Renal cell carcinoma. Ultrasound image **(A)** shows a solid echo-filled mass measuring approximately 10 × 9 cm in a 55-year-old woman with hematuria. Axial **(B)** and coronal **(C)** CT images demonstrate an inhomogeneous mass in the middle pole of the right kidney. The left kidney mass in the superior pole exhibits inhomogeneous attenuation and a decreased central density, indicating areas of necrosis.

Figure 5-40 Necrotic renal cell carcinoma. CT image shows huge, nonenhancing, cystlike mass *(M)* with irregular margins (especially on its medial and posterior aspects).

Figure 5-41 Renal cell carcinoma with left renal vein invasion. CT scan after administration of contrast shows dilated left renal vein filled with tumor thrombus *(arrowheads).* The thrombus extends to inferior vena cava *(arrow).* (From McClennan BL, Lee JKT: Kidney. In Lee JKT, Sagel SS, Stanley RJ, editors: *Computed body tomography,* New York, 1983, Raven Press.)

Figure 5-42   Renal cell carcinoma. **A,** Sagittal T1-weighted MR image through the left kidney demonstrates a large renal cell carcinoma *(straight arrow)* arising from the posterior aspect of the kidney and displacing Gerota's fascia outward *(curved arrows).* **B,** Transverse MR image at the level of the renal veins *(arrows)* and inferior vena cava *(I)* demonstrates normal signal from flowing blood without evidence of a tumor thrombus. This modality is especially useful for staging renal cell carcinoma because of its multiplanar capability and its ability to allow assessment of vascular invasion. *A,* Aorta.

Figure 5-43   Wilms' tumor. Huge mass in right kidney distorts and displaces pelvicalyceal system. (From Friedland GW et al, editors: *Uroradiology: an integrated approach,* New York, 1983, Churchill Livingstone.)

the extrarenal neuroblastoma is to displace the entire kidney downward and laterally. Because the kidney itself is usually not invaded, there is no distortion of the pelvicalyceal system.

Ultrasound is of value in distinguishing Wilms' tumor from hydronephrosis, another major cause of a palpable renal mass in a child. Wilms' tumors typically have a solid appearance with gross distortion of the renal structure (Figure 5-44), which is not like the precise organization of symmetrically positioned fluid-filled spaces in hydronephrosis. Ultrasound can also demonstrate the intrarenal location of Wilms' tumor, which is different from the extrarenal origin of a neuroblastoma.

Although it entails the use of ionizing radiation, CT can show the full extent of the tumor (including invasion of the inferior vena cava) and can detect any recurrence of the neoplasm after surgical removal (Figure 5-45). Coronal T1-weighted MR images can accurately differentiate Wilms' tumor from renal or hepatic lesions (Figure 5-46). This is also extremely useful in defining the extent of the lesion and showing possible tumor thrombus within the renal vein or the inferior vena cava. Because MRI has no ionizing radiation, it is an ideal modality for follow-up evaluation after surgical removal of the tumor.

Figure 5-44 Wilms' tumor. Ultrasound image of the right kidney shows a large, complex mass measuring 12.6 × 9.95 cm. The kidney hilum is pushed medially.

Figure 5-45 Wilms' tumor. CT scan of a 3-year-old child with a large nonfunctioning mass pushing the functioning right kidney anteriorly *(arrow)*.

Treatment

Surgery, radiation therapy, and chemotherapy result in an 85% cure rate in patients with Wilms' tumor.

Carcinoma of the bladder

Bladder carcinoma is usually seen in men more than 50 years of age. Many industrial chemicals have been implicated as factors in the development of carcinoma of the bladder. Cigarette smoking has also been associated with bladder tumors, presumably because of carcinogenic metabolites being excreted in the urine. The incidence of bladder cancer is especially high in

Figure 5-46 T1-weighted coronal MRI scan shows sharply margined infrahepatic mass *(W)* that is clearly distinct from the liver. The inferior vena cava *(arrowheads)*, although displaced by the mass, shows no evidence of tumor extension into it. *L*, Liver. (From Merten DE, Kirks DR: In Eisenberg RL, editor: *Diagnostic imaging: an algorithmic approach,* Philadelphia, 1988, Lippincott.)

Egypt, most likely related to the high prevalence of the parasitic infection schistosomiasis in that country.

Radiographic appearance

Carcinoma of the bladder may produce fingerlike projections into the lumen or it may infiltrate the bladder wall. Plain radiographs may demonstrate punctate, coarse, or linear calcifications that are usually encrusted on the surface of the tumor but occasionally lie within it. On excretory urograms, bladder cancer appears as one or more polypoid defects arising from the bladder wall or as focal bladder wall thickening (Figure 5-47). However, urography can detect only about 60% of bladder carcinomas because most are small when first symptomatic and are located on the trigone, where they can be difficult to visualize. Therefore all patients with lower urinary tract hematuria should undergo cystoscopy to exclude a bladder neoplasm.

CT with full distention of the bladder demonstrates a neoplasm as a mass projecting into the bladder lumen or as focal thickening of the bladder wall (Figure 5-48, *A*). This modality is excellent when MRI is not available for preoperative staging because it can determine the presence and degree of extravesical ex-

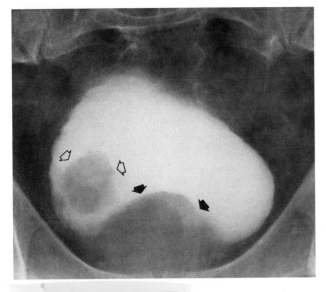

Figure 5-47   Bladder carcinoma. An irregular tumor *(open arrows)* is associated with a large filling defect *(solid arrows),* representing benign prostatic hypertrophy, at the base of the bladder.

Figure 5-48   CT scan of bladder carcinoma. **A,** Focal thickening of the posterior wall *(arrows).* **B,** Extensive bladder cancer *(m)* has extended to involve the sidewall of the pelvis *(arrow).* (From Friedland GW et al, editors: *Uroradiology: an integrated approach,* New York, 1983, Churchill Livingstone.)

tension, involvement of the pelvic sidewalls (Figure 5-48, *B*), and enlargement of pelvic or paraaortic lymph nodes.

MRI can demonstrate the depth of bladder wall invasion by showing a high-signal-intensity tumor disruption on T2-weighted images. The extension in the perivesical fat appears as a low signal intensity on T1-weighted images. MRI is equal to or better than CT for this purpose.

Treatment

Many carcinomas of the bladder have a low grade of malignancy, although they tend to recur repeatedly after surgical removal. More invasive tumors require removal of the entire bladder with transplantation of the ureters into a loop of ileum.

■ Renal Vein Thrombosis

Renal vein thrombosis occurs most frequently in children who are severely dehydrated. In the adult, thrombosis is most often a complication of another renal disease (e.g., chronic glomerulonephritis, amyloidosis, pyelonephritis), trauma, the extension of a thrombus from the inferior vena cava, or direct invasion or extrinsic pressure resulting from renal tumors.

Radiographic appearance

Renal vein thrombosis may be unilateral or bilateral. The clinical and radiographic findings are greatly in-

fluenced by the rapidity with which venous occlusion occurs. Sudden total occlusion causes striking kidney enlargement with minimal or no opacification on excretory urograms (Figure 5-49). If unresolved, this acute venous occlusion leads to the urographic appearance of a small, atrophic, nonfunctioning kidney.

When venous occlusion is partial or accompanied by adequate collateral formation, the kidney enlarges and appears smooth, and there is some degree of contrast excretion. The collecting system is stretched and thinned as a result of surrounding interstitial edema. Enlargement of collateral pathways (e.g., gonadal and ureteric veins) for renal venous outflow produces characteristic notching of the upper ureter.

Diagnostic ultrasound images show enlarged kidneys in acute renal vein thrombosis; the kidneys become increasingly atrophic as the disease slowly progresses. Doppler sonography may permit direct visualization of the clot within the renal vein. CT does not allow visualization of a clot-filled renal vein on

- -

Summary of Findings for Cysts and Tumors

DISORDER	LOCATION	RADIOGRAPHIC APPEARANCE	TREATMENT
Renal cyst	Renal parenchyma	US—fluid-filled cyst, echo free CT—region with lack of contrast enhancement	Percutaneous drainage; if indicated, an injection to collapse the cyst
Polycystic kidney	Renal parenchyma	IVU—mottled presence of multiple lucent lesions US—enlarged and hyperechoic kidneys, multiple anechoic lesions CT—hemorrhagic cyst with increased attenuation MRI—hemorrhagic cyst with increased signal intensity on both T1- and T2-weighted images	Unilateral—removal of lesions Loss of kidney function—dialysis and renal transplantation
Renal carcinoma	Kidney	Nephrotomogram—indistinct outlines; tumor density similar to that of normal tissue; cystic type surrounded by thick irregular walls US—solid mass with internal echoes CT—heterogeneous attenuation values increase with contrast MRI—determines extent of involvement and staging of tumor	Nephrectomy
Wilms' tumor	Embryonic renal tissue	IVU—kidney displacement inferiorly and laterally US—solid structure with gross distortion of the renal structure CT—tumor and extent of invasion MRI—differentiates Wilms' from other renal or hepatic tumors	Surgical removal, with chemotherapy and radiation therapy
Bladder carcinoma	Wall of bladder	KUB—punctate, coarse, or linear calcifications IVU—polypoid defects with wall thickening CT—mass projecting into bladder lumen, focal thickening of bladder wall MRI—predicts depth of wall invasion	Surgical removal of tumor Surgical removal of bladder and redirection of ureters into the ileum

IVU, Intravenous urography; *KUB,* kidney–ureter–bladder radiograph; *US,* ultrasound.

contrast-enhanced images. MRI can detect an abnormally strong signal from the renal veins, suggesting stasis (no flow) of blood. A renal vein with a slow flow caused by partial obstruction by a clot produces a lower signal. Ultrasound and MRI are the modalities used more frequently because they do not require an iodinated contrast agent to demonstrate the anatomy.

The confirmation of renal vein thrombosis requires venographic demonstration of vessel occlusion or a localized filling defect (Figure 5-50). An examination of the inferior vena cava with a catheter placed well below the renal veins is often performed initially to exclude caval thrombosis with proximal extension before the renal veins are catheterized directly.

Treatment

Anticoagulants are generally given to prevent new clots from forming. To reduce the possibility of emboli,

Figure 5-49 Acute renal vein thrombosis. Radiograph of the right kidney taken 5 minutes after injection of contrast material shows a dense nephrogram (*arrows*) and an absence of calyceal filling.

Figure 5-50 Renal vein thrombosis. Renal venogram demonstrates a large filling defect in the left renal vein (*arrows*) that extends into the vena cava. (From Cohn LH et al: The treatment of bilateral renal vein thrombosis and nephrotic syndrome, *Surgery* 64:387-396, 1968.)

the patient assumes bed rest and limited activity. Medications can be given intravenously or directly injected into the clot to lyse it. Renal vein thrombosis usually resolves without permanent damage to the kidneys.

▪ Acute Renal Failure

Acute renal failure refers to a rapid deterioration in kidney function that is sufficient to result in the accumulation of nitrogen-containing wastes in the blood and a characteristic odor of ammonia on the breath. In prerenal failure, there is decreased blood flow to the kidneys caused by low blood volume (e.g., because of hemorrhage, dehydration, surgical shock), cardiac failure, or obstruction of both renal arteries.

Postrenal failure is caused by obstruction of the urine outflow from both kidneys, most commonly a result of prostatic disease or functional obstruction of the bladder neck. Acute renal failure may also be the result of specific kidney diseases, such as glomerulonephritis, bilateral acute pyelonephritis, and malignant (severe) hypertension. Other causes of acute renal failure include nephrotoxic agents (antibiotics, radiographic contrast material, anesthetic agents, heavy metals, organic solvents), intravascular hemolysis, and large amounts of myoglobin (muscle protein) in the circulation resulting from muscle trauma or ischemia. Urine output may decrease to less than 400 ml per 24-hour period (oliguria).

Radiographic appearance

Because it is independent of renal function, ultrasound is especially useful in the evaluation of patients with acute renal failure. In addition to demonstrating dilatation of the ureters and pelves caused by postobstructive hypernephrosis, ultrasound can assess renal size and the presence of focal kidney lesions or diffuse renal cystic disease. In the patient with prerenal failure, ultrasound can aid in distinguishing low blood volume from right-sided heart failure. In the latter, there is dilatation of the inferior vena cava and hepatic veins that does not occur in patients with low circulating blood volume.

Plain film tomography can often demonstrate renal size and contours. Bilaterally enlarged, smooth kidneys are suggestive of acute renal parenchymal dysfunction; small kidneys usually indicate chronic, preexisting renal disease. Plain film tomograms can also demonstrate bilateral renal calcification, which may indicate either secondary hyperparathyroidism caused by chronic renal disease or bilateral stones that have obstructed both ureters to produce postrenal failure.

Excretory urography in the patient with acute renal failure demonstrates bilateral renal enlargement with a delayed and prolonged nephrogram (Figure 5-51); vicarious excretion of contrast material by the liver occasionally results in opacification of the gallbladder. However, in most instances excretory urography is unnecessary in the patient with acute renal failure, especially as many authors believe that intravenous contrast material can cause further damage to the kidneys in this condition.

Sonography is the modality of choice because it does not require the use of intravenous contrast agents. Ultrasound can assess renal size, identify renal parenchymal disease, and exclude hydronephrosis. Renal parenchymal disease appears as a diffuse increase in echogenicity, with loss of corticomedullary differentiation. If a vascular cause is suggested clinically, color Doppler studies allow visualization of

Figure 5-51 Acute renal failure. Excretory urogram 20 minutes after injection of contrast material shows bilateral persistent nephrograms with no calyceal filling.

patency or occlusion. If this is unsuccessful, a radionuclide scan or an MRI study may show these vessels without the use of an intravenous contrast agent.

Treatment

Treatment of predisposing conditions reduces the risk of acute renal failure becoming chronic or continued. Some physicians use diuretics to increase urine flow, and vasodilators to increase renal blood flow to help prevent the likelihood of more severe renal failure. Dietary modifications, including decreasing potassium and protein intake and increasing carbohydrates, can decrease the load on the kidneys. Antibiotics may be used to prevent or treat infections because of the high associated risk of sepsis with renal failure. In some cases, renal dialysis provides time for the kidneys to recover.

■ Chronic Renal Failure

Like acute renal failure, chronic kidney dysfunction may reflect prerenal, postrenal, or intrinsic kidney disease. Therefore, underlying causes of chronic renal failure include bilateral renal artery stenosis, bilateral ureteral obstruction, and intrinsic renal disorders such as chronic glomerulonephritis, pyelonephritis, and familial cystic diseases.

A failure to clear nitrogen-containing wastes adequately from the circulation leads to the accumulation of excessive blood levels of urea and creatinine (waste products of protein metabolism) in the blood. This condition, called **uremia,** produces toxic effects on many body systems. Irritation of the gastrointestinal tract produces nausea, vomiting, and diarrhea. In the nervous system, uremia causes drowsiness, dim vision, decreased mental ability, convulsions, and eventually coma. A decreased ability of the kidney to synthesize erythropoietin, which helps regulate the production of red blood cells, leads to the development of anemia. In the skin, uremia causes intense itching (pruritus) and a sallow (yellowish) coloring resulting from the combined effects of anemia and retention of a variety of pigmented metabolites (urochromes).

Because of the kidney's role in maintaining water balance and regulating acid–base balance and electrolyte levels, chronic renal failure causes abnormalities involving all these vital functions. Retention of sodium leads to increased water retention and the development of generalized edema and congestive heart failure. An elevated serum potassium level is potentially life threatening because of its direct effect on cardiac muscle contractility and the possibility of causing an arrhythmia or cardiac arrest. A reduction of serum calcium can produce the muscle twitching commonly seen in uremic patients. Low calcium levels also lead to increased activity of the parathyroid glands, which results in the removal of calcium from bones and a high incidence of renal stones.

Radiographic appearance

Because it is independent of renal function, ultrasound is most often the initial procedure in the evaluation of patients with chronic renal failure (Figure 5-52). It is of special value in diagnosing treatable diseases such as hydronephrosis and intrarenal or perirenal infections. This modality can also allow assessment of renal size and the presence of focal kidney lesions or diffuse renal cystic disease, and it can be used to localize the kidneys for percutaneous renal biopsy.

Even in patients with chronic renal failure and uremia, excretory urography with tomography may produce sufficient opacification of the kidneys to be of diagnostic value. However, excretory urography is infrequently required because similar information can be provided by ultrasound or retrograde pyelography. An initial plain abdominal radiograph may demonstrate bilateral renal calcifications (nephrocalcinosis) or obstructing ureteral stones (see Figure 5-25). Small kidneys with smooth contours are suggestive of chronic glomerulonephritis (see Figure 5-10), nephrosclerosis, or bilateral renal artery stenosis. Small kidneys with irregular contours, thin cortices, and typical clubbing of the calyces are consistent with chronic pyelonephritis (see Figure 5-11). Large kidneys are suggestive of obstructive disease, infiltrative processes (lymphoma, myeloma, amyloidosis), renal vein thrombosis (see Figure 5-49), or polycystic kidney disease (see Figure 5-35).

Figure 5-52 Ultrasound of patient with chronic renal failure. The right kidney is very small, measuring less than 6 cm, which suggests irreversible end-stage renal disease.

Summary of Findings for Renal Disorders

DISORDER	LOCATION	RADIOGRAPHIC APPEARANCE	TREATMENT
Renal vein thrombosis	Renal vein	IVU—kidney enlarged, appearing smooth with some contrast excretion; collecting system stretches and thins; notching of upper ureter US—acute: enlarged kidneys; chronic: atrophic kidneys Doppler—visualization of clot CT—lack of visualization of renal vein MRI—abnormally high signal intensity, suggesting stasis	Prevention of new clots—anticoagulants Bed rest and limited activity to reduce risk of clot travel Usually resolves without permanent injury
Acute renal failure	Nephron function	Tomography—acute: enlarged smooth kidneys; chronic: small kidneys IVU—prolonged nephrogram US—renal size, parenchymal disease, and hydronephrosis	Prevention—treat predisposing conditions Drug and dietary intervention Short-term dialysis
Chronic renal failure	Renal parenchyma	US—renal size, lesions, and cysts; hydronephrosis, intrarenal or perirenal infections	Slow destructive process Correct fluid imbalances Dialysis and transplantation

IVU, Intravenous urography; *US,* ultrasound.

Treatment

The initial goal of treatment is to slow the nephron loss and minimize complications. Antihypertensive drugs assist in preventing the continuation of this process. It is essential to properly balance intake and output of fluids as well as electrolyte levels. The inevitable occurrence of kidney failure requires dialysis to maintain the balance of body fluids. At this point, kidney transplant may be suggested.

QUESTIONS

1. The imaging criteria for pyelography are the same as for an abdominal radiograph but must include the area from the _____ to the _____.
   A. Diaphragm; kidneys
   B. Kidneys; pelvis
   C. Kidneys; superior pubis
   D. A and B

2. What organ of the body plays an essential role in maintaining the acid–base balance of the blood and body fluids, as well as the electrolyte balance?
   A. Nephron
   B. Glomerulus
   C. Bladder
   D. Kidney

3. A bacterial inflammation of the kidney and renal pelvis is termed _____.
   A. Renitis
   B. Pyelonephritis
   C. Glomerulitis
   D. None of the above

4. The medical term used to describe dilated calyces and renal pelvis is _____.
   A. Hydronephrosis
   B. Pyelonephritis
   C. Nephrosis
   D. None of the above

5. What is the name for the most common abdominal neoplasm of infants and children?
   A. Polycystic disease
   B. Pyelonephritis
   C. Wilms' tumor
   D. Hypernephroma

6. What is the name of the most common fusion anomaly of the kidneys?
   A. Complete fusion
   B. Crossed ectopia
   C. Pelvic kidney
   D. Horseshoe kidney

7. What is the name for a cystic dilatation of the distal ureter near the bladder?
   A. Compensatory hypertrophy
   B. Renal agenesis
   C. Ureterocele
   D. Hypoplasty

8. Name the first portion of the kidney to become visible after injection of a contrast agent.
   A. Nephron
   B. Glomerulus
   C. Bowman's capsule
   D. Calyces

9. What term is used to describe a kidney not in the normal area of the abdomen?
   A. Horseshoe
   B. Duplex
   C. Ectopic
   D. Ectopic ureterocele

10. The medical term for painful urination is _____.
    A. Dysuria
    B. Anuria
    C. Micturition
    D. Exacerbation

BIBLIOGRAPHY

Davidson AJ: *Radiology of the kidney,* Philadelphia, 1985, Saunders.

Pollack HM: *Clinical urography: an atlas and textbook of urological imaging,* Philadelphia, 1990, Saunders.

CHAPTER 6

Cardiovascular System

■ **Prerequisite Knowledge**

The student should have a basic knowledge of the anatomy and physiology of the cardiovascular system. In addition, proper learning and understanding of the material will be facilitated if the student has some clinical experience in chest radiography and film evaluation, including a concept of the changes in technique required to compensate for density differences produced by the underlying pathologic conditions. Experience in a cardiac or a vascular catheterization laboratory would be beneficial.

■ **Goals**

To acquaint the student radiographer with the pathophysiology and radiographic manifestations of all of the common and some of the unusual disorders of the cardiovascular system

■ **Objectives**

1. To understand and be able to define or describe all bold-faced terms in this chapter
2. To be able to describe the physiology of the cardiovascular system
3. To be able to identify anatomic structures on both diagrams and radiographs of the cardiovascular system
4. To be able to describe the various pathologic conditions affecting the cardiovascular system and their radiographic manifestations
5. To be familiar with the special procedures that are used when imaging particular pathologic conditions

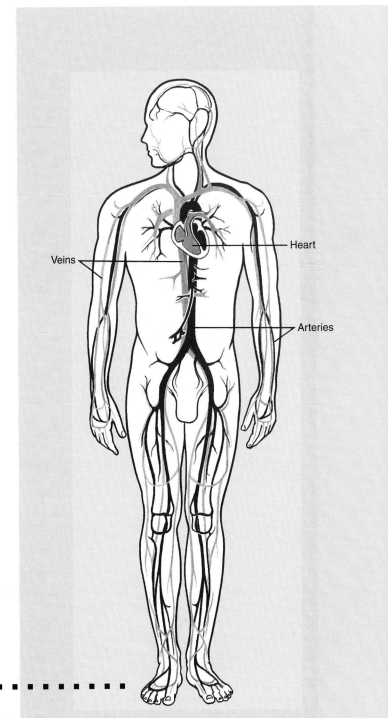

Heart

Veins

Arteries

▪ ▪ ▪ ▪ ▪ ▪ ▪ ▪ ▪ Radiographer Notes

Plain chest radiography and fluoroscopy of the cardiovascular system are used to identify abnormalities in the size and shape of the heart and to detect calcification of heart valves, coronary arteries, or the pericardium. The presence and extent of functional disorders are better demonstrated using angiography, ultrasound, radionuclide imaging, and magnetic resonance imaging.

As for all chest radiographs, it is essential that the radiographer perform cardiovascular studies with the patient positioned correctly and using proper technical factors. To this end, it would be helpful for the reader to review the radiographer notes at the beginning of the chapter on the respiratory system. An abnormality identified on a chest radiograph may be the first evidence of cardiovascular disease in an asymptomatic patient.

Radiographers can specialize in invasive diagnostic and therapeutic cardiovascular procedures, gain advanced certification in cardiovascular interventional technology, and be employed by cardiac or vascular catheterization laboratories. Angiocardiography is a diagnostic procedure performed to identify the exact anatomic location of an intracardiac disorder. Coronary angioplasty is a therapeutic procedure in which a narrowed coronary artery is dilated by inflation of a balloon that is attached to a catheter and manipulated fluoroscopically to the site of the stenosis. Because both angiocardiography and angioplasty involve the use of contrast material in patients who often have severe preexisting medical conditions, it is essential that the radiographer be always alert to the possibility of cardiac or respiratory arrest and be prepared to immediately assist with basic and advanced life support.

The injection of contrast material into arteries (arteriograms) and veins (venograms) can be performed in almost any portion of the body. As in the heart, these invasive studies use potentially dangerous substances, so the radiographer must be alert for possible complications and be prepared to assist in cardiorespiratory emergencies. In addition, these examinations require that the radiographer be trained in sterile technique, be able to use specialty equipment, and be familiar with the various types of catheters that are inserted into the vascular system for the delivery of contrast material.

Ultrasound, Doppler ultrasound, CT, and MRI are quickly becoming preferred initial modalities in imaging the vascular system.

▪ Physiology of the Cardiovascular System

The function of the cardiovascular system is to maintain an adequate supply of blood to all the tissues of the body. This is accomplished by the rhythmic contractions of the heart, the rate of which is controlled by the autonomic nervous system. The vagus nerve slows heart action by transmitting the chemical acetylcholine, whereas the sympathetic nervous system stimulates the release of epinephrine that accelerates the heart rate and increases the force of its contractions.

The heart consists of four chambers whose walls are composed of smooth muscle (myocardium), and it is lined with a smooth delicate membrane (endocardium) that is continuous with the inner surface of the blood vessels. The heart consists of two atria and two ventricles, with a partition (the septum) separating the right and left sides of the heart. The ventricles are considerably larger and thicker walled than the atria because they have a substantially heavier pumping load. Between each atrium and its associated ventricle are the atrioventricular valves (one on the right and one on the left side of the heart) that permit blood to flow in only one direction. These valves consist of flaps (or cusps) of endocardium that are anchored to the papillary muscles of the ventricles by cordlike structures called the chordae tendineae. The **mitral,** or bicuspid, **valve** between the left atrium and the left ventricle has two cusps, whereas the **tricuspid valve** between the right atrium and the right ventricle has three cusps. The semilunar valves separate the ventricles from the great vessels leaving the heart. The **pulmonary valve** lies between the right ventricle and the pulmonary artery, whereas the **aortic valve** separates the aorta from the left ventricle.

Deoxygenated venous blood is returned to the heart from the body through the superior and inferior venae cavae, which empty into the right atrium. Blood flows from the right atrium across the tricuspid valve into the right ventricle, which then pumps blood through the pulmonary valve into the pulmonary artery. Within the capillaries of the lungs, the red blood cells take up oxygen and release carbon dioxide. The freshly oxygenated blood then passes through the pulmonary veins into the left atrium, from which it flows across the mitral valve into the left ventricle. Contraction of the left ventricle forces oxygenated blood through the aortic valve into the aorta and the rest of the arterial tree to provide oxygen and nourishment to tissues throughout the body. The general circulation of the body is termed the **systemic circulation,** whereas the circulation of blood through the lungs is the pulmonary circulation. Because greater pressure is needed to pump blood through the systemic circulation than through the pulmonary circulation, the wall of the left ventricle is considerably thicker than that of the right ventricle.

The atria and ventricles alternately contract and relax. The contraction phase is called **systole;** the heart chambers relax and fill with blood during **diastole** (the relaxation phase). The normal cardiac impulse that stimulates mechanical contraction of the heart arises in the sinoatrial (SA) node, or pacemaker, which is situated in the right atrial wall near the opening of the superior vena cava. The impulse passes slowly through the atrioventricular (AV) node, which is located in the right atrium along the lower portion of the interatrial septum, and then spreads quickly throughout the ventricles by way of the fibrous bundle of His. The bundle of His terminates in Purkinje's fibers that can conduct impulses throughout the muscle of both ventricles and stimulate them to contract almost simultaneously. Specialized pacemaker cells in the SA node possess an **intrinsic rhythm,** so that even without any stimulation by the autonomic nervous system the node itself initiates impulses at regular intervals (about 70 to 75 beats per minute).

If the SA node is for some reason unable to generate an impulse, pacemaker activity shifts to another excitable component of the conduction system. These **ectopic pacemakers** also generate impulses rhythmically, although at a much slower rate. For example, if the AV node were to control pacemaker activity, the heart would beat 40 to 60 times per minute. If the conduction system of the heart is unable to maintain an adequate rhythm, the patient may receive an artificial pacemaker that electrically stimulates the heart, either at a set rhythm or only when the heart rate decreases below a preset minimum.

The heart muscle is supplied with oxygenated arterial blood by way of the right and left coronary arteries. These small vessels arise from the aorta just above the aortic valve. Unoxygenated blood from the myocardium drains into the coronary veins, which lead into the coronary sinus before opening into the right atrium.

The heart is surrounded by a double membranous sac termed the **pericardium.** The pericardium has a well-lubricated lining that protects against friction and permits the heart to move easily during contraction.

Figure 6-1 Atrial septal defect. Frontal projection of the chest demonstrates cardiomegaly along with an increase in pulmonary vascularity reflecting a left-to-right shunt. Small aortic knob *(white arrow)* and descending aorta *(small arrows)* are dwarfed by enlarged pulmonary outflow tract *(open arrow)*.

■ Congenital Heart Disease
Left-to-right shunts

The most common congenital cardiac lesions are left-to-right shunts, which permit mixing of blood in the systemic and pulmonary circulations. Because blood is preferentially shunted from the high-pressure systemic circulation to the relatively low pressure pulmonary circulation, the lungs become overloaded with blood. The magnitude of the shunt depends on the size of the defect and the differences in pressure on both sides. An increased load on the heart produces enlargement of specific cardiac chambers, depending on the location of the shunt.

The most common congenital cardiac lesion is **atrial septal defect,** which permits free communication between the two atria as a result of the lack of closure of the foramen ovale after birth or improper closure during gestation. Because the left atrial pressure is usually higher than the pressure in the right atrium, the resulting shunt is from left to right and causes increased pulmonary blood flow and overloading of the right ventricle. This produces the *radiographic appearance* of enlargement of the right ventricle, right atrium, and the pulmonary outflow tract (Figure 6-1).

In a patient with a **ventricular septal defect,** the resulting shunt is also from left to right because the left ventricular pressure is usually higher than the pressure in the right ventricle. The shunt causes increased pulmonary blood flow and, consequently, increased pulmonary venous return (Figure 6-2). This leads to diastolic overloading and enlargement of the left

Figure 6-2   Ventricular septal defect. Heart is enlarged and somewhat triangular, and there is increased pulmonary vascular volume. Pulmonary trunk is very large and overshadows normal-size aorta, which seems small by comparison. (From Cooley RN, Schreiber MH: *Radiology of the heart and great vessels,* Baltimore, 1978, Williams & Wilkins.)

atrium and left ventricle. Because shunting occurs primarily in systole and any blood directed to the right ventricle immediately goes into the pulmonary artery, there is no overloading of the right ventricle and *radiographically* no right ventricular enlargement is seen.

The third major type of left-to-right shunt is **patent ductus arteriosus.** The ductus arteriosus is a vessel that extends from the bifurcation of the pulmonary artery to join the aorta just distal to the left subclavian artery. It serves to shunt blood from the pulmonary artery into the systemic circulation during intrauterine life. Persistence of the ductus arteriosus, which normally closes soon after birth, results in a left-to-right shunt. The flow of blood from the higher-pressure aorta to the lower-pressure pulmonary artery causes increased pulmonary blood flow, and an excess volume of blood is returned to the left atrium and left ventricle. Radiographically, there is enlargement of the left atrium, the left ventricle, and the central pulmonary arteries, along with a diffuse increase in pulmonary vascularity (Figure 6-3). The increased blood flow through the aorta proximal to the shunt produces a prominent aortic knob, in contrast to the small or normal-size aorta seen in atrial and ventricular septal defects.

All left-to-right shunts can be complicated by the development of pulmonary hypertension **(Eisenmenger's syndrome).** This is caused by increased vascular resistance within the pulmonary arteries related to chronic increased flow through the pulmonary circulation. Pulmonary hypertension appears *radiographically* as an increased fullness of the central pulmonary arteries with abrupt narrowing and pruning

Figure 6-3   Patent ductus arteriosus. **A,** Frontal chest radiograph demonstrates cardiomegaly with enlargement of left atrium, left ventricle, and central pulmonary arteries. There is diffuse increase in pulmonary vascularity. **B,** In another patient, aortogram shows patency of ductus arteriosus *(arrow).* (From Cooley RN, Schreiber MH: *Radiology of the heart and great vessels,* Baltimore, 1978, Williams & Wilkins.)

of peripheral vessels (Figure 6-4). The elevation of pulmonary arterial pressure tends to balance or even reverse the left-to-right shunt, thus easing the volume overloading of the heart.

Radiographic appearance

Chest radiographs provide an initial assessment of pulmonary vasculature, size of the main pulmonary arteries, size and position of the aorta, and size and contour of the cardiac silhouette. In the preceding paragraphs, specific descriptions appear with each septal defect.

Magnetic resonance imaging (MRI) cine studies are becoming the primary modality for imaging in most congenital heart diseases because both the morphologic and the functional anomalies may be demonstrated in multiple planes.

Angiocardiography is the most definitive imaging technique for demonstrating the atria and ventricles of the heart, but it is also the most invasive.

Treatment

Small defects may not require treatment and may spontaneously close. Surgery may be necessary to correct a large defect.

Tetralogy of Fallot

Tetralogy of Fallot is the most common cause of cyanotic congenital heart disease. It consists of four (thus "tetra") abnormalities: (1) high ventricular septal defect, (2) pulmonary stenosis, (3) overriding of the aortic orifice above the ventricular defect, and (4) right ventricular hypertrophy. Pulmonary stenosis causes an elevation of pressure in the right ventricle and hypertrophy of that chamber. Because of the narrow opening of the pulmonary valve, an inadequate amount of blood reaches the lungs to be oxygenated. The ventricular septal defect and the overriding of the aorta produce right-to-left shunting of unoxygenated venous blood into the left ventricle and then into the systemic circulation, thus increasing the degree of cyanosis.

Radiographic appearance

Enlargement of the right ventricle causes upward and lateral displacement of the apex of the heart (Figure 6-5). This results in the classic **coeur en sabot** appearance resembling the curved-toe portion of a wooden shoe. In about one fourth of patients with tetralogy of Fallot, the aorta is on the right side.

Treatment

Without surgical repair, most patients die before reaching puberty. Although operative repair provides some chance of recovery, the outcome depends on the severity of the defect and other extenuating circumstances.

Coarctation of the aorta

Coarctation refers to a narrowing, or constriction, of the aorta that most commonly occurs just beyond the

Figure 6-4 Eisenmenger's syndrome in atrial septal defect. There is slight but definite cardiomegaly and great increase in size of the pulmonary trunk. Right and left pulmonary artery branches are huge, but peripheral pulmonary vasculature is relatively sparse. Long-standing pulmonary hypertension has produced degenerative changes in the walls of the pulmonary arteries, which have become densely calcified. (From Cooley RN, Schreiber MH: *Radiology of the heart and great vessels*, Baltimore, 1978, Williams & Wilkins.)

Figure 6-5 Tetralogy of Fallot. Plain chest radiograph demonstrates characteristic lateral displacement and upward tilting of prominent cardiac apex. There is also decreased pulmonary vascularity and flat pulmonary outflow tract.

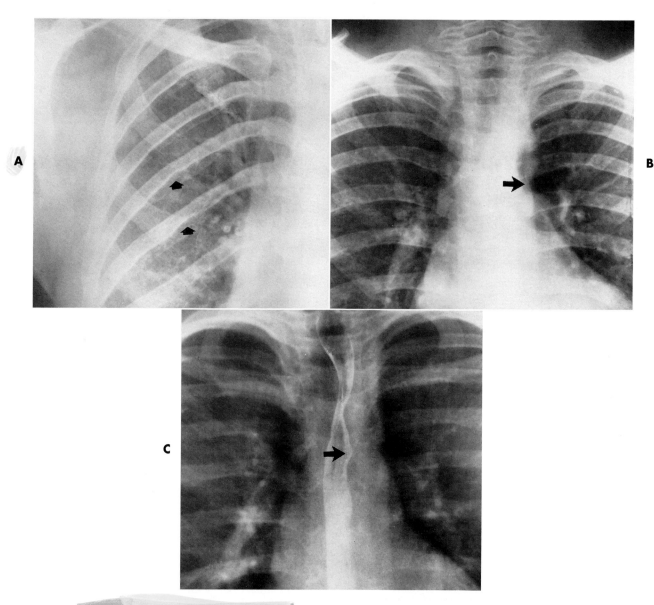

Figure 6-6 Coarctation of the aorta. **A,** There is notching of the fourth through eighth posterior ribs *(arrows).* **B,** Plain chest radiograph demonstrates a figure-3 sign *(arrow pointing to its center).* Upper bulge represents prestenotic dilatation; lower bulge represents poststenotic dilatation. **C,** Esophagram demonstrates reverse figure-3 sign *(arrow pointing to its center).* (From Swischuk LE: *Plain film interpretation in congenital heart disease,* Baltimore, 1979, Williams & Wilkins.)

branching of the blood vessels to the head and arms. Although the blood supply and pressure to the upper extremities is normal, there is decreased blood flow through the constricted area to the abdomen and legs. Classically, the patient has normal blood pressure in the arms but very low blood pressure in the legs.

The relative obstruction of aortic blood flow leads to the progressive development of collateral circulation—the enlargement of normally tiny vessels in an attempt to compensate for the inadequate blood supply to the lower portion of the body.

Radiographic appearance

Coarctation of the aorta is often seen radiographically as rib notching (usually involving the posterior fourth to eighth ribs) resulting from pressure erosion by dilated and pulsating intercostal collateral vessels, which run along the inferior margins of these ribs (Figure 6-6, *A*). Notching of the posterior border of the sternum may be produced by dilatation of mammary artery collaterals.

Coarctation of the aorta often causes two bulges in the region of the aortic knob that produce a charac-

Figure 6-7   Coarctation of aorta. Sagittal MR image demonstrates coarctation *(straight arrow)* of thoracic aorta with associated poststenotic dilatation of proximal descending thoracic aorta *(curved arrow)*. L, Left subclavian artery.

teristic figure-3 sign on plain chest radiographs (see Figure 6-6, *B*) and a reverse figure-3 (or figure-E) impression on the barium-filled esophagus (see Figure 6-6, *C*). The more cephalic bulge represents dilatation of the proximal aorta and the base of the subclavian artery (prestenotic dilatation); the lower bulge reflects poststenotic aortic dilatation.

Aortography can accurately localize the site of obstruction, determine the length of the coarctation, and identify any associated cardiac malformations. More recently, MRI has been used to demonstrate aortic narrowing (Figure 6-7) and to check the appearance of the aorta after corrective surgery.

Treatment

Uncorrected aortic coarctation has a dismal prognosis, and surgical repair is required for patient survival.

■ Acquired Vascular Disease

Coronary artery disease

Narrowing of the coronary arteries causes oxygen deprivation of the myocardium and ischemic heart disease. In most patients, narrowing of the lumen of one or more of the coronary arteries is attributable to the deposition of fatty material on the inner arterial wall (atherosclerosis). Factors predisposing to the devel-

opment of coronary artery disease include hypertension, obesity, smoking, a high-cholesterol diet, and lack of exercise.

The speed and degree of luminal narrowing determine whether an atherosclerotic lesion causes significant and clinically evident ischemia. Temporary oxygen insufficiency causes angina pectoris, a feeling of severe chest pain that may radiate to the neck, jaw, and left arm and is often associated with the sensation of chest tightness or suffocation. Attacks of angina pectoris are often related to a sudden increase in the demand of the myocardium for oxygen, as after strenuous exercise, a heavy meal, emotional stress, or exposure to severe cold. The placing of a nitroglycerin tablet under the tongue causes dilatation of the coronary arteries, which permits an adequate flow to the myocardium.

Occlusion of a coronary artery deprives an area of myocardium of its blood supply and leads to the death of muscle cells **(myocardial infarction)** in the area of vascular distribution. The size of the coronary artery that is occluded determines the extent of heart muscle damage. The greater the area affected, the poorer the prognosis because of the increased loss of pumping function that may result in congestive heart failure. A favorable prognostic factor is the development of collateral circulation, through which blood from surrounding vessels is channeled into the damaged tissue. If the patient survives, the infarcted region heals with fibrosis. Long-term complications include the development of thrombi on the surface of the damaged area and the production of a local bulge (ventricular aneurysm) at the site of the weakness of the myocardial wall.

Radiographic appearance

Radionuclide thallium perfusion scanning is the major noninvasive study for assessment of regional blood flow to the myocardium. Focal decreases in thallium uptake that are observed immediately after exercise but are no longer identified on delayed scans usually indicate transient ischemia associated with significant coronary artery stenosis or spasm. After exercise, focal defects that remain unchanged on delayed scans more frequently reflect scar formation. A normal thallium exercise scan makes the diagnosis of myocardial ischemia unlikely, although in about 10% of patients with significant obstructive disease the presence of sufficient collateral vessels can prevent the radionuclide demonstration of regional ischemia.

Radionuclide scanning (single photon emission computed tomography, or SPECT), using technetium pyrophosphate or other compounds that are taken up by acutely infarcted myocardium, is a new noninvasive technique for detecting, localizing, and classifying

■ ■

Summary of Findings for Congenital Heart Disease

DISORDER	LOCATION	RADIOGRAPHIC APPEARANCE	TREATMENT
Atrial septal defect	Communication between atria	Enlarged right ventricle, right atrium, and pulmonary outflow tract	Small defects may spontaneously close and not require treatment Large defects require surgical repair
Ventricular septal defect	Communication between ventricles	No right ventricular enlargement	
Patent ductus arteriosus	Vascular connection between pulmonary artery and aorta	Enlargement of left atrium, left ventricle, and pulmonary arteries with an increase in pulmonary vascularity	
Tetralogy of Fallot	High ventricular septal defect Pulmonary stenosis Overriding of the aortic orifice above the ventricular defect Right ventricular hypertrophy	Enlarged right ventricle Operative repair Upward and lateral displacement of the heart apex	
Coarctation of the aorta	Constriction of aorta at the distal arch	Rib notching, figure 3 or E on barium-filled esophagus Aortography—localizes obstruction, determines length of coarctation, and identifies an associated malformation MRI—demonstrates narrowing; used for follow-up of corrective surgery	Surgical repair

■ ■

myocardial necrosis (Figure 6-8). On CT, areas of myocardial ischemia appear as regions of decreased attenuation because of the increased water content resulting from intramyocardial cellular edema. Initial studies have indicated that MRI will also be of value in detecting early signs of muscular necrosis in myocardial infarction (Figure 6-9) and may help determine whether the infarction is acute or remote.

Plain chest radiographs are usually normal or nonspecific in most patients with ischemic heart disease. Calcification of a coronary artery, although infrequently visualized on routine chest radiographs and usually requiring cardiac fluoroscopy, strongly suggests of the presence of hemodynamically significant coronary artery disease (Figure 6-10). Plain chest radiographs are also entirely normal in many, if not most, patients after myocardial infarction. They are primarily of value in detecting evidence of pulmonary

venous congestion in patients who develop congestive heart failure as a result of an inability of the remaining heart muscle to propel blood through the circulation adequately.

Coronary arteriography is generally considered the definitive test for determining the presence and assessing the severity of coronary artery disease. About 30% of significant stenoses involve a single vessel, most commonly the anterior descending artery. Another 30% involve two vessels, and significant stenosis of the three main vessels can be demonstrated in the remaining 40%. About 50% of coronary artery disease occurs in the left coronary, 35% in the right coronary, and 15% in the left circumflex (Figure 6-11).

Intravascular ultrasound is a new technique that provides the most precise anatomic information to guide interventional procedures. The severity of arterial stenosis, measurement of lesion length, lumen

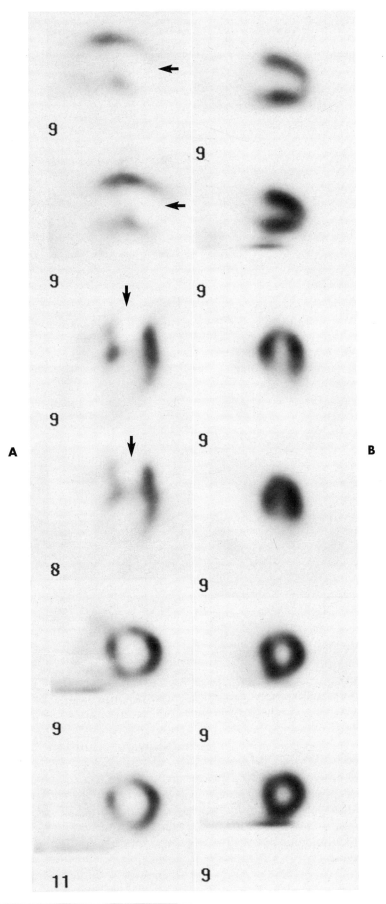

A

B

9

9

9

9

9

9

9

9

8

9

9

9

11

9

Figure 6-8 Myocardial stress/rest perfusion SPECT scan. **A,** Apical defect is demonstrated on the stress images because of the lack of uptake in the cardiac apex *(arrows).* **B,** The defect on rest images shows perfusion to the apex of the heart, indicating ischemia.

Figure 6-9 MR image of acute myocardial infarction. **A,** T2-weighted coronal image obtained in patient 10 days after acute myocardial infarction demonstrates area of increased signal intensity (indicating edema associated with muscle necrosis) in subendocardial regions of lateral wall *(arrowhead).* **B,** Short-axis view of another patient shows acute transmural infarction *(arrow)* of anterolateral wall. (From Stark DD, Bradley WG, editors: *Magnetic resonance imaging,* St Louis, 1988, Mosby.)

Figure 6-10 Ischemic heart disease. Frontal projection of chest demonstrates cardiomegaly with typical linear calcification in coronary artery *(arrows).*

dimension, and any unusual morphology can be determined. This modality is especially helpful in demonstrating the origin of the left main coronary artery, which may be obscured by the catheter in angiography. However, this equipment is not readily available because of its expense.

Treatment

Aortocoronary bypass grafting, usually using sections of saphenous vein, is an increasingly popular procedure in patients with ischemic heart disease. Arteriography has been the procedure of choice for demonstrating the patency and functional efficiency of aortocoronary bypass grafts. Patent functioning grafts demonstrate prompt clearing of contrast material and good filling of the grafted artery. Stenotic or malfunctioning grafts demonstrate areas of narrowing, filling defects, and slow flow with delayed washout of contrast material.

Percutaneous transluminal angioplasty (PTA) using a balloon catheter is now a recognized procedure for the treatment of patients with narrowing of one or more coronary arteries (Figure 6-12). As in other types of PTA, a catheter is placed under fluoroscopic guidance into the affected coronary artery, and an arteriogram is performed for localization. The angioplasty balloon is then positioned at the level of the stenosis and inflated. After dilatation, coronary arteriography is repeated to show the resulting appearance of the stenosis and to detect any complications of the procedure. Symptomatic improvement occurs in 50% to 70% of dilatations. About 3% to 8% of patients who undergo PTA develop either persistent coronary insufficiency or sudden occlusion of a coronary artery at the site of dilatation at the time of the procedure. Therefore the procedure should be performed at a time when an operating room, an anesthetist, and a cardiac surgeon are available so that immediate coronary bypass surgery can be performed if necessary. The mortality of coronary angioplasty is less than 1%. In conjunction with PTA, deployment

Figure 6-11   Coronary angiography. **A,** PA cranial projection of the left main coronary artery shows a lesion involving the left anterior descending artery. **B,** Right anterior oblique cranial projection of left main coronary artery shows a lesion in the diagonal artery. **C,** Left anterior oblique projection of the right coronary artery demonstrates an ostial lesion at the origin.

of a stent helps in many cases to maintain the open lumen (Figure 6-13). Other interventional procedures include endovascular stent, atherectomy, and laser-assisted angioplasty.

Congestive heart failure

Congestive heart failure (CHF) refers to the inability of the heart to propel blood at a rate and volume sufficient to provide an adequate supply to the tissues. Causes of CHF include an intrinsic cardiac abnor-

mality, hypertension, or any obstructive process that abnormally increases the peripheral resistance to blood flow.

Radiographic appearance

Left-sided heart failure produces a classic radiographic appearance of cardiac enlargement, redistribution of pulmonary venous blood flow (enlarged superior pulmonary veins and decreased caliber of the veins draining the lower lungs), interstitial edema, alveolar

Figure 6-12 Percutaneous transluminal coronary angioplasty. **A,** Initial right coronary angiogram shows severe narrowing *(arrow)* of the mid-portion of the right coronary artery. **B,** During percutaneous transluminal coronary angioplasty, a steerable guide wire *(G)* is passed down the coronary artery and through the coronary stenosis. The tip lies within the distal right coronary artery. Radiopaque markers *(M)* identify the balloon portion of the dilating catheter that has been advanced over the guide wire through the coronary stenosis. **C,** Immediately after angioplasty, the previous site of stenosis *(arrow)* is now patent. (From Fischell TA, Block PC: *Cardiovasc Reviews Reports* 6:89-99, 1985.)

Figure 6-13 **A,** Angiogram of left coronary artery with a stenotic lesion in the circumflex artery *(arrow)*. **B,** Angiogram demonstrating the left circumflex artery after PTA and stent placement with no evidence of a stenotic lesion.

edema (irregular, poorly defined patchy densities), and pleural effusions (Figure 6-14). In acute left ventricular failure resulting from coronary thrombosis, however, there may be severe pulmonary congestion and edema with very little cardiac enlargement. Pulmonary congestion and edema may require a change in technique to compensate for the increased fluid in the lungs. The major causes of left-sided heart failure include coronary heart disease, valvular disease, and hypertension.

Figure 6-14 Left-sided heart failure. Diffuse perihilar alveolar densities.

In right-sided heart failure, dilatation of the right ventricle and right atrium is present (Figure 6-15). The transmission of increased pressure may cause dilatation of the superior vena cava, widening of the right superior mediastinum, and edema of the lower extremities. The enlargement of a congested liver may elevate the right hemidiaphragm. Common causes of right-sided heart failure include pulmonary valvular stenosis, emphysema, and pulmonary hypertension resulting from pulmonary emboli.

Many patients with CHF have cardiomegaly. A simple test to evaluate the heart size is the cardiothoracic ratio (C/T ratio), with greater than 50% indicating cardiomegaly. In these cases, the radiologist relies on information provided by the technologist about the images: erect versus recumbent, posteroanterior (PA) versus anteroposterior (AP), and source-image-to-receptor distance, all of which influence the heart size. Lack of (or inaccurate) information can result in misdiagnosis.

Pulmonary edema

Pulmonary edema refers to an abnormal accumulation of fluid in the extravascular pulmonary tissues. The most common cause of pulmonary edema is an elevation of the pulmonary venous pressure. This is most often attributable to left-sided heart failure but may also be caused by pulmonary venous obstruction

A   **B**

Figure 6-15 Right-sided heart failure. Frontal **(A)** and lateral **(B)** projections of the chest in a patient with primary pulmonary hypertension show pronounced globular cardiomegaly with prominence of the pulmonary trunk and central pulmonary arteries. Peripheral pulmonary vascularity is strikingly reduced. Right ventricular enlargement has obliterated retrosternal air space on the lateral projection.

(mitral valve disease, left atrial tumor) or lymphatic blockade (fibrotic, inflammatory, or metastatic disease involving the mediastinal lymph nodes). Other causes of pulmonary edema include uremia, narcotic overdose, exposure to noxious fumes, excessive oxygen, high altitudes, fat embolism, adult respiratory distress syndrome, and various neurologic abnormalities.

Radiographic appearance

Transudation of fluid into the interstitial spaces of the lungs is the earliest stage of pulmonary edema. However, in patients with CHF or pulmonary venous hypertension, increased pulmonary venous pressure first appears as a redistribution of blood flow from the lower to the upper lung zones. This phenomenon, probably caused by reflex venous spasm, causes prominent enlargement of the superior pulmonary veins and decreased caliber of the veins draining the inferior portions of the lung. Edema fluid in the interstitial space causes a loss of the normal sharp definition of pulmonary vascular markings (Figure 6-16). Accentuation of the vascular markings about the hila produces a perihilar haze. Fluid in the interlobular septa produces characteristic thin horizontal lines of increased density at the axillary margins of the lung inferiorly (Kerley B lines).

A further increase in pulmonary venous pressure leads to the development of alveolar or pleural transudates. Alveolar edema appears as irregular, poorly defined patchy densities scattered throughout the lungs. The classic radiographic finding of alveolar pulmonary edema is the butterfly (or bat's-wing) pattern, a diffuse, bilaterally symmetric, fan-shaped infiltration that is most prominent in the central portion of the lungs and fades toward the periphery (Figure 6-17).

Figure 6-17 Butterfly pattern of severe pulmonary edema. Diffuse bilateral symmetric infiltration of the central portion of lungs along with relative sparing of the periphery produces a butterfly pattern. (From Fraser RG, Pare JAP: *Diagnosis of diseases of the chest*, Philadelphia, 1979, Saunders.)

Figure 6-16 Interstitial pulmonary edema. Edema fluid in the interstitial space causes loss of the normal sharp definition of pulmonary vascular markings and a perihilar haze. At the bases, notice the thin horizontal lines of increased density (Kerley B lines), which represent fluid in interlobular septa.

Figure 6-18 Unilateral pulmonary edema. Diffuse alveolar pattern limited to the left lung because of the effect of gravity on the patient lying on the left side.

Pleural effusion associated with pulmonary edema usually occurs on the right side (Figure 6-18). When bilateral, the effusion tends to be more noticeable on the right. There is often an associated thickening of the interlobar fissures.

After adequate treatment of pulmonary edema, the interstitial, alveolar, and pleural abnormalities may disappear within several hours. Loculated pleural fluid within a fissure (especially the minor fissure)

may resorb more slowly and appear as a sharply defined, elliptical or circular density that simulates a solid parenchymal mass (Figure 6-19).

Most patients with pulmonary edema caused by congestive failure or other heart disease have evidence of cardiomegaly. When the cause of the pulmonary edema is noncardiogenic, the heart often remains normal in size (Figure 6-20).

Treatment of congestive heart failure and pulmonary edema

The nonpharmacologic approach includes avoiding excessive physical stress, decreasing dietary salt, and wearing compressive stockings to decrease deep vein thrombosis. Pharmocologic therapy includes some combination of the following drugs: diuretics, angiotensin-converting enzyme inhibitors, digoxin (digitalis), parenteral inotropic agent, calcium channel blocker, beta blocker, and antithrombotic therapy.

Hypertension

Hypertension, or high blood pressure, is the leading cause of strokes and CHF. The blood pressure is a function of cardiac output (the amount of blood pumped per minute by the heart) and the total peripheral resistance, which reflects the condition of the walls of the blood vessels throughout the body. Although the peripheral resistance and cardiac output may fluctuate rapidly, depending on such factors as whether a person sits or stands and is quiet or excited, the systemic blood pressure remains remarkably constant in a healthy person.

Figure 6-19 Loculated pleural fluid (phantom tumors). **A,** Frontal chest radiograph taken during an episode of congestive heart failure demonstrates pronounced cardiomegaly with bilateral pleural effusions. Note fluid collections along the lateral chest wall *(solid arrow),* in minor fissure *(open arrow),* and in left major fissure *(arrowhead).* **B,** With improvement in the patient's cardiac status, phantom tumors have disappeared. Bilateral small pleural effusions persist.

Figure 6-20 After a near-drowning event, the patient has a normal-size heart and a pattern of diffuse pulmonary edema.

A blood pressure reading consists of two parts. The systolic pressure is the highest pressure in the peripheral arteries that occurs when the left ventricle contracts. The diastolic pressure is the pressure in the peripheral arteries when the left ventricle is relaxing and filling with blood from the left atrium. High blood pressure is defined as elevation of the systolic pressure above 140 millimeters of mercury (mm Hg) and of the diastolic pressure above 90 mm Hg. In patients older than 40 years, the systolic pressure may be somewhat higher and still be considered within normal limits. As a rough rule of thumb, a person is allowed an additional 10 mm Hg in systolic pressure for each decade over 40 years of age.

Most patients with elevated blood pressure have essential, or idiopathic, hypertension. The benign form of essential hypertension is characterized by a gradual onset and a prolonged course, often of many years. In the much less common malignant form, the elevated blood pressure has an abrupt onset, runs a rapid course, and often leads to renal failure or cerebral hemorrhage.

About 6% of patients have secondary hypertension resulting from another disease. Although some patients in this group have adrenal abnormalities (Cushing's syndrome, primary aldosteronism, pheochromocytoma) in which there is an abnormality of the regulation of salt and water content (and thus the blood volume), and others have an abnormality involving the secretion of a substance that increases vascular tone and peripheral arterial resistance, most have renal parenchymal or vascular disease as the underlying cause of hypertension.

Radiographic appearance

Arteriography is the most accurate screening examination for detecting renovascular lesions. If a noninvasive screening test is desired, a radionuclide renogram with captopril is performed. The most common cause of renal artery obstruction is arteriosclerotic narrowing, which usually occurs in the proximal portion of the vessel close to its origin from the aorta (Figure 6-21). Bilateral renal artery stenoses are noted in up to one third of these patients. Oblique projections, which demonstrate the vessel origins in profile, are often required to demonstrate renal artery stenosis. CT angiography can detect renal artery stenosis including fibromuscular dysplasia. MR angiography (MRA) can detect stenosis but the resolution is still inadequate to visualize segmental renal branches. One of the advantages of MRA is that iodinated contrast agents are not required to visualize the vessel anatomy.

The other major cause of renovascular hypertension is **fibromuscular dysplasia.** This disease is most frequent in young adult women and is often bilateral.

A

B

Figure 6-21 Renovascular hypertension. **A,** Radiograph shows diminished size of right kidney. **B,** Arteriography demonstrates that the cause is renal artery stenosis *(arrow).* (From Burko H et al: In Eisenberg RL, Amberg JR, editors: *Critical diagnostic pathways in radiology: an algorithmic approach,* Philadelphia, 1981, Lippincott.)

The most common radiographic appearance of fibromuscular dysplasia is the string-of-beads pattern, in which there are alternating areas of narrowing and dilatation (Figure 6-22). Smooth, concentric stenoses occur less frequently.

The mere presence of a renovascular lesion does not mean that it is the cause of hypertension; indeed, many patients with normal blood pressure have severe renal artery disease. Therefore bilateral renal vein catheterization for the measurement of plasma renin activity is used to assess the functional significance of any stenotic lesion. A renal vein renin concentration on the abnormal side that is more than 50% greater than the renin level in the renal vein on the normal side indicates the functional significance of a lesion with an accuracy rate of about 85%.

Prolonged high blood pressure forces the heart to overwork, causing the left ventricle to enlarge and eventually fail. Since high blood pressure affects all arteries of the body, including the coronary and

Figure 6-22 Renovascular hypertension. String-of-beads pattern of fibromuscular dysplasia bilaterally.

carotid vessels, this condition increases the risk of coronary occlusion and myocardial infarction, as well as carotid narrowing leading to a stroke.

Decreased function of the kidneys leads to the retention of water and salt, which increases the blood volume and elevates the blood pressure. Long-standing hypertension causes atherosclerosis of the renal artery, which reduces blood flow to the kidneys and causes further damage.

Treatment

Medical treatment includes some combination of diuretics and beta, alpha, and calcium blockers to control blood pressure. Surgery has traditionally been the treatment for a patient with arteriographically demonstrated renal artery lesions and confirmatory renal vein renin studies. Recently, PTA, with stent placement, has been shown to be effective in dilating renal artery stenoses (Figure 6-23). Although insufficient time has elapsed to compare the long-term results of renal transluminal angioplasty with corrective surgical procedures, initial studies demonstrate the improvement or cure of hypertension in about 80% of patients treated with angioplasty. Stenosis recurs in 10% to 20%, usually because of incomplete dilatation.

Hypertensive heart disease

Long-standing high blood pressure causes narrowing of systemic blood vessels and an increased resistance to blood flow. The left ventricle is forced to assume an increased work load, which initially causes hypertrophy (double thickness of normal wall) and little if any change in the radiographic appearance of the cardiac silhouette.

Radiographic appearance

Eventually, the continued strain on the heart leads to dilatation and enlargement of the left ventricle (Figure 6-24), along with downward displacement of the cardiac apex, which often projects below the left hemidiaphragm. Aortic tortuosity with prominence of the ascending portion commonly occurs (Figure 6-25). Failure of the left ventricle leads to increased pulmonary venous pressure and congestive failure (40%).

Treatment

Therapy includes treating the high blood pressure and complications such as CHF.

Aneurysm

An aneurysm is a localized dilatation of an artery that most commonly involves the aorta, especially its abdominal portion. A **saccular** aneurysm involves only one side of the arterial wall, whereas bulging of the entire circumference of the vessel wall is termed a **fusiform** aneurysm. An aneurysm represents a weakness in the wall of a blood vessel caused by atherosclerosis, syphilis or other infection, trauma, or a congenital defect such as Marfan's syndrome. The presence of multiple small aneurysms is suggestive of a generalized arterial inflammation (arteritis). In the abdominal aorta, most aneurysms occur below the origin of the renal arteries, and thus the aneurysm can be surgically replaced by a prosthetic graft without injuring the kidneys. The danger of an aneurysm is its tendency to increase in size and rupture, leading to massive hemorrhage, which may be fatal if it involves a critical organ such as the brain.

Figure 6-23 Percutaneous transluminal angioplasty for renovascular hypertension. **A,** Abdominal aortogram demonstrates severe bilateral stenoses of main renal arteries *(straight arrows)* and stenoses at origins of early bifurcations *(curved arrows).* **B,** Aortogram after angioplasty of both renal arteries shows irregularities in areas of previous atherosclerotic narrowing *(arrows)* but an improved residual lumen in both main renal arteries. After the procedure, the patient's previous severe hypertension was controllable to normal levels with only minimal dosages of diuretic medication. (From Waltman AC: In Athanasoulis CA et al, editors: *Interventional radiology,* Philadelphia, 1982, Saunders.)

Figure 6-24 Hypertensive heart disease. Lateral projection of chest shows prominence of left ventricle *(arrows).*

Figure 6-25 Hypertensive heart disease. Generalized tortuosity and elongation of ascending aorta *(open arrows)* and descending aorta *(solid arrows).*

Figure 6-26   Calcification in walls of aneurysms of lower abdominal aorta and both common iliac arteries *(arrows)*. Of incidental note is calcified uterine fibroid *(arrowhead)* in pelvis. (From Eisenberg R: *Gastrointestinal radiology: a pattern approach*, Philadelphia, 1990, Lippincott.)

Radiographic appearance

Although plain abdominal radiographs can demonstrate curvilinear calcification in the wall of an aneurysm (Figure 6-26), ultrasound is the modality of choice for detection of an abdominal aortic aneurysm. The sonographic definition of aneurysmal dilatation of the abdominal aorta is an enlargement of the structure to a diameter greater than 3 cm. Ultrasound can demonstrate an intraluminal clot (Figure 6-27, *A*), and the noninvasive nature of ultrasound permits an evaluation of the enlargement of an aneurysm on serial studies.

CT angiography (CTA) and MRA also can demonstrate the location and extent of an aneurysm, and these modalities have begun to replace catheter angiography. CTA can identify a retroperitoneal hematoma secondary to leaking or acute rupture of the aneurysm. With helical CT, three-dimensional reformation permits demonstration of the abdominal aorta in multiple planes, improving visualization of the origin of the aneurysm as well as its relationship to the renal arteries (see Figure 6-27, *B*). MRA may be the better choice if the patient has depressed renal function, because the contrast agent used is not nephrotoxic.

The major value of arteriography in patients with abdominal aortic aneurysm is as a presurgical road map to define the extent of the lesion and whether the renal arteries or other major branches are involved. Because the lumen of an aneurysm may be filled with clot, aortography often produces an underestimation of the extent of aneurysmal dilatation.

Figure 6-27   Abdominal aortic aneurysm. **A,** Ultrasound shows large aneurysm with echogenic thrombus *(t)* filling the outer margins of the aorta, creating a false lumen 2.25 cm in diameter. **B,** CT axial scan of an abdominal aortic aneurysm in another patient shows a low-density thrombus *(t)* surrounding a blood-filled lumen *(L)*. The wall of the aneurysm contains high-density calcification *(arrows)*. **C,** CT coronal reconstruction of third patient shows an abdominal aortic aneurysm beginning below the renal arteries and extending below the iliac bifurcation.

Figure 6-28 MR image of aortic aneurysm. Transverse scan with cardiac gating permits differentiation of large mural thrombus *(arrow)* from signal void of rapidly flowing intraluminal blood. *aa,* Ascending aorta; *da,* descending aorta; *svc,* superior vena cava. (From Thoeni RF, Margulis AR: In Eisenberg RL, editor: *Diagnostic imaging: an algorithmic approach,* Philadelphia, 1988, Lippincott.)

Figure 6-29 CT angiography of an abdominal aortic stent placed for an abdominal aortic aneurysm. Posterior perspective demonstrates the stent placed in the aorta and a second stent placed in the right iliac artery.

In the chest, CT after the intravenous injection of contrast material is the most efficient technique for demonstrating the size and extent of an aortic aneurysm and for differentiating this vascular lesion from a solid mediastinal mass. Unlike aortography, CT is relatively noninvasive and can directly identify an intraluminal thrombus (seen as a soft-tissue density separating the contrast-filled portion of the lumen from the aortic wall), which can only be inferred on contrast examination (see Figure 6-27, *B* and *C*). CT can also demonstrate aortic mural calcification and effects of the aneurysm on adjacent structures, such as displacement of the mediastinum or bone erosion. Because of its ability to demonstrate flowing blood as a signal void, and clot as a heterogeneous collection of signal intensities, MRI can provide information about an aneurysm that is comparable to that obtained from CT without the need for intravenous contrast material (Figure 6-28).

Treatment

An abdominal aortic aneurysm may require surgical graft placement to maintain circulation to the inferior part of the abdomen and lower extremity. Currently, a patient may be a candidate for percutaneous stent placement (Figure 6-29) to strengthen the abdominal aorta and prevent rupture and growth of the aneurysm.

Traumatic rupture of the aorta

Traumatic rupture of the aorta is a potentially fatal complication of closed chest trauma (rapid deceleration, blast, compression). In almost all cases the aortic tear occurs just distal to the left subclavian artery at the site of the ductus arteriosus.

Radiographic appearance

On plain chest radiographs, hemorrhage into the mediastinum causes widening of the mediastinal silhouette and loss of a discrete aortic knob shadow. Associated rib or sternal fractures may be apparent. However, because nonspecific mediastinal widening is a frequent finding, especially on the supine, AP portable radiographs taken after trauma, other plain film signs are of diagnostic importance (Figure 6-30). These include displacement of an opaque nasogastric tube to the right (because of a hematoma that displaces the esophagus), widening of the right paratracheal stripe (Figure 6-31), and a collection of blood over the apex of the left lung (apical pleural cap sign). Emergency aortography is the definitive examination for the evaluation of possible laceration or rupture of the aorta.

Treatment

Immediate surgical intervention to repair the aortic laceration or rupture is required to prevent morbidity.

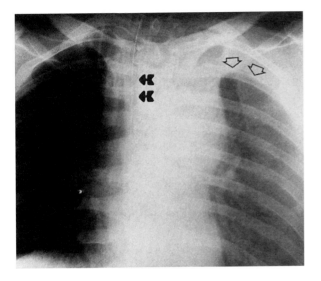

Figure 6-30 Traumatic aneurysm of the aorta. There is widening of the mediastinum and deviation of the nasogastric tube to right *(solid arrows)*. Open arrows point to the collection of fluid over the left apex (apical pleural cap) in this patient who suffered severe blunt chest trauma. (From Fisher RG, Hadlock FP, Ben-Menachem Y: *Radiol Clin North Am* 19:91-112, 1981.)

Dissection of the aorta

Dissection of the aorta is a potentially life-threatening condition in which disruption of the intima (the inner layer) permits blood to enter the wall of the aorta and separate its layers. Most aortic dissections occur in patients with arterial hypertension. Some are a result of trauma, whereas others are attributable to a congenital defect such as Marfan's syndrome. An acute dissection typically causes sudden sharp or excruciating pain in the chest or abdomen. Although the pain passes, death frequently occurs some days later from rupture of the aneurysm into the chest or abdominal cavity.

Most aortic dissections begin as a tear in the intima immediately above the aortic valve. In two thirds of these (type I), the dissection continues into the descending aorta, often extending as far as the level of the iliac bifurcation. In the remainder (type II), the dissection is limited to the ascending aorta and stops at the origin of the innominate artery. In type III disease, the dissection begins in the thoracic aorta distal to the subclavian artery and extends for a variable distance proximally and distally to the original site.

Radiographic appearance

On plain chest radiographs, aortic dissection causes progressive widening of the aortic shadow, which

Figure 6-31 Traumatic aneurysm of the aorta. **A,** Supine chest radiograph in a patient with blunt chest trauma shows thickening of the right paratracheal stripe *(arrows)*, which measures 1 cm in width. **B,** Aortogram demonstrates pseudoaneurysm at the level of the aortic isthmus *(arrows)*. Arrowhead indicates intimal flap. (From Woodring JH, Pulmano CM, Stevens RK: The right paratracheal stripe in blunt chest trauma. *Radiology* 143:605-608, 1982.)

may have an irregular or wavy outer border (Figure 6-32) that most likely represents the site of origin of the dissection. However, this is a nonspecific appearance and a definite diagnosis of dissection must be made on the basis of aortography or CT. In the patient with a suspected acute dissection of the thoracic aorta, aortography is the procedure of choice. The diagnosis of aortic dissection depends on the demonstration of two channels separated by a thin radiolucent intimal flap (Figure 6-33). The false channel may be filled with clot and impossible to opacify with contrast material. In this case, the diagnosis can be made by demonstration of narrowing and compression of the true channel. When both

Figure 6-32 Aortic dissection. Plain chest radiograph shows diffuse widening of descending aorta with irregular, wavy outer border *(arrows)*. (From Ovenfors CO, Godwin JD: In Eisenberg RL, editor: *Diagnostic imaging: an algorithmic approach,* Philadelphia, 1988, Lippincott.)

Figure 6-33 Aortic dissection. Aortogram demonstrates thin radiolucent intimal flap *(arrows)* separating true and false aortic channels.

true and false lumina fill with contrast material, it is important to demonstrate the distal reentry point where the false lumen joins the true lumen. If the dissection extends below the diaphragm, arteriography can provide presurgical information about which major vessel branches from the aorta are blocked and which remain patent.

In the patient in whom nonacute aortic dissection is being considered in the differential diagnosis of chest pain, CT and MRI offer low-risk alternative diagnostic methods to aortography. CT demonstrates an aortic dissection as a double channel with an intimal flap. With dynamic scanning and the rapid injection of a bolus of contrast material, differential filling of the true and false channels can be observed as with aortography (Figure 6-34). The major limitation of CT in the patient with suspected acute dissection is that only a single level can be evaluated on a given slice, as opposed to the rapid series of images covering a large portion of the aorta that can be obtained with aortography. With the development of helical CT, multiplane images are available to quickly visualize the classic double-barrel aorta and the linear filling defect within the aortic lumen.

The high contrast between rapidly flowing blood, vessel wall, and adjacent soft-tissue structures permits identification of vessels by MRI without the need for intravenous injection of contrast material. This technique can demonstrate aortic dissections and show their extent. The intimal flap is usually detected as a linear, medium-signal-intensity structure separating the true and false lumina (Figure 6-35). Rapidly flowing blood in these lumina appears as a signal void. If the false lumen is thrombosed, or even if it is open but the flow is slow, the intimal flap may not be visualized. In this situation, aortic dissection is difficult to differentiate from an aortic aneurysm with mural thrombus, and aortography may be required to make this distinction.

Treatment

Proximal aortic dissections are fatal if not immediately treated surgically (by graft placement). Many other dissections require only medical management (80% survival rate).

Atherosclerosis

Arteriosclerosis occurs when arteries become marked by thickening, hardening, and loss of elasticity in the arterial wall. Atherosclerosis is one form of arteriosclerosis. The major cause of vascular disease of the extremities is atherosclerosis, in which fatty deposits called plaques develop in the intima and produce progressive narrowing and often complete occlusion of large and medium-size arteries. In the abdomen, the

Figure 6-34 CT image of aortic dissection. The ascending aorta is dilated and has a radiolucent intimal flap *(arrow).* The descending aorta demonstrates a much larger tear and hemorrhage *(h)* surrounding the aorta.

Figure 6-36 Atherosclerosis. Lateral projection of chest demonstrates calcification of anterior and posterior walls of ascending aorta *(arrows).* Descending thoracic aorta is tortuous.

Figure 6-35 MR image of aortic dissection. Axial scan at level of main and right pulmonary arteries clearly shows intimal flap *(arrow)* in descending aorta. (From Ovenfors CO, Godwin JD: In Eisenberg RL, editor: *Diagnostic imaging: an algorithmic approach,* Philadelphia, 1988, Lippincott.)

disease primarily involves the aorta and the common iliac arteries, often sparing the external iliac vessels. In the lower extremities, atherosclerotic narrowing most commonly affects the superficial femoral artery just above the knee. Plaque formation and luminal narrowing often involve the coronary and cerebral arteries, thus decreasing the blood flow to the heart muscle and the brain and leading to a myocardial infarction or stroke (cerebrovascular accident).

Radiographic appearance

Atherosclerotic plaques often calcify and appear on plain radiographs as irregularly distributed densities along the course of an artery (Figure 6-36). Small vessel calcification, especially in the hands and feet, is often seen in patients with accelerated arteriosclerosis, especially those with diabetes mellitus.

Doppler ultrasound is an effective and preferred noninvasive technique for screening patients with clinically suspected peripheral arteriosclerotic disease. Color Doppler demonstrates the presence of atherosclerotic plaques and assesses the degree of luminal stenosis. Definitive diagnosis requires arteriographic demonstration of the peripheral vascular tree. Evidence of arteriosclerosis includes diffuse vascular narrowing, irregularity of the lumen, and filling defects. In patients with severe stenosis or obstruction, arteriography demonstrates the degree and source of collateral circulation and the status of the vessels distal to an area of narrowing (Figure 6-37). As MRA evolves, it may become the standard for imaging, replacing catheter angiography. Currently, the two-dimensional time-of-flight method is preferred for evaluation of the pelvis and thighs.

Treatment

Percutaneous transluminal angioplasty using a balloon catheter is now a recognized procedure for the alleviation of symptoms of peripheral ischemia in patients with arteriosclerosis (Figure 6-38). In addition, a stent may be placed to aid in keeping the vessel open. The results of this interventional approach (95% success for the iliac artery and 50% to 60% for the thigh and calf) are similar to those of bypass grafting, but with a much lower morbidity rate. It is of special value in patients who are extremely ill and those who would not benefit from reconstructive arterial surgery.

Figure 6-37   Bilateral atherosclerotic occlusion of superficial femoral arteries. Arteriogram demonstrates occlusion of both distal superficial femoral arteries *(open arrows)* with reconstitution by collateral vessels *(solid arrows).*

Figure 6-38   Percutaneous transluminal angioplasty of right external iliac artery stenosis. **A,** Initial film in patient with claudication demonstrates narrowing of proximal right external iliac artery *(arrow).* **B,** After angioplasty, there is relief of stenosis *(arrow)* and of symptoms. (From Waltman AC: In Athanasoulis CA et al, editors: *Interventional radiology,* Philadelphia, 1982, Saunders.)

Thrombosis and embolism

The blood-clotting mechanism is the major protective device of the body in response to the escape of blood from a vessel (hemorrhage). This same mechanism can occur in intact blood vessels, leading to the development of an intravascular clot called a **thrombus.** Three factors lead to the development of intravascular thrombosis. Clots tend to form where blood flow is slow and thus develop much more commonly in veins than in arteries. Thrombi occur especially in areas of stasis (slow circulation) in patients who are inactive or immobilized, as after abdominal surgery.

Changes in the wall of blood vessels can lead to thrombosis. Normally, the inner wall of a blood vessel has a very smooth lining (endothelium), and platelets cannot stick, or adhere, to it. However, when the endothelium is destroyed by injury or inflammation, platelets rapidly adhere to the rough spot, and a clot begins to form from the blood as it flows past. Arteriosclerosis is the major cause of endothelial irregularity and subsequent thrombosis. Nodules of vegetation on heart valves caused by rheumatic heart disease are also important predisposing factors for thrombus formation.

Changes in the blood itself can lead to thrombosis. A low level of oxygen within the blood, as in some forms of heart disease, forces the body to compensate by increasing the number of red blood cells (polycythemia). This causes the blood to become more viscous and increases the risk of thrombosis. Changes in the clotting and fibrinolytic mechanisms also may increase the risk of thrombus formation.

Once a thrombus is formed, it may follow one of three courses. The thrombus may contract or become canalized so that blood can once again flow through the lumen. The thrombus may continually enlarge or become converted into fibrous tissue, resulting in permanent occlusion of the vessel. A potentially catastrophic event is the production of an **embolus,** which refers to part or all of a thrombus that becomes detached from the vessel wall and enters the bloodstream. Embolization is especially likely to occur if there is infected tissue around the thrombus or if there is a sudden movement caused by rough handling of the involved area. An embolism may lodge at any of several points, depending on the size of the vessels through which it travels. Since veins become larger as they approach the heart, an embolism arising from a thrombus in a leg vein flows easily to the heart and typically gets stuck in a pulmonary artery (pulmonary embolism). An embolism arising from a mitral valve damaged by rheumatic heart disease flows through the left ventricle and aorta and lodges in a smaller artery in the brain, kidney, or other organ. A septic embolism contains infected material from pyogenic bacteria, whereas tumor emboli are groups of cancer cells that have invaded a vein, become detached, and are then carried to the lungs or other organs where they form metastases. Fat emboli are the result of trauma, especially leg fractures, in which marrow fat enters torn peripheral veins and is trapped by the pulmonary circulation. An air embolism refers to bubbles of air introduced into a vein during surgery, trauma, or an improperly administered intravenous injection.

Regardless of its type or source, an embolism blocks the vascular lumen and cuts off the blood supply to the organ or parts supplied by that artery. The effect of an embolism depends on the size of the embolus and on the extent of collateral circulation, which can bring blood to an affected part by an alternate route.

Radiographic appearance

Acute embolic occlusion of an artery most commonly affects the lower extremities. The success of therapy depends on the rapid recognition of the clinical problem and the institution of appropriate treatment. Arteriography is the procedure of choice to confirm the clinical diagnosis and to demonstrate the extent of occlusion, the degree of collateral circulation, and the condition of the distal vessels. Embolic occlusion typically appears as an abrupt termination of the contrast column, along with a proximal curved margin reflecting the nonopaque embolus protruding into the contrast-filled lumen (Figure 6-39). In acute occlusion, there is usually little if any evidence of collateral circulation.

Treatment

Anticoagulants such as heparin and Coumadin are often used to prevent intravascular clotting. Heparin prevents platelets from sticking together and to the vessel wall, helping prevent thrombus formation. Coumadin acts by antagonizing the action of vitamin K, which is necessary for blood clotting. However, these medications also interfere with the person's normal ability to stop bleeding and may lead to severe hemorrhage from relatively minor trauma or to potentially fatal bleeding in the brain and gastrointestinal tract. Recent reports have suggested the value of aspirin to prevent intravascular clotting because of its inhibition of platelet aggregation.

Although emergency surgery to remove the embolus (embolectomy) has been the traditional treatment

Figure 6-39   Acute embolic occlusion of left renal artery. There is abrupt termination of contrast column *(arrow)*. Note irregular infrarenal aortic contour, which represents atherosclerotic disease.

A

B

Figure 6-40   Streptokinase therapy for acute arterial occlusion. **A,** After angioplasty of right external iliac artery, there was loss of right common femoral pulse. Repeat arteriogram from left femoral approach shows complete occlusion of external iliac artery at its origin. **B,** After 8 hours of streptokinase administration, arteriogram demonstrates lysis of thrombus and reestablishment of lumen. One year after angioplasty, patient had normal femoral pulse and patent artery. (From Katzen BT, van Breda A: Low dose streptokinase in the treatment of arterial occlusions. *AJR Am J Roentgenol* 136:1171-1178, 1981.)

for acute arterial occlusion, the intraarterial infusion of streptokinase by means of a catheter placed immediately proximal to the occlusion is becoming a more common alternative therapy, especially in patients who are poor surgical risks (Figure 6-40). The tissue plasminogen activator (TPA) Activase, produced by recombinant DNA technology, has been administered intravenously to lyse thrombi obstructing coronary arteries in the treatment of acute myocardial infarction.

Summary of Findings for Acquired Vascular Disease

DISORDER	LOCATION	RADIOGRAPHIC APPEARANCE	TREATMENT
Coronary artery disease	Blood vessels supplying the heart	Chest film—vessel calcifications CT—decreased attenuation in affected myocardial tissue MRI—increased T2-weighted signal intensity in affected myocardial tissue NM—focal defects (cold spots) IVUS—vessel size and length of lesion Angiogram—strictures or narrowings present as filling defects	Surgery—bypass graft procedure Interventional—PTCA, PTCA with stent placement, percutaneous atherectomy
Congestive heart failure	Insufficient cardiac output	Chest film—C/T ratio greater than 50% —Left sided: cardiac enlargement, pulmonary edema, and pulmonary effusion —Right sided: widened mediastinum and elevated right hemidiaphragm	Oxygen Diuretics Digoxin
Pulmonary edema	Extravascular fluid in the lungs	Chest film—vascular markings not sharp Butterfly pattern	Treat cause of edema
Hypertension	Increased pressure in the systemic vascular system	Arteriography—detects renovascular lesions Radionuclide renogram—noninvasive screening to demonstrate lesions	Drug therapy to control vascular volume and heart rates Interventional—PTA with or without stent
Hypertensive heart disease	Left ventricle enlargement	Chest film—enlarged left ventricle, inferior displacement of cardiac apex, aortic tortuosity	Therapy for high blood pressure and/or congestive heart failure
Aneurysm	Dilation of artery; fusiform or saccular	Radiograph—calcification outlining vessel US—abdominal aortic enlargement, diameter greater than 3 cm CTA—aneurysm extent and size, evidence of leak or rupture by retroperitoneal hematoma MRA—same as CTA, but used when iodinated contrast agents are contraindicated	Surgical graft placement Percutaneous stent placement
Traumatic aortic rupture	Aortic tear distal to left subclavian artery	Widened mediastinum Deviation of NG tube to right Apical pleural cap	Surgical repair
Aortic dissection	Disruption of aortic intima	Chest film—widening of aortic shadow, which may be irregular CT—double-barrel channel with linear filling defect within lumen (intimal flap) MRI—intimal flap causes medium-intensity signal separating true and false lumina; blood flow causes signal void	Proximal or continuous dissection—immediate surgical repair Other dissections—medical management

CTA, CT angiography; *IVUS,* intravascular ultrasound; *MRA,* MR angiography; *NM,* nuclear medicine; *PTA,* percutaneous transluminal angioplasty; *US,* ultrasound.

Continued

Summary of Findings for Acquired Vascular Disease—cont'd

DISORDER	LOCATION	RADIOGRAPHIC APPEARANCE	TREATMENT
Atherosclerosis	Plaques develop in the intima of the artery	Radiograph—calcification demonstrating "hardening" of the artery Color Doppler—demonstrates plaque and degree of luminal stenosis MRA—two-dimensional time-of-flight view demonstrates narrowing and flow changes in the pelvis and thighs	PTA with or without stent placement Surgical bypass
Thrombus and embolism	Blockage of a vessel	Arteriography—extent of occlusion, degree of collateral circulation, and distal vessel condition	Surgical removal Medical treatment to reduce thrombus or emboli

CTA, CT angiography; *IVUS,* intravascular ultrasound; *MRA,* MR angiography; *NM,* nuclear medicine; *PTA,* percutaneous transluminal angioplasty; *US,* ultrasound.

■ Valvular Disease

The valves of the heart permit blood to flow in only one direction through the heart. When the valve is closed, a heart chamber fills with blood; when the valve opens, blood can move forward and leave the chamber. There are four heart valves. The **tricuspid valve** separates the right atrium and the right ventricle, and the **mitral valve** separates the left atrium and the left ventricle. The **pulmonary valve** lies between the right ventricle and the pulmonary artery, and the **aortic valve** is situated between the left ventricle and the aorta.

The malfunction of a heart valve alters the normal blood flow through the heart. Too small an opening (stenosis) does not permit sufficient blood flow. In contrast, too large an opening or failure of the valve to properly close permits backflow of blood (regurgitation) and the condition of valvular insufficiency. Both stenosis and insufficiency of valves cause heart murmurs with characteristic sounds that indicate the nature of the defect. Although valvular heart disease once invariably forced a patient to restrict activity and was associated with a limited life span, surgical reconstruction or replacement of a diseased valve (Figure 6-41) can offer a patient the prospect of a normal life.

Rheumatic heart disease

Rheumatic fever is an autoimmune disease that results from a reaction of the patient's antibodies against antigens from a previous streptococcal infection. The disease is much less common today because of the frequent use of antibiotics to treat streptococcal throat or ear infections. The symptoms of rheumatic fever (fever, inflamed and painful joints, rash) typically develop several weeks after the streptococcal infection.

The major damage of rheumatic fever is to the valves of the heart, most frequently the mitral and aortic valves. Indeed, it is the major cause of acquired cardiac valve disease. The allergic response causes inflammation of the valves. Deposits of blood platelets and fibrin from blood flowing over the valve produce small nodules **(vegetations)** along the margin of the valve cusps. The thickened valves may stick together, so that the valvular opening remains permanently narrowed **(stenosis)** rather than opening properly when blood flows through. In contrast, fibrous scarring may cause retraction of the valve cusps so that the cusps are unable to meet when the valve tries to close; this is **insufficiency,** and blood leaks through the valve when it should be closed.

Treatment

Prevention of rheumatic fever and subsequent heart disease by treating the streptococcal infection with a full course of antibiotic therapy is the best approach. If the infection progresses into rheumatic heart disease, antibiotics, antiinflammatory drugs, and restricted activity are the appropriate interventions.

Mitral stenosis

Stenosis of the mitral valve, almost always a complication of rheumatic disease, results from diffuse thickening of the valve by fibrous tissue, calcific deposits, or both.

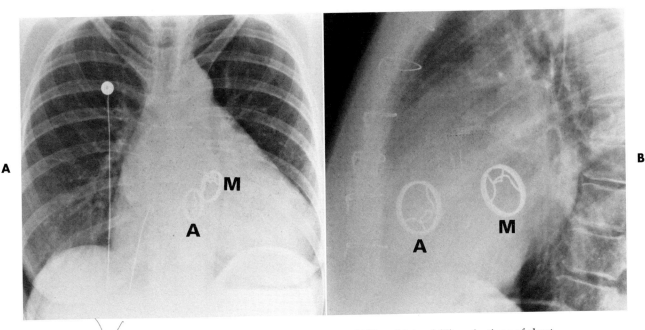

Figure 6-41 Prosthetic aortic and mitral valves. Frontal **(A)** and lateral **(B)** projections of chest show anteromedially located prosthetic aortic valve *(A)* and posterolaterally situated prosthetic mitral valve *(M)*.

Figure 6-42 Mitral stenosis. Frontal **(A)** and lateral **(B)** projections of chest demonstrate cardiomegaly with enlargement of right ventricle and left atrium. Right ventricular enlargement causes obliteration of retrosternal air space, whereas left atrial enlargement produces convexity of upper left border of heart *(arrow)*.

Radiographic appearance

The obstruction of blood flow from the left atrium into the left ventricle during diastole causes increased pressure in the left atrium and enlargement of this chamber (Figure 6-42). The enlarged left atrium produces a characteristic anterior impression on and posterior displacement of the barium-filled esophagus that is best seen on lateral and right anterior oblique projections. Other radiographic signs of left atrial enlargement include posterior

Figure 6-43 Left atrial calcification in mitral stenosis. Lateral projection with barium in esophagus shows enlargement of left atrium and calcification of the wall of its chamber *(arrows)*. (From Vickers SCW et al: *Radiology* 72:569-575, 1959.)

Figure 6-44 Echocardiogram of mitral stenosis. There is thickening of the mitral valve with decreased slope *(arrows)*.

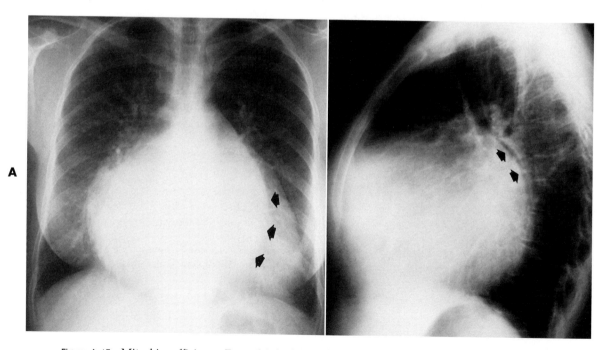

Figure 6-45 Mitral insufficiency. Frontal **(A)** and lateral **(B)** projections of chest demonstrate gross cardiomegaly with enlargement of left atrium and left ventricle. Note striking double-contour configuration *(arrows)* on frontal film and elevation of left main-stem bronchus *(arrows)* on lateral film, characteristic signs of left atrial enlargement.

displacement of the left main-stem bronchus, widening of the tracheal bifurcation (carina), and a characteristic "double-contour" configuration caused by the projection of the enlarged left atrium through the normal right atrial silhouette. The increased left atrial pressure is transmitted to the pulmonary veins and produces the appearance of chronic venous congestion.

Calcification of the mitral valve or left atrial wall (Figure 6-43), best demonstrated by fluoroscopy, can develop in patients with long-standing severe mitral stenosis. A thrombus may form in the dilated left atrium and be the source of emboli to the brain or elsewhere in the systemic circulation.

Echocardiography is the most sensitive and most specific noninvasive method for diagnosing mitral stenosis (Figure 6-44). Echocardiography demonstrates chamber enlargement or wall thickening and permits measurement of the valvular orifices. More recently, cine MRI has been used to demonstrate and quantitate the abnormal pattern of flow between the left atrium and the left ventricle in mitral stenosis without the use of contrast agents.

Mitral insufficiency

Although most often caused by rheumatic heart disease, mitral insufficiency may also be caused by the rupture of the chordae tendineae or by the dysfunction of the papillary muscles that are attached to the underside of the valve cusps and normally prevent them from swinging up into the atrium when the ventricles contract. Regurgitation of blood into the left atrium during ventricular systole causes overfilling and dilatation of this chamber, which leads to a decrease in ventricular stroke volume and cardiac output.

In most cases, the left atrium is considerably larger in mitral insufficiency than in mitral stenosis (Figure 6-45); occasionally, an enormous left atrium can form both the right and left borders of the heart on frontal projections. An increased volume of blood flowing from the dilated left atrium to the left ventricle in diastole increases the left ventricular workload and leads to dilatation and hypertrophy of this chamber. CHF, pulmonary congestion, and pulmonary hypertension may result. This causes downward displacement of the cardiac apex and rounding of the lower left border of the heart.

Treatment of mitral stenosis and insufficiency

Surgical valvular replacement or correction of the stenosis may be performed to correct flow insufficiency. CHF resulting from stenosis or insufficiency may require treatment.

Aortic stenosis

Aortic stenosis may be caused by rheumatic heart disease, a congenital valvular deformity (especially of a bicuspid valve), or a degenerative process of aging (idiopathic calcific stenosis). The obstruction to left ventricular outflow in aortic stenosis increases the workload of the left ventricle.

Initially, this causes left ventricular hypertrophy without dilatation, which produces only some rounding of the cardiac apex on frontal chest radiographs and slight backward displacement on lateral projections. The overall size of the heart remains within normal limits until left ventricular failure develops. Significant aortic stenosis is usually associated with lateral bulging (poststenotic dilatation) of the ascending aorta caused by the jet of blood forced under high pressure through the narrowed valve (Figure 6-46). Aortic valve calcification, best demonstrated on fluoroscopic examination, is a common finding and indicates that the aortic stenosis is severe (Figure 6-47).

Aortic insufficiency

Although most commonly caused by rheumatic heart disease, aortic insufficiency may be attributable to syphilis, infective endocarditis, dissecting aneurysm, or Marfan's syndrome. Reflux of blood from the aorta during diastole causes volume overloading of the left ventricle and dilatation of this chamber.

Radiographic appearance

Aortic insufficiency causes downward, lateral, and posterior displacement of the cardiac apex (Figure 6-48). Pronounced left ventricular dilatation causes relative mitral insufficiency, which leads to left atrial enlargement and signs of pulmonary edema.

Treatment of aortic stenosis and aortic insufficiency

Congestive heart failure should be treated if the patient is symptomatic. Surgical valvular replacement or repair to correct stenosis can reestablish correct pressures and flow.

Infective endocarditis

Infective endocarditis refers to the development of nodules or vegetations forming on heart valves caused by deposits of bacteria or fungi. Unlike the smaller nodules in rheumatic fever, the vegetations of infective endocarditis are filled with bacteria and tend to break apart easily (they are friable) to enter the bloodstream and form septic emboli that travel to the brain, kidney, lung, or other vital

Figure 6-46   Aortic stenosis. **A,** Frontal projection shows downward displacement of cardiac apex with poststenotic dilatation of ascending aorta *(arrowheads).* Aortic knob and descending aorta *(arrows)* are normal. **B,** On lateral projection in another patient, bulging of the lower half of the posterior cardiac silhouette causes a broad indentation on the barium-filled esophagus *(arrows).*

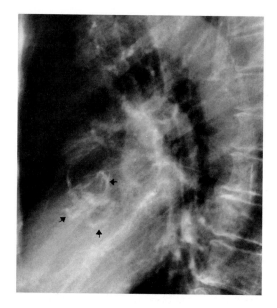

Figure 6-47   Aortic stenosis. Calcification in three leaflets of the aortic valve *(arrows).*

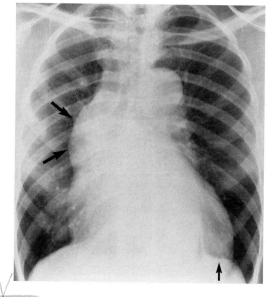

Figure 6-48   Aortic insufficiency. Frontal chest radiograph shows left ventricular enlargement with downward and lateral displacement of the cardiac apex. Notice that the cardiac shadow extends below the dome of the left hemidiaphragm *(small arrow).* Ascending aorta is strikingly dilated *(large arrows),* suggestive of some underlying aortic stenosis.

Summary of Findings for Valvular Disease

DISORDER	LOCATION	RADIOGRAPHIC APPEARANCE	TREATMENT
Rheumatic heart disease	Most frequently in mitral and aortic valves	None	Prevention—antibiotics for streptococcal infections Therapy—antibiotics, antiinflammatory drugs, and restricted activity
Mitral stenosis	Mitral valve	Left atrium enlargement Lateral, RAO—posterior displacement of esophagus, posterior displacement of left main bronchus, calcification of valves Echocardiography—chamber enlargement, wall thickness, and size of valvular orifices Cine MRI—demonstrates and quantitates abnormal flow pattern Cardiomegaly—enlarged left atrium and left ventricle	Surgical—valvular replacement, correction of stenosis Treat for congestive heart failure if needed
Mitral insufficiency	Valve dysfunction, rupture, or muscular dysfunction		
Aortic stenosis	Obstruction of flow exiting the heart	Enlargement of left ventricle Rounding of cardiac apex Posterior displacement of cardiac apex in lateral projection Lateral bulging of ascending aorta Aortic valve calcification	
Aortic insufficiency	Reflux of blood causing volume overload of left ventricle	Cardiac apex—inferior, lateral, and posterior displacement	
Infective endocarditis	Nodules on heart valves	Echocardiography—shaggy echoes produced by irregular thickening of affected valves Electron-beam CT—vegetations in valve, valvular calcifications, distorted orifices	Bacterial—treat with antibiotics Surgically replace severely damaged valves

RAO, Right anterior oblique.

Figure 6-49 Infective endocarditis. Echocardiogram demonstrates vegetations as masses of shaggy echoes producing irregular thickening of the aortic valve *(arrows)*.

Figure 6-50 Pericardial effusion. Globular enlargement of cardiac silhouette.

organs. Emboli lodging in the skin may cause rupture of small blood vessels and characteristic tiny hemorrhagic red spots (petechiae).

Radiographic appearance

Plain radiography is of little value in patients with infective endocarditis. The cardiac silhouette may be normal or demonstrate evidence of previous valvular heart disease or CHF. Echocardiography is the only noninvasive procedure that can detect the valvular vegetations that are the hallmark of infective endocarditis. On the echocardiogram, these vegetations appear as masses of shaggy echoes producing an irregular thickening of the affected valves (Figure 6-49). Electron-beam CT demonstrates the vegetations as well as the valvular calcifications, distorted orifices, and possible aneurysms.

Treatment

Antibiotics are taken until there is complete eradication of the bacterial infections. Severely damaged valves must be surgically replaced with artificial valves.

■ Pericardial Effusion

Pericardial effusion refers to the accumulation of fluid within the pericardial space surrounding the heart. The effusion may result from bacteria, viruses, or neoplastic involvement. In some cases, the cause cannot be determined (idiopathic pericardial effu-

sion). Rapid accumulation of effusion interferes with cardiac function because of an increase in pericardial pressure. A slow accumulation of fluid allows the pericardium to expand, so that the pericardial pressure usually remains within the normal range.

Radiographic appearance

Echocardiography is the most effective imaging technique for demonstrating pericardial effusions and has largely replaced other methods. With this modality, a pericardial effusion is seen as a posterior sonolucent collection, and as little as 50 ml of fluid can be detected. Plain chest radiographs, on the other hand, which show a pericardial effusion as an enlargement of the cardiac silhouette (Figure 6-50), require at least 200 ml of fluid to be present before the effusion can be detected. Rapid enlargement of the cardiac silhouette, especially in the absence of pulmonary vascular engorgement indicating CHF, is highly suggestive of pericardial effusion.

Angiocardiography, intravenous carbon dioxide injection, and a pericardial tap with air injection have been used in the past to demonstrate pericardial effusion by showing an excessive distance (greater than 5 mm) between the contrast- or air-filled atrium and the outer border of the cardiac silhouette. CT can detect loculated pericardial effusions (Figure 6-51), whereas MRI may be able to characterize the fluid as serous or hemorrhagic by characteristic changes in the signal intensity. Gated MRI (Figure 6-52) shows a peri-

Summary of Findings for Pericardial Effusion

DISORDER	LOCATION	RADIOGRAPHIC APPEARANCE	TREATMENT
Pericardial effusion	Increased fluid accumulation in pericardial sac	Chest film—enlargement of cardiac silhouette Echocardiography—posterior sonolucent fluid collection CT—loculated fluid accumulations MRI—differentiates serous from hemorrhagic fluid	Pericardiocentesis Pericardiectomy Administration of drugs into pericardial sac

A   **B**

Figure 6-51 CT images demonstrating pericardial effusion. **A,** Heart is seen with a dark halo surrounded by fluid. **B,** A CT-guided catheter was placed in this patient for drainage.

Figure 6-52 MR image of pericardial effusion. Pericardium *(arrows)* is displaced away from the heart by a huge pericardial effusion that has a very low signal intensity. Effect of gravity is seen in the posterior location of both pericardial and right pleural effusions. (From Miller SW et al: Cardiac magnetic resonance imaging: the Massachusetts General Hospital experience. *Radiol Clin North Am* 23:745-764, 1985.)

Figure 6-53   Pericardial effusion. Echocardiogram demonstrates an apical four-chamber heart image with fluid around the heart *(f)* producing back-wall enhancement *(arrow)*. *LA,* Left atria; *LV,* left ventricle; *RA,* right atrium; *RV,* right ventricle.

Figure 6-54   Deep vein thrombosis. **A,** Initial contrast venogram demonstrates early nonocclusive thrombus extending from valve cusp. Arrow points to thrombus tail, the portion most likely to embolize. **B,** Subsequent contrast venogram demonstrates growth and proximal extension of thrombus, which has resulted in occlusion of popliteal vein at adductor hiatus. (From Holden RW, Mail JT, Becker GJ: In Eisenberg RL, editor: *Diagnostic imaging: an algorithmic approach,* Philadelphia, 1988, Lippincott.)

cardial effusion as a region of decreased signal intensity between the myocardium and the fat on the surface of the parietal pericardium (which is usually invisible when it is in direct contact with the heart). However, echocardiography has effectively replaced these invasive techniques (Figure 6-53).

Treatment

The treatment depends on the cause. Pericardiocentesis is performed to remove fluid buildup, and insertion of a drain may be required. If the pericardial effusion recurs, a pericardiectomy may be necessary. An interventional technique includes administration of drugs into the pericardial sac.

■ Venous Disease

Deep venous thrombosis

Deep venous thrombosis (DVT), which primarily involves the lower extremities, is the major source of potentially fatal pulmonary embolism. Precipitating factors in the development of venous thrombosis include trauma, bacterial infection, prolonged bed rest, and oral contraceptives. At times, DVT may be the earliest symptom of an unsuspected malignancy of the pancreas, lung, or gastrointestinal system.

Radiographic appearance

A precise diagnosis of deep vein thrombosis requires contrast venography, which can demonstrate the major venous channels and their tributaries from the foot to the inferior vena cava. During venography, the patient's leg should not be massaged to decrease edema. If DVT exists, the pressure applied could cause a thrombus to break free, becoming an embolus. The identification of a constant filling defect, representing the actual thrombus, is conclusive evidence of deep vein thrombosis (Figure 6-54). Venographic findings that are highly suggestive of, although not conclusive for, the diagnosis of DVT include the abrupt ending of the opaque column in a vein, the nonfilling of one or more veins that are normally opacified, and extensive collateral venous circulation.

Because venography is an invasive technique, other modalities have been developed for detecting DVT. Duplex color Doppler ultrasound, which demonstrates changes in the velocity of venous blood flow with 95% accuracy, is now the preferred initial imaging modality. It is of special value in demonstrating thrombotic occlusion of major venous pathways in the popliteal and femoral regions. Ultrasound demonstrates lack of compressibility of the vein, an indication of the presence of a thrombus (Figure 6-55). Color Doppler allows visualization of

A **B**

Figure 6-55 Doppler image of deep vein thrombosis. The left leg was swollen with some discoloration. The deep venous system shows abnormal intraluminal echoes involving the distal superficial femoral vein (SFV) **(A)** and popliteal vein **(B);** both areas show no compressibility, which is consistent with a diagnosis of thrombosis.

the intraluminal thrombus itself as well as the characteristic changes in spontaneous flow that occur because of obstruction. However, an abnormal Doppler ultrasound examination is not specific for thrombosis, since similar changes in venous blood flow may be caused by CHF, extensive leg edema, local soft-tissue masses, and decreased inflow of arterial blood into the extremity.

Treatment

An anticoagulant drug is prescribed to prevent the formation of more thrombi. The patient receives an intravenous thrombolytic agent to lyse the already formed clot. If the lower extremity is involved, many recommend bed rest to prevent the possibility of emboli.

Varicose veins

Varicose veins are dilated, elongated, and tortuous vessels that most commonly involve the superficial veins of the leg just under the skin (Figure 6-56). If the venous dilatation becomes extreme, the valves that normally prevent backflow of blood because of gravity become incompetent and cease to function, thus increasing the volume of blood in these slow-flowing vessels.

Although heredity plays some role in the development of varicose veins, the underlying cause is increased pressure in an affected vein. Varicose veins can be an occupational hazard for people who stand or sit for long periods. Normally, the action of leg muscles helps move blood upward toward the heart from one venous valve to the next. If this "milking action" of the muscles is absent, the blood puts pressure

Figure 6-56   Varicose veins. Lower extremity venogram shows multiple tortuous, dilated venous structures.

Figure 6-57   Varicose veins. Multiple round and oval calcifications in soft tissues (phleboliths) represent calcified thrombi, some of which have characteristic lucent centers *(black arrows)*. Extensive new bone formation along the medial aspect of the tibial shaft *(white arrows)* is caused by long-standing venous stasis.

Summary of Findings for Venous Disease

DISORDER	LOCATION	RADIOGRAPHIC APPEARANCE	TREATMENT
Deep venous thrombosis	Primarily involves the lower extremities	Venography—constant filling defect or abrupt ending of the opaque column in a vein; nonfilling of one or more veins; extensive collateral venous circulation Color Doppler—visualization of thrombus and flow changes due to obstruction	Anticoagulants to prevent new thrombus formation Thrombolytic to lyse clot Bed rest to decrease possible emboli
Varicose veins	Commonly involve superficial veins of the leg	Venography—demonstrates patency of the deep venous system and degree of collateral circulation from the superficial to deep veins	Therapeutic—weight reduction; elevation of legs; support hose and exercise Surgical—vein stripping or cauterization; removing superficial veins

on the closed valves and the thin walls of the veins, resulting in venous dilatation, incompetence of the valves, and stasis of blood in the stagnant lower extremity veins. Increased pressure on a vein can also be attributable to a pregnant uterus or a pelvic tumor.

Stasis of blood within varicose veins may lead to the development of phleboliths, calcified clots within a vein that appear radiographically as rounded densities that often contain lucent centers (Figure 6-57). Chronic venous stasis may also lead to periosteal new bone formation along the tibial and fibular shafts and the development of plaquelike calcifications in the chronically congested subcutaneous tissues. The poor venous flow can lead to the development of superficial ulcers, and the distended veins can rupture, causing hemorrhage into the surrounding tissues.

Radiographic appearance

Although the diagnosis of varicose veins is primarily based on the clinical observation of the multiple bluish nodules just under the skin, venography is of value in demonstrating the patency of the deep venous system and the degree of collateral circulation from the superficial to the deep veins, especially if there is consideration of surgical intervention (tying off and removing the superficial veins). After the application of a tourniquet to occlude superficial flow, the peripheral injection of contrast material opacifies the deep venous system. Filling of the superficial veins indicates that the perforating veins above the level of the tourniquet are incompetent.

Treatment

Treatment consists of various ways to decrease the pressure in the lower extremities. If the varices are related to excess weight, weight reduction helps alleviate symptoms; if they are related to standing all day, then elevating the legs to assist blood flow return is recommended. Support hose and exercise to strengthen contractibility of the leg muscles may also aid in blood flow return. When nonsurgical treatment is not successful, vein stripping or cauterization may be performed.

QUESTIONS

1. Heart rate is controlled by the _____ nervous system.
   A. Psychogenic   C. Peripheral
   B. Central   D. Autonomic

2. The _____ valve is located between the left atrium and the left ventricle, whereas the _____ valve is located between the right atrium and right ventricle.
   I. Tricuspid
   II. Mitral
   III. Pulmonary
   IV. Aortic
   A. II, I   C. IV, I
   B. III, I   D. I, II

3. The general circulation of the body is termed the _____ circulation.
   A. Pulmonary   C. General
   B. Systemic   D. Autonomic

4. The contracting phase of the heart is termed _____, whereas the relaxation phase is termed _____.
   I. Autonomic
   II. Diastole
   III. Systemic
   IV. Systole
   A. I, III   C. II, III
   B. II, IV   D. IV, II

5. Contraction of which chamber of the heart forces oxygenated blood into the aorta?
   A. Right atrium   C. Left atrium
   B. Right ventricle   D. Left ventricle

6. Oxygenated blood reaches the heart muscle by way of the _____.
   I. Right coronary artery
   II. Left coronary artery
   III. Left coronary vein
   IV. Right coronary vein
   A. I, III   C. II, I
   B. IV, I   D. II, III

7. The heart has a specialized pacemaker named the _____.
   A. Bundle of His   C. Purkinje fibers
   B. Sinoatrial node   D. Atrioventricular node

8. Which factor(s) lead to coronary artery disease?
   A. Lack of exercise   C. Smoking, high-cholesterol diet
   B. Obesity, hypertension   D. All of the above

9. Temporary oxygen insufficiency to the heart muscle causes severe chest pain termed _____.
   A. Angina pectoris   C. Myocardial pectoris
   B. Myocardial occlusion   D. Angina occlusion

10. Arterial disease caused by fatty deposits on the inner arterial wall is termed _____.
    A. Arteriosclerosis   C. Aneurysm
    B. Myocardial   D. Myocardial
       infarction   ischemia

11. What radiographic procedure is used to determine the presence of coronary artery disease?
    A. Angioplasty   C. Coronary
    B. Chest film   arteriogram
                              D. CT

12. The procedure in which a balloon is used to dilate narrowed coronary arteries is named _____.
    A. Aortocoronary   C. Percutaneous
       bypass   transluminal
    B. Coronary   angioplasty
       arteriography   D. Fluoroscopy

13. Which term refers to an inability of the heart to propel blood at a sufficient rate and volume?
    A. Congestive   C. Valvular disease
       heart failure   D. Valvular stenosis
    B. Pulmonary edema

14. An elevation of the pulmonary venous pressure is the most common cause of _____.
    A. Congestive   C. Valvular disease
       heart failure   D. Valvular stenosis
    B. Pulmonary edema

15. The leading cause of strokes and congestive heart failure is _____.
    A. Hypertension   C. Hypotension
    B. Low blood   D. Cor pulmonale
       pressure

16. A localized bulging or dilatation of an artery is termed _____.
    A. Edema   C. Aneurysm
    B. Effusion   D. Fat emboli

17. What is the modality of choice for demonstration of an abdominal aortic aneurysm?
    A. MRI   C. CT
    B. Ultrasonography   D. Plain film
                                 radiography

18. A congenital narrowing or constriction of the thoracic aorta is referred to as _____.
    A. Embolism   C. Coarctation
    B. Plaque   D. Tetralogy

19. The _____ of the heart is/are the major site of damage from rheumatic fever.
    A. Myocardium   C. Septum
    B. Valves   D. Endocardium

20. The most sensitive and specific noninvasive method of diagnosing mitral stenosis is _____.
    A. Ultrasonography   C. Cardiac
    B. Echocardiography   arteriography
                              D. CT

21. The accumulation of fluid within the pericardial space surrounding the heart is termed _____.
    A. Pericardial   C. Pulmonary edema
       thrombosis   D. Pulmonary
    B. Pericardial   effusion
       effusion

22. The invasive procedure for determining deep vein thrombosis is _____.
    A. Doppler   C. CT
       ultrasound   D. Arteriography
    B. Venography

23. The most accurate screening procedure for assessing renovascular lesions is _____.
    A. Doppler   C. CT
       ultrasound   D. Arteriography
    B. Venography

24. A potentially life-threatening condition that usually begins as a tear in the intima above the aortic valve is an _____.
    A. Aortic stenosis   C. Aortic thrombosis
    B. Aortic coarctation   D. Aortic dissection

BIBLIOGRAPHY

Cooley RN, Schreiber MH: *Radiology of the heart and great vessels*, Baltimore, 1978, Williams & Wilkins.

Mintz G: *Intravenous ultrasound imaging: practical considerations*, Paris Course on Revascularization, 2000, Europa Organization.

Swischuk LE: *Plain film interpretation in congenital heart disease*, Baltimore, 1979, Williams & Wilkins.

CHAPTER 7

Nervous System

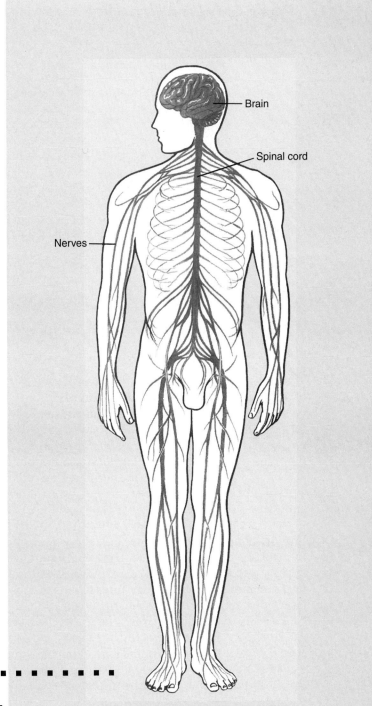

■ Prerequisite Knowledge

The student should have a basic knowledge of the anatomy and physiology of the skull and nervous system. In addition, proper learning and understanding of the material will be facilitated if the student has some clinical experience in skull radiography and film evaluation, including a concept of the newer imaging modalities: computed tomography (CT), CT angiography (CTA), magnetic resonance imaging (MRI), MR angiography (MRA), and positron emission tomography (PET).

■ Goals

To acquaint the student radiographer with the pathophysiology and radiographic manifestations of all of the common and some of the unusual disorders of the skull and nervous system

■ Objectives

1. To understand and be able to define or describe all bold-faced terms in this chapter
2. To be able to describe the physiology of the nervous system
3. To be able to identify anatomic structures on both diagrams and radiographs of the skull and nervous system
4. To be able to describe the various pathologic conditions affecting the skull and nervous system as well as their radiographic manifestations

■ Radiographer Notes

Proper positioning is critical in skull and spine radiography to ensure bilateral symmetry and to permit an evaluation of the complex anatomy and structural relationships. The demonstration of asymmetry or a shift in the normal location of a structure in a patient who is positioned correctly may be indicative of an underlying pathologic condition. Proper positioning and correct angulation of the central ray may allow visualization of otherwise superimposed structures. When evaluating such anatomic areas as the sinuses or facial bones, it is often necessary to place the patient in the erect position (either standing or sitting) and to use a horizontal beam to demonstrate an air–fluid level indicative of underlying inflammatory disease or fracture. If the patient's condition prohibits placement in an erect position, air–fluid levels can be demonstrated only by obtaining a cross-table lateral projection using a horizontal beam with the patient in a dorsal decubitus position.

Exposure factors should produce a scale of contrast that provides maximal detail (definition), especially when imaging vascular structures and when looking for subtle changes in bone density such as result from fractures of the skull or spine. Advanced stages of certain pathologic conditions may require changes in technique to maintain the proper level of density, contrast, and visibility of detail (see the Box in Chapter 1, p. 3, Relative Attenuation of X-rays in Advanced Stages of Diseases). If contrast material is used, the kilovolts-peak level must remain in the low to mid range to provide enough radiographic contrast to properly show the contrast-filled vessels.

The administration of radiographic contrast material is an essential component of many examinations of the skull and nervous system. Therefore it is essential that the radiographer be familiar with the use of these agents and be extremely alert to the development of possible allergic reactions. Currently the radiographic scope of practice includes venous access and pharmacology of contrast agents. Some facilities may require the technologist to inject agents, especially for CT and MRI. After contrast administration, the radiographer is often left alone in the room with the patient and must be able to immediately recognize an allergic reaction to contrast material and be able to initiate and maintain basic life-support techniques until advanced life-support personnel have arrived. Although departmental policy varies, it is usually the radiographer's responsibility to assist during resuscitation procedures. Therefore it is essential that the radiographer be familiar with the contents of the emergency cart and be responsible for ensuring that the cart is completely stocked with all appropriate medications.

■ Physiology of the Nervous System

The divisions of the nervous system can be classified by location or by the type of tissue supplied by the nerve cells in the division. The **central nervous system** (CNS) consists of the brain and spinal cord. The remaining neural structures, including 12 pairs of cranial nerves, 31 pairs of spinal nerves, autonomic nerves, and ganglia, make up the **peripheral nervous system** (PNS). The PNS consists of afferent and efferent neurons. Afferent **(sensory)** neurons conduct impulses from peripheral receptors to the CNS. Efferent **(motor)** neurons conduct impulses away from the CNS to the peripheral effectors. The **somatic nervous system** supplies the striated skeletal muscles, whereas the **autonomic nervous system** supplies smooth muscle, cardiac muscle, and glandular epithelial tissue.

The basic unit of the nervous system is the **neuron,** or nerve cell. A neuron consists of a cell body and two types of long, threadlike extensions. A single **axon** leads from the nerve cell body, and one or more **dendrites** lead toward it. Axons are insulated by a fatty covering called the **myelin sheath,** which increases the rate of transmission of nervous impulses. Deterioration of this fatty myelin sheath (demyelination) is a characteristic abnormality in multiple sclerosis.

The impulse conduction route to and from the CNS is termed a **reflex arc.** The basic reflex arc consists of an afferent, or sensory, neuron, which conducts impulses to the CNS from the periphery, and an efferent, or motor, neuron, which conducts impulses from the CNS to peripheral effectors (muscles or glandular tissue).

Impulses pass from one neuron to another at a junction called the **synapse.** Transmission at the synapse is a chemical reaction in which the termini of the axon release a neurotransmitter substance that produces an electrical impulse in the dendrites of the next axon. Once the neurotransmitter has accomplished its task, its activity rapidly terminates so that subsequent impulses can be conducted along this same route.

The largest part of the brain is the **cerebrum,** which consists of two cerebral hemispheres. The surface of the cerebrum is highly convoluted with elevations called **gyri** and shallow grooves called **sulci.** Deeper grooves called **fissures** divide each cerebral hemisphere into lobes. The outer portion of the cerebrum, termed the **cortex,** consists of a thin layer of gray matter where the nerve cell bodies are concentrated. The inner area consists of white matter, which is composed of the nerve fiber tracts.

The cerebral cortex is responsible for receiving sensory information from all parts of the body, and for triggering impulses that govern all motor activity. Just posterior to the central sulcus, the cerebral cortex has specialized areas to receive and precisely localize sensory information from the PNS. Visual impulses are transmitted to the posterior portion of the brain; olfactory (smell) and auditory impulses are received in the lateral portions. The primary motor cortex is just anterior to the central sulcus. Because efferent motor fibers cross over from one side of the body to the other at the level of the medulla and spinal cord, stimulation on one side of the cerebral cortex causes contraction of muscles on the opposite side of the body. The premotor cortex, which lies anterior to the primary motor cortex, controls coordinate movements of muscles by stimulating groups of muscles that work together. This region also contains the portion of the brain responsible for speech, which is usually on the left side in right-handed people. The cerebral cortex also is the site of all higher functions, including memory and creative thought.

The two cerebral hemispheres are connected by a mass of white matter called the **corpus callosum.** These extensive bundles of nerve fibers lie in the midline just above the roofs of the lateral ventricles.

Deep within the white matter are a few islands of gray matter that are collectively called the **basal ganglia.** These structures help control position and automatic movements and consist of the caudate nuclei, the globus pallidus, and the putamen.

Between the cerebrum and spinal cord lies the brainstem, which is composed of (from top down) the **midbrain** (mesencephalon), the **pons,** and the **medulla.** In addition to performing sensory, motor, and reflex functions, the brainstem contains the nuclei of the 12 cranial nerves and the vital centers controlling cardiac, vasomotor, and respiratory function. Centers in the medulla are responsible for such nonvital reflexes as vomiting, coughing, sneezing, hiccuping, and swallowing.

The **cerebellum,** the second largest part of the brain, is located just below the posterior portion of the cerebrum. It is composed of two large lateral masses, the cerebellar hemispheres, and a central section **(vermis)** that resembles a worm coiled on itself. The cerebellum acts with the cerebral cortex to produce skilled movements by coordinating the activities of groups of

muscles. It coordinates skeletal muscles used in maintaining equilibrium and posture by functioning below the level of consciousness to make movements smooth rather than jerky, steady rather than trembling, and efficient and coordinated rather than ineffective and awkward. Therefore cerebellar disease produces such characteristic symptoms as ataxia (muscle incoordination), tremors, and disturbances of gait and equilibrium.

The **diencephalon** lies between the cerebrum and the midbrain. It consists of several structures located around the third ventricle, primarily the thalamus and hypothalamus. The **thalamus** primarily functions as a relay station that receives and processes sensory information of almost all kinds of sensory impulses before sending this information on to the cerebral cortex. The tiny **hypothalamus** is an extremely complex structure that functions as a link between the mind and body and is the site of "pleasure" or "reward" centers for such primary drives as eating, drinking, and mating. It plays a major role in regulating the body's internal environment by coordinating the activities of the autonomic nervous system and secreting the **releasing hormones** that control the secretion of hormones by the anterior and posterior portions of the pituitary gland. The hypothalamus is also important in helping to maintain a normal body temperature and in keeping the individual in a waking state.

The spinal cord lies within the vertebral column and extends from its junction with the brainstem at the foramen magnum to approximately the lower border of the first lumbar vertebra. It consists of an inner core of gray matter surrounded by white matter tracts. The basic function of the spinal cord is to conduct impulses up the cord to the brain (ascending tracts) and down the cord from the brain to spinal nerves (descending tracts). It also serves as the center for spinal reflexes, and involuntary responses such as the knee jerk (patellar reflex).

The delicate, yet vital, brain and spinal cord are protected by two layers of coverings. The outer bony coverings are the cranial bones of the skull encasing the brain, and the vertebrae surrounding the spinal cord. The inner coverings consist of three distinct layers of **meninges.** The innermost layer adhering to the outer surface of the brain and spinal cord is the transparent **pia mater,** and the tough outermost covering is termed the **dura mater.** Between these layers is the delicate, cobweb-like **arachnoid membrane.** Inflammation of these three protective layers is called **meningitis.**

Three extensions of the dura mater separate portions of the brain. The **falx cerebri** projects downward into the longitudinal fissure to separate the cerebral hemispheres. Similarly, the **falx cerebelli** separates the two cerebellar hemispheres. The

tentorium cerebelli forms a tentlike covering over the cerebellum that separates it from the occipital lobe of the cerebrum.

In addition to bony and membranous coverings, the brain and spinal cord are further protected by a cushion of fluid both around them and within them. The ventricles are four spaces within the brain that contain cerebrospinal fluid (CSF). There are two large lateral ventricles, one located in each cerebral hemisphere. The slitlike third ventricle lies between the right and left thalamus. The anterior parts of the lateral ventricles (frontal horns) are connected by a Y-shaped canal that extends downward to open into the upper part of the third ventricle at the **foramen of Monro.** The fourth ventricle is a diamond-shaped space between the cerebellum posteriorly and the medulla and pons anteriorly. It is continuous inferiorly with the central canal of the spinal cord. The third and fourth ventricles are connected by the **aqueduct of Sylvius** (cerebral aqueduct), a narrow canal that runs through the posterior part of the midbrain.

CSF is formed by the filtration of plasma from blood in the **choroid plexuses,** networks of capillaries that project from the pia mater into the lateral ventricles and into the roofs of the third and fourth ventricles. After flowing through the ventricular system, the fluid circulates in the **subarachnoid space** around the brain and spinal cord before being absorbed into venous blood through **arachnoid villi.** Obstruction of CSF circulation results in hydrocephalus.

■ Infections of the Central Nervous System

With the widespread availability of antibiotics, infectious disease of the CNS is now much less common than previously. Nevertheless, bacterial, fungal, viral, and protozoal organisms can infect the brain parenchyma, meningeal linings, and bones of the skull.

Meningitis

Meningitis is an acute inflammation of the pia mater and arachnoid, the membranes covering the brain and spinal cord. Infecting organisms can reach the meninges from a middle ear, the upper respiratory tract, or a frontal sinus infection, or they can be spread through the bloodstream (hematogenously) from an infection in the lungs or other site. **Bacterial meningitis** is most commonly caused by *Haemophilus influenzae* in neonates and young children, and by meningococci and pneumococci in adolescents and adults. **Viral meningitis** may be caused by mumps, poliovirus, and occasionally by herpes simplex. A chronic form of meningitis can be caused by tuberculous infection. Bacterial meningitis is the most common form. The bacteria release toxins that destroy the meningeal cells, thus stimulating immune and inflammatory reactions.

Radiographic appearance

Although the meninges initially demonstrate vascular congestion, edema, and minute hemorrhages, the underlying brain remains intact. MRI and CT scans are normal during most acute episodes of meningitis and remain normal if appropriate therapy is promptly instituted. If the infection extends to involve the cortex of the brain and the ependymal lining of the ventricles, contrast studies may show characteristic meningeal enhancement in the basal cisterns, interhemispheric fissure, and choroid plexus (Figure 7-1). Diffuse brain swelling may symmetrically compress the lateral and third ventricles. MRI and CT are also of value in the early detection of such complications of acute meningitis as arterial or venous vasculitis or thrombosis with infarction, hydrocephalus caused by adhesions or thickening of the arachnoid at the base of the brain, subdural effusion or empyema, and brain abscess.

Although MRI and CT are best for evaluating acute bacterial meningitis, plain films of the sinuses and skull can demonstrate cranial osteomyelitis, paranasal sinusitis, or a skull fracture as the underlying cause of meningitis. Chest radiographs may show a silent area of pneumonia or a lung abscess.

Treatment

A sample of CSF is collected for culture, and when the organism is identified, specific antibiotics are given to

Figure 7-1 Meningitis. Subarachnoid enhancement in the basal cisterns and left sylvian fissure in a patient with cysticercosis. (From Ross MR, Davis DO, Mark AS: *MRI Decisions* 4:24-33, 1990.)

eradicate the bacteria. Even before these results are available, the patient is immediately treated with a broad-spectrum antibiotic to prevent morbidity. If secondary encephalitis develops, the patient receives antiviral drugs. Any increased intracranial pressure is appropriately treated.

Encephalitis

Encephalitis, a viral inflammation of the brain and meninges, produces symptoms ranging from mild headache and fever to severe cerebral dysfunction, seizures, and coma. About 30% of cases occur in children. Encephalitis caused by herpes simplex is an often fatal, fulminant process.

Radiographic appearance

The earliest and predominant findings in herpetic encephalitis are poorly marginated areas (with a patchy parenchymal pattern) in the temporal lobes, which have high signal intensity on T2-weighted MR images and demonstrate low density on CT scans. These changes probably represent a combination of tissue necrosis and focal brain edema. A mass effect is common and may be seen as a midline shift or as a focal mass compressing the ventricles or the sylvian cisterns. Compromise of the blood–brain barrier in areas of rapid, more progressive hemorrhagic necrosis results in a nonhomogeneous pattern of contrast enhancement. CT reveals abnormalities 3 to 5 days after the onset of symptoms, when the patient may be comatose. MRI is the preferred modality even though in acute cases a contrast-enhanced scan may appear negative. Follow-up scans typically demonstrate widespread low-density encephalomalacia involving the temporal and frontal lobes.

Treatment

In addition to confirming the clinical diagnosis of herpes simplex encephalitis and excluding the presence of an abscess or a tumor, MRI and CT are important because they can indicate the best site for biopsy. A definitive diagnosis of herpes infection is essential before beginning treatment with adenine arabinoside, a chemotherapeutic agent that may be neurotoxic, mutagenic, and carcinogenic. Acyclovir, a new antiviral drug used in treating herpes infection, interferes with the DNA synthesis and inhibits viral replication.

Brain abscess

Brain abscesses are usually a result of chronic infections of the middle ear, paranasal sinuses, or mastoid air cells, or of systemic infections (pneumonia, bacterial endocarditis, osteomyelitis). The most common organisms causing brain abscesses are streptococci. In patients with acquired immunodeficiency syndrome

(AIDS), unusual organisms such as toxoplasmosis and cryptococcosis often cause brain abscesses. The microorganisms lodge preferentially in the gray matter and spread to the adjacent white matter.

Radiographic appearance

The earliest sign of brain abscess on an MR or CT image is an area of abnormal density with poorly defined borders and a mass effect reflecting vascular congestion and edema. Further progression of the inflammatory process leads to cerebral softening, which may undergo necrosis and liquefaction and result in a true abscess. MRI is considered superior for demonstrating a brain abscess, although CT can be employed when MRI is unavailable. On T1-weighted MR images, an abscess appears as a hypointense mass with an isointense capsule surrounded by low-signal-intensity edema (Figure 7-2, A). Both the mass and the edema are hyperintense on T2-weighted images (Figure 7-2, B). After the intravenous administration of contrast material, an oval or circular peripheral ring of contrast enhancement outlines the abscess capsule. Although the wall is usually thin and of uniform thickness, an irregularly thick wall, resulting from the formation of granulation tissue, may mimic a malignant glioma. Multiple abscesses indicate the possibility of septic emboli from a systemic infection (Figure 7-3).

Plain skull radiographs may show evidence of underlying sinusitis, mastoiditis, or osteomyelitis, although this is better evaluated by CT scanning with bone-window settings. Infection by gas-forming organisms occasionally produces an air–fluid level within the abscess cavity.

Treatment

A broad-spectrum antibiotic is given to fight the infection. A craniotomy to totally excise the abscess is most successful in cases of a multiloculated abscess. Image-directed stereotactic aspiration to provide a specimen for microbial evaluation is better because it is less invasive. In some cases, the patient may require medication to reduce increased intracranial pressure.

MRI and CT can be used to assess the results of therapy for a brain abscess and to document complications. These modalities can demonstrate the often fatal intraventricular rupture of an abscess and the development of increased intracranial pressure, which may lead to brain herniation.

Subdural empyema

Subdural empyema is a suppurative process in the space between the inner surface of the dura and the outer surface of the arachnoid. Approximately 25% of intracranial infections are subdural empyemas. The most common cause of subdural empyema is the

Figure 7-2   Brain abscess. **A,** T1-weighted MRI scan shows a central hypointense necrotic mass with an isointense capsule surrounded by low-signal-intensity edema. **B,** On the T2-weighted image, the hypointense capsule is highlighted by increased signal centrally and peripherally. (From Edelman RR, Hesselink JR, editors: *Clinical magnetic resonance imaging,* Philadelphia, 1990, Saunders.)

Figure 7-3   Pyogenic brain abscesses. CT scan shows one frontal and two occipital lesions *(arrows)* with relatively thin, uniform rings of enhancement.

spread of infection from the frontal or ethmoid sinuses. Less frequently, subdural empyema may result from mastoiditis, middle ear infection, purulent meningitis, penetrating wounds to the skull, craniectomy, or osteomyelitis of the skull. Subdural empyema is often bilateral and associated with a high mortality even if properly treated. The most common location of a subdural empyema is over the cerebral convexity; the base of the skull is usually spared.

Radiographic appearance

MRI is the procedure of choice in evaluating the patient with suspected subdural empyema. Unlike CT, MRI is free from bony artifacts adjacent to the inner table of the skull. In addition, signal characteristics may permit differentiation between benign effusions and infected empyemas. Noncontrast scans demonstrate a crescentic or lentiform (lenslike), extraaxial fluid collection (representing pus) adjacent to the inner border of the skull or the falx (Figure 7-4). There is compression and displacement of the ipsilateral ventricular structures. After the intravenous administration of contrast material, a narrow zone of enhancement of relatively uniform thickness separates the extracerebral collection from the brain surface. MRI can also demonstrate involvement of the adjacent parenchyma by means of

Figure 7-4 Subdural empyema. T2-weighted MRI scan demonstrates high signal intensity of the fluid collections along the falx. (From Stark DD, Bradley WG: *Magnetic resonance imaging*, ed 2, St Louis, 1991, Mosby.)

Figure 7-5 Epidural empyema. Black rim of dura delineates the epidural fluid collection in the right frontal region. (From Stark DD, Bradley WG: *Magnetic resonance imaging*, ed 2, St Louis, 1991, Mosby.)

retrograde thrombophlebitis with resultant infarction or abscess formation, signs associated with a poor prognosis.

Epidural empyema

Epidural empyema (Figure 7-5) is almost invariably associated with osteomyelitis in a cranial bone originating from an infection in the ear or paranasal sinuses. The infectious process is localized outside the dural membrane and beneath the inner table of the skull. The frontal region is most frequently affected because of its close relationship to the frontal sinuses and the ease with which the dura can be stripped from the bone.

Radiographic appearance

Noncontrast CT scans demonstrate the epidural infection as a poorly defined area of low density adjacent to the inner table of the skull. An adjacent area of bone destruction or evidence of paranasal sinus or mastoid infection (fluid, soft-tissue thickening) can often be demonstrated on CT or plain skull radiographs. After the intravenous administration of contrast material, the inflamed dural membrane appears as a thickened zone of enhancement on the convex inner side of the lesion. If the collection lies in the mid-

line, the attachment of the falx is displaced inward and separated from the adjacent skull, thus identifying its extradural location.

Treatment of subdural and epidural empyemas

Subdural and epidural empyemas should be treated as medical emergencies. Immediate surgical drainage of an empyema and the underlying sinus infection aids in preventing recurrence. Craniotomy provides the most complete evacuation. The broad-spectrum antibiotic regimen used for a brain abscess is utilized here also.

Osteomyelitis of the skull

Osteomyelitis of the skull is most commonly caused by direct extension of a suppurative process from the paranasal sinuses, mastoid air cells, or scalp. As with osteomyelitis elsewhere in the skeleton, the radiographic changes often develop 1 to 2 weeks after the onset of clinical symptoms and signs.

Radiographic appearance

Acute osteomyelitis first appears radiographically as multiple small, poorly defined areas of lucency (Figure 7-6). Over the next several weeks, the lucencies enlarge and coalesce centrally with an expanding perimeter of

●　●

Summary of Findings for Infections of the Central Nervous System

DISORDER	LOCATION	RADIOGRAPHIC APPEARANCE	TREATMENT
Meningitis	Acute inflammation of meninges	CT/MRI—arterial and venous vasculitis or thrombosis, hydrocephalus, subdural effusion, and brain abscess Radiographs—osteomyelitis, sinusitis, or fracture	Immediate broad-spectrum antibiotics followed by specific antibiotics determined by culture results
Encephalitis	Viral inflammation of brain and meninges	MRI—hyperintensity on T2-weighted images with mass effect CT—low-attenuation regions without focal enhancement; mass effect	Herpes infection—adenine arabinoside
Brain abscess	Microorganism infection of gray and white matter	MRI—T1-weighted images show hypointense mass with isointense capsule; T2-weighted images show hyperintensity of both the mass and surrounding edema CT—contrast-enhanced scan identifies a high-attenuation capsule surrounding a hypodense necrotic center	Broad-spectrum antibiotics Craniotomy to totally excise the multiloculated abscess Image-directed stereotactic aspiration provides a specimen for microbial evaluation Medication to reduce increased intracranial pressure if symptoms occur
Subdural empyema	Infection located between the dura and the arachnoid	MRI—characteristic crescentic or lentiform extraaxial fluid collection that is mildly hyperintense to CSF on T2-weighted images	Craniotomy for immediate surgical drainage of empyema and underlying sinus empyema; aids in preventing recurrence Same broad-spectrum antibiotic regimen as for brain abscess
Epidural empyema	Infectious process above the dura and beneath the inner skull table	CT (noncontrast)—shows low-density area adjacent to the inner table of the skull, with possible bone destruction CT (contrast enhanced)—dural membrane appears as a thickened zone of enhancement on the convex inner side of the lesion	Craniotomy for immediate surgical drainage of empyema and underlying sinus empyema; aids in preventing recurrence Same broad-spectrum antibiotic regimen as for brain abscess
Osteomyelitis of the skull	Cranial bones	Radiograph—multiple small poorly defined areas of lucency, 1-2 weeks after onset of symptoms	See Chapter 3

●　●

CSF, Cerebrospinal fluid.

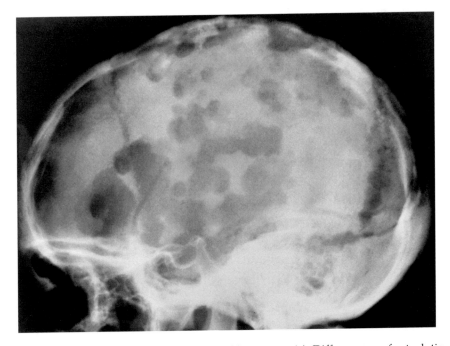

Figure 7-6 Osteomyelitis of skull (resulting from blastomycosis). Diffuse areas of osteolytic destruction affect most of the calvaria.

small satellite foci. As the infection becomes more chronic (especially with syphilis, tuberculosis, or fungal infections), attempts at bone regeneration produce multiple areas of poorly defined reactive sclerosis.

Treatment
(Refer to the discussion on bacterial osteomyelitis in Chapter 3.)

■ Tumors of the Central Nervous System

Intracranial neoplasms present clinically with seizure disorders or gradual neurologic deficits (difficulty thinking, slow comprehension, weakness, headache). About 50% of CNS tumors are primary lesions, and the others represent metastases.

Radiographic appearance
The clinical presentation and radiographic appearance depend on the location of the tumor and the site of the subsequent mass effect. MRI is generally considered to be the most sensitive technique for detecting most suspected brain tumors. In general, both the tumor and its surrounding edema demonstrate high signal intensity on T2-weighted images. After the intravenous injection of contrast material, the enhancing tumor can usually be distinguished from nonenhancing edema on T1-weighted scans (Figure 7-7). In addition to its exquisite sensitivity in detecting patho-

Figure 7-7 Glioblastoma multiforme. Axial T1-weighted MRI scan shows intense contrast enhancement of this complex necrotic mass. (From Eisenberg RL: *Clinical imaging: an atlas of differential diagnosis*, Gaithersburg, Md, 1992, Aspen.)

logic alteration of normal tissue constituents, MRI provides excellent delineation of tumor extent and can show associated abnormalities such as hydrocephalus. This modality is of special value in imaging neoplasms of the brainstem and posterior fossa, which may be poorly seen on CT because of bone artifact. CT with contrast enhancement is an excellent examination for evaluating a patient with suspected brain tumor. It is of special value for detecting punctate or larger calcification that cannot be shown by MRI. Although skull radiographs were used in the past to demonstrate tumoral calcification, bone erosion, and displacement of the calcified pineal gland, plain films are no longer indicated, as this information can be more effectively obtained on CT scans.

Before the advent of CT, cerebral arteriography was used to demonstrate evidence of brain tumors, such as mass effect, contralateral displacement of midline arteries and veins, abnormal vessels with tumor staining, and early venous filling. At present, the major use of arteriography is for precise delineation of the arterial and venous anatomy before surgical therapy and for evaluation of those cases in which a vascular anomaly is a strong consideration in the differential diagnosis of a tumor. Radionuclide brain scans have a relatively high rate of detection of cerebral tumors but are far less specific than CT or MRI. PET scans demonstrate metabolic activity and specific location of a lesion for presurgical planning (Figure 7-8).

Treatment

Therapy depends on the location and histology of the tumor. If possible, the tumor is surgically resected, followed by radiation therapy if the tumor is not completely removed. In some cases, radiation therapy and chemotherapy are utilized when the tumor is inoperable.

Glioma

Gliomas, the most common primary **malignant** brain tumors, consist of glial cells that still have the ability to multiply. They spread by direct extension and can cross from one cerebral hemisphere to the other through connecting white matter tracts such as the corpus callosum. Gliomas have a peak incidence in middle adult life and are infrequent in persons less than 30 years of age.

Glioblastomas are highly malignant lesions that are predominantly cerebral, although similar tumors may occur in the brainstem, cerebellum, or spinal cord. **Astrocytomas** (70% of all gliomas) are slowly growing tumors that have an infiltrative character and can form large cavities or pseudocysts. Favored sites are the cerebrum, cerebellum, thalamus, optic chiasm, and pons.

Less frequent types of gliomas are **ependymoma, medulloblastoma,** and **oligodendrocytoma.** Ependymomas most commonly arise from the walls of the fourth ventricle, especially in children, and usually

Figure 7-8 Low-grade brain tumor studied by three-dimensional reconstruction of a PET cerebral study using ¹¹C-methionine. **A,** Mass effect near the thalamus is evident when the increased uptake *(open arrow)* is compared with a cystic component showing lack of uptake *(solid arrow).* **B,** The greatest activity is noted in the right temporal lobe corresponding to receptive and expressive language areas.

from the lateral ventricles in adults. Medulloblastomas are rapidly growing tumors, disseminating throughout the spinal fluid, that develop in the posterior portion of the vermis in children and, rarely, in the cerebellar hemisphere in adults. The tumor tends to spread through the subarachnoid space, with metastatic deposits occurring anywhere within the brain or spinal column. Oligodendrocytomas are slow-growing lesions that usually arise in the cerebrum and have a tendency to calcify.

Radiographic appearance

On MRI scans (Figure 7-9), gliomas typically appear as masses of high signal intensity on T2-weighted images. They may be of low intensity or isointense on T1-weighted sequences. MR spectroscopy has a typical spectral pattern with a strongly increased choline peak, which indicates myelin or the breakdown of myelin (the chemical structure that goes into making white matter). In MR spectroscopy, a highly elevated choline level, a drastically lower level of *N*-acetylaspartate (a neuronal marker), and a drastically lower creatine/phosphocreatine confirm an infiltrating glioma (Figure 7-10). Ependymomas, often partially calcified and cystic, have a heterogeneous signal intensity and show enhancement.

On noncontrast CT scans, gliomas are most commonly seen as single, nonhomogeneous masses. Low-grade astrocytomas tend to be low-density lesions showing little or no enhancement (Figure 7-11); glioblastomas most frequently contain areas of both increased and decreased density, although a broad spectrum of CT appearances can occur. Edema is often seen in the adjacent subcortical white matter. After the intravenous injection of contrast material, virtually all gliomas show enhancement, with the most malignant lesions tending to be enhanced to the greatest degree (see Figure 7-7). In MR spectroscopy, an elevated choline/creatine ratio suggests a malignant neoplasm. The most common pattern is an irregular ring of contrast enhancement, representing solid vascularized tumor, surrounding a central low-density area of necrosis. Contrast enhancement also can appear as patches of increased density distributed irregularly throughout a low-density lesion or as rounded nodules of increased density within the mass.

Treatment

Therapy depends on the location and histology of the tumor. Astrocytomas have a good 5-year survival rate after surgery and radiation therapy. For ependymomas of the filum terminale, surgical removal provides a favorable prognosis.

Meningioma

Meningioma is a benign tumor that arises from arachnoid lining cells and is attached to the dura. The most common sites of meningioma are the convexity of the calvaria, the olfactory groove, the tuberculum sellae, the parasagittal region, the sylvian fissure, the cerebellopontine angle, and the spinal canal. Seizures and neurologic defects are most often caused by mass effect.

Figure 7-9 Brainstem glioma. Sagittal MRI scans show enlargement of brainstem involving pons and midbrain. Notice that various imaging techniques alter the appearance of the tumor *(T).* **A,** On T1-weighted image, tumor is gray (low-intensity signal). **B,** On T2-weighted image, tumor appears white (high-intensity signal).

Figure 7-10 Infiltrating glioma. **A,** T2-weighted image demonstrates a 3-cm hypointense lesion in the deep right parietal lobe with a hyperintense peripheral rim. A poorly defined hyperintense lesion is seen within the deep white matter of the left temporal and parietal lobes. **B,** On the T1-weighted coronal image, the hyperintense periphery is seen surrounding a low-signal-intensity and a high-signal-intensity lesion. **C,** On MR spectroscopy, the left frontal lobe demonstrates an elevated choline (first) peak, a slightly lower creatine/phosphocreatine (second) peak, and a mildly depressed *N*-acetylaspartate (third) peak. These findings help confirm a low-grade, diffuse infiltrating glioma. (Courtesy Bartram J. Pierce RT(R)(MR), Good Samaritan Regional Medical Center, Corvallis, Ore.)

Figure 7-11   Cystic astrocytoma. CT scan shows hypodense mass with thin rim of contrast enhancement.

A   **B**

Figure 7-12   Meningioma. **A,** Huge mass *(arrowheads)* appears hypointense on T1-weighted coronal MRI scan. **B,** The mass appears hyperintense on T2-weighted image. Notice the dramatic shift of the ventricle *(v)* caused by mass effect of tumor. *Black arrows* point to areas of hemorrhage within the neoplasm *(white arrowheads).*

Radiographic appearance

Because meningiomas tend to be isointense with brain on both T1- and T2-weighted images, anatomic distortion is the key to the MRI diagnosis (Figure 7-12). A thin rim of low intensity, consisting of a CSF cleft, the vascular rim, or dura, may separate the tumor from adjacent brain. Calcification within a meningioma may produce nonuniform signal or focal signal void. Surrounding edema may make the lesion easier to identify. Just as the detection of meningiomas by CT is facilitated by the use of iodinated contrast material, paramagnetic contrast agents can enhance the detection of meningiomas on MRI. MR spectroscopy has a typical spectral pattern with a strongly increased choline peak; creatine is a marker of energy metabo-

lism. Alanine is another specific amino acid marker producing a unique peak in meningiomas. CT typically shows a meningioma as a rounded, sharply delineated, isodense (25%) or hyperdense (75%) tumor abutting a dural surface. Calcification often is seen

Figure 7-13 Meningioma. **A,** CT scan after intravenous injection of contrast material shows uniformly enhancing mass *(arrow)* with surrounding low-density edema attached to falx. **B,** Venous phase of carotid arteriogram shows characteristic prominent vascular blush *(arrow)* of meningioma. Note that the superior sagittal sinus *(arrowheads)* is patent.

Figure 7-14 Parietal meningioma. **A,** Plain skull film shows dense calcification in tumor. **B,** CT scan of another patient, demonstrating a midline calcified meningioma.

within the mass on noncontrast scans. After the intravenous injection of contrast material, there is intense homogeneous enhancement, which reflects the highly vascular nature of the tumor (Figure 7-13).

Pronounced dilatation of meningeal and diploic vessels, which provide part of the blood supply to the tumor, may produce prominent grooves in the calvaria on plain films of the skull. Calvarial hyperostosis (increased density) may develop because of invasion of the bone by tumor cells that stimulate osteoblastic activity. Dense calcification or granular psammomatous deposits may be seen within the tumor (Figure 7-14).

Arteriography can demonstrate the feeding arteries, which most commonly arise from both the internal and the external carotid artery circulation. Preoperative embolization of the external carotid artery supply can decrease the amount of blood loss at surgery.

Treatment

Surgical resection is very successful because of the superficial position of the tumor and the lack of tumor infiltration. Incomplete resection results in a lobulated and mushroom pattern of tumor growth.

Acoustic neuroma

Acoustic neuroma is a slowly growing benign tumor that may occur as a solitary lesion or as part of the syndrome of neurofibromatosis. The tumor arises from Schwann's cells in the vestibular portion of the auditory (eighth cranial) nerve. It usually originates in the internal auditory canal and extends into the cerebellopontine angle cistern.

Radiographic appearance

MRI scans (T1-weighted), the preferred modality, exquisitely show the tumor as a focal or generalized enlargement of the eighth cranial nerve. This technique can even demonstrate small intracanalicular tumors confined to the internal auditory canal, which may be impossible to show on CT unless contrast material (nonionic water-soluble material, or air) is administered into the ventricular system (Figure 7-15). CT scans demonstrate enlargement and erosion of the internal auditory canal and a uniformly enhancing mass in the cerebellopontine angle (Figure 7-16). Very large tumors may compress the fourth ventricle and lead to the development of hydrocephalus.

Treatment

Surgical excision of the lesion or gamma knife radiosurgery improves symptoms.

Pituitary adenoma

Pituitary adenomas, almost all of which arise in the anterior lobe, constitute more than 10% of all intracranial tumors. Most are nonsecreting **chromo-**

Figure 7-15   Acoustic neuroma. MRI scan shows considerable contrast enhancement of the left-sided lesion *(arrowheads)*. Notice the normal neural structures on the right. (From Eisenberg RL: *Clinical imaging: an atlas of differential diagnosis,* Gaithersburg, Md, 1992, Aspen.)

Figure 7-16   Acoustic neuroma. CT scan shows widening and erosion of right internal auditory canal *(open arrows)* associated with large extraaxial mass *(white arrows)* in right cerebellopontine angle. Solid black arrows point to normal internal auditory canal on left. (From Williams AL, Haughton VM: *Cranial computed tomography,* St Louis, 1985, Mosby.)

phobe adenomas. As chromophobe tumors enlarge, the adjoining secreting cells within the sella turcica are compressed, leading to diminished secretion and decreased levels of growth hormone, gonadotropins, thyrotropic hormone, and adrenocorticotropic hormone (ACTH). Large chromophobe adenomas can extend upward to distort the region of the optic chiasm, whereas lateral expansion of tumor can compress the cranial nerves passing within the cavernous sinus.

Hormone-secreting pituitary tumors can cause clinical symptoms even if too small to produce mechanical

Figure 7-17 Pituitary adenoma. Coronal CT scan shows enhancing mass filling and extending out from pituitary fossa. Note erosion of base of sella.

Figure 7-18 Pituitary adenoma. Sagittal **(A)** and coronal **(B)** MRI scans demonstrate large mass *(m)* that arises from sella turcica and extends upward to fill suprasellar cistern.

mass effect. Hypersecretion of growth hormone results in gigantism in adolescents (before the epiphyses have closed) and acromegaly in adults (after the epiphyses have closed). Excess secretion of ACTH by a pituitary tumor results in the hypersecretion of steroid hormones from the adrenal cortex and symptoms of Cushing's disease. Hypersecretion of thyroid-stimulating hormone (TSH) leads to hyperthyroidism; excess secretion of prolactin by a pituitary tumor in women causes the amenorrhea/galactorrhea syndrome.

Radiographic appearance

Thin-section CT and MRI are the examinations of choice for evaluating a patient with a suspected pituitary tumor. After the intravenous administration of contrast material, large pituitary tumors are typically homogeneous and hyperdense with respect to surrounding brain tissue. Most pituitary microadenomas are of lower density than the normal pituitary gland. CT can also demonstrate adjacent bone erosion, tumor extension beyond the confines of the sella, and impression on nearby structures such as the third ventricle, optic nerves, or optic chiasm (Figure 7-17).

The preferred modality for detecting and defining the extent of a pituitary tumor is MRI because of its superior sensitivity and multiplanar capability. Thin section coronal and sagittal T1-weighted

MRI scans show a microadenoma as a low-signal-intensity focal lesion associated with contralateral deviation of the pituitary stalk and an upwardly convex contour of the gland (Figure 7-18). The intravenous injection of paramagnetic contrast material significantly improves diagnostic sensitivity in patients with tiny secreting pituitary tumors. Immediately after injection, small microadenomas appear hypointense relative to the normally enhancing pituitary gland. On delayed scans, the neoplasm may become hyperintense relative to the normal gland.

Although plain skull radiographs can show enlargement of the sella turcica, erosion of the dorsum sellae, and a double floor resulting from the unequal downward growth of the mass, this imaging modality is now of value only in the incidental detection of sellar enlargement on films taken for other purposes.

Treatment

The size of the pituitary adenoma determines the extent of the treatment. For pituitary tumors not extending beyond the gland, surgical transsphenoidal resection has a good prognosis. Adenomas extending beyond the pituitary require surgical resection followed by radiation therapy for best results. The new gamma knife radiosurgery is another therapeutic alternative.

Craniopharyngioma

Craniopharyngioma is a benign tumor that contains both cystic and solid components and usually occurs before the age of 20 years. The lesion generally originates above the sella turcica, from embryonic remnants, depressing the optic chiasm and extending up into the third ventricle. Less commonly, a craniopharyngioma lies within the sella, where it compresses the pituitary gland and may erode adjacent bony walls.

Radiographic appearance

Most craniopharyngiomas have calcification that can be detected on plain skull films or CT scans (Figure 7-19). In cystic lesions, the shell-like calcification lies along the periphery of the tumor; in mixed or solid lesions, the calcification is nodular, amorphous, or cloudlike. CT clearly demonstrates the cystic and solid components of the multilobulated mass. After the intravenous administration of contrast material, there is variable enhancement, depending on the type of calcification and the amount of cystic component within the tumor (Figure 7-20). CT can also demonstrate hydrocephalus if the tumor has expanded to obstruct one or both of the foramina of Monro.

The MRI appearance of craniopharyngioma depends on the tissue components of the tumor. Cystic areas have low signal intensity on T1-weighted scans and high signal intensity on T2-weighted scans; fat-containing regions have high signal intensity on T1-weighted images and show moderate signal intensity on T2-weighted scans (Figure 7-21). Large areas of calcification appear dark on all imaging sequences.

Treatment

A new treatment is MR-guided stereotactic resection via microsurgery. Some tumors are completely resectable; for others, surgical debulking and radiation therapy are performed. Surgery and radiation, either

Figure 7-19   Craniopharyngioma. Plain skull radiograph shows large suprasellar calcified mass in a child.

Figure 7-20   Craniopharyngioma. CT scan shows rim-enhancing tumor that contains dense calcification *(straight arrows)* and large cystic component *(curved arrows)* that extends into the posterior fossa. Note the associated hydrocephalus. (From Williams AL, Haughton VM: *Cranial computed tomography,* St Louis, 1985, Mosby.)

alone or in combination, may provide long-term control in many patients.

Pineal tumors

The most common tumors of the pineal gland are germinomas and teratomas, rapidly growing germ cell tumors, both of which occur predominantly in males

Figure 7-21   Craniopharyngioma. Sagittal MRI scan demonstrates large multiloculated suprasellar mass with cystic (C) and lipid (L) components. c, Cerebellum; p, pons.

Figure 7-22   Pineal germinoma. Sagittal T1-weighted MRI scan shows a large isointense mass (white arrowheads) that compresses the midbrain (black arrowhead) and elevates the splenium of the corpus callosum. (From Eisenberg RL: Clinical imaging: an atlas of differential diagnosis, Gaithersburg, Md, 1992, Aspen.)

less than 25 years of age and may be associated with precocious puberty.

Radiographic appearance

Sagittal MRI scans are ideal for showing pineal tumors, which typically compress the midbrain from above and lift up the splenium of the corpus callosum (Figure 7-22). Although most germinomas are isointense to brain on both T1- and T2-weighted images, teratomas may have mixed signal intensity because they contain cystic components and fat.

On CT, germinomas appear as hyperdense or isodense masses that tend to deform or displace the posterior aspect of the third ventricle and often obliterate the quadrigeminal cistern. Punctate calcification can often be detected within the mass. Intense enhancement of the tumor occurs after the injection of contrast material. Teratomas in the pineal region typically appear as hypodense masses with internal calcification (Figure 7-23). Occasionally, other formed elements (e.g., teeth) can occur. Contrast enhancement is usually much less pronounced than with germinomas. Large pineal tumors may cause obstructive hydrocephalus with ventricular dilatation.

A small number of tumors with the histologic appearance of pinealomas appear elsewhere in the brain at some distance from the normal pineal gland. These "ectopic pinealomas" generally occur in the anterior aspect of the third ventricle or within the suprasellar

cistern. They may produce the clinical triad of bitemporal hemianopsia, hypopituitarism, and diabetes insipidus that simulates a craniopharyngioma.

Treatment

Surgery is the initial therapy of choice for pineal tumors. Radiation therapy following surgery may be helpful. Chemotherapy is used with radiation therapy if surgery is not a viable option.

Chordoma

Chordomas are tumors that arise from remnants of the notochord (the embryonic neural tube). Although any part of the vertebral column and base of the skull can be involved, the most common sites are the clivus and the lower lumbosacral region. The tumors are locally invasive but do not metastasize. Chordomas arising at the base of the skull produce the striking clinical picture of multiple cranial nerve palsies on one or both sides combined with a retropharyngeal mass and erosion of the clivus.

Radiographic appearance

On plain radiographs, a chordoma tends to be a bulky mass causing ill-defined bone destruction or cortical expansion. Flocculent (fluffy or cloudlike) calcification

Figure 7-23 Pineal teratoma. Nonenhanced CT scan shows inhomogeneous mass containing a large amount of calcification.

may develop within a large soft-tissue mass (Figure 7-24, *A*). On CT scans, chordomas at the base of the skull tend to appear as lesions that are slightly denser than brain tissue and often demonstrate moderate contrast enhancement (Figure 7-24, *B*). Sagittal MRI scans well demonstrate the clival origin of the mass and its effect on surrounding structures (Figure 7-25).

Treatment

Chordomas of the clivus region are difficult to completely remove surgically, and thus the patient usually is also treated with radiation. For chordomas of the lumbar region, complete surgical resection is usually possible.

Metastatic carcinoma

Carcinomas usually reach the brain by hematogenous spread. Infrequently, epithelial malignancies of the nasopharynx can spread into the cranial cavity through neural foramina or by direct invasion through bone. The most common neoplasms that metastasize to the brain arise in the lung and breast. Melanomas, colon carcinomas, and testicular and kidney tumors also cause brain metastases.

Figure 7-24 Chordoma. **A,** Plain skull radiograph shows dense calcification *(arrows)* within a large soft-tissue mass that has an eroded dorsum sellae and upper portion of the clivus. **B,** In another patient, CT scan shows enlarging mass with destruction of the entire clivus *(short arrows)* and only small bone fragments remaining. Left petrous pyramid is also destroyed *(long arrow).* (**B** from Levine HL, Kleefield J, Rao KCVG: In Lee SH, Rao KCVG, editors: *Cranial computed tomography,* New York, 1983, McGraw-Hill.)

Radiographic appearance

On T2-weighted MRI scans, metastases appear as single or multiple masses of high signal intensity that are most commonly situated at the junction between gray matter and white matter (Figure 7-26). Additional lesions can often be demonstrated after the injection of

Figure 7-25 Clival chordoma. Sagittal MRI scan shows a low-intensity multilobulated mass deforming and displacing the brainstem, destroying the clivus, and extending into the sella turcica *(upper arrowhead)* and nasopharynx *(two lower arrowheads)*. (From Bilaniuk LT: Adult infratentorial tumors, *Semin Roentgenol* 25:155-173, 1990.)

Figure 7-26 Metastases. Axial MRI scan demonstrates three large masses *(arrows)* surrounded by extensive high-signal-intensity edema.

a paramagnetic contrast agent. On CT, brain metastases typically appear as multiple enhancing lesions of various sizes with surrounding amounts of low-density edema (Figures 7-27 and 7-28). On noncontrast scans, metastatic deposits may be hypodense, hyperdense, or similar in density to normal brain tissue, depending on

Figure 7-27 Metastases. CT scan shows multiple enhancing masses of various shapes and sizes representing hematogenous metastases from carcinoma of the breast.

such factors as cellular density, tumor neovascularity, and degree of necrosis. In general, metastases from lung, breast, kidney, and colon tend to be hypodense or isodense; hyperdense metastases often reflect hemorrhage or calcification within or adjacent to the tumor.

Single metastatic deposits in the brain may be indistinguishable from primary tumors. However, because primary brain neoplasms are unusual in older patients, single lesions in this population should suggest metastatic disease.

Treatment

The number of lesions determines the choice of therapy. Single metastatic lesions or second-year postprimary (residual or regrowth) lesions require surgical intervention, which may provide relief from symptoms. Multiple metastases require radiation or chemotherapy. Radiation therapy can be to the whole brain or by the gamma knife. Systemic chemotherapy is used if metastasis occurs after radiation treatment. Surgery combined with whole-brain radiation therapy is the most successful treatment.

■ Traumatic Processes of the Brain and Skull

In the patient with head trauma, the purpose of radiographic imaging is to detect a surgically correctable

Figure 7-28 Metastases. CT shows enhancing metastases from squamous cell carcinoma of lung that are both ring enhancing *(open arrow)* and solid *(solid arrow)*.

Summary of Findings for Tumors of the Central Nervous System (CNS)

DISORDER	LOCATION	RADIOGRAPHIC APPEARANCE	TREATMENT
Glioma	Glial cells in CNS	MRI—masses of high signal intensity on T2-weighted images, low signal intensity or isodense on T1-weighted images CT (nonenhanced)—a single heterogeneous mass (isodense to hypodense) CT (contrast enhanced)—a homogeneous lesion with an irregular ring of enhancement	Depends on location and histology Astrocytomas—good 5-year survival rate with surgery and radiation therapy Ependymomas of the filum terminale—surgical removal provides the most favorable prognosis
Meningioma	Arises from arachnoid lining and is attached to the dura	MRI—isodense lesion on T1- and T2-weighted images CT—rounded, sharply delineated, hyperdense (75%) tumor	Surgical resection is very successful because of the superficial position of the tumor and the lack of tumor infiltration
Acoustic neuroma	Schwann's cells of cranial nerve VIII	MRI—T1-weighted images show focal or generalized enlargement of cranial nerve VIII CT—best demonstrates bone involvement	Surgical excision of the lesion, or gamma knife radiosurgery, to improve symptoms
Pituitary adenoma	Most commonly from anterior lobe of the pituitary gland	CT—large tumor typically homogeneous and hyperdense in comparison to normal brain tissue, bone erosion and tumor extension MRI—T1-weighted images show hypointense mass associated with contralateral deviation MRI (contrast-enhanced)—the microadenoma becomes hypointense initially; delayed scans demonstrate hyperintensity of the tumor	Surgical resection by transsphenoidal approach Radiation therapy if tumor extends beyond pituitary gland Gamma knife radiosurgery—a new alternative

Continued

Summary of Findings for Tumors of the Central Nervous System (CNS)—cont'd

DISORDER	LOCATION	RADIOGRAPHIC APPEARANCE	TREATMENT
Cranio-pharyngioma	Usually superior to sella turcica	CT—cystic and solid mass with possible calcification MRI—cysts produce low signal intensity on T1-weighted images, high signal intensity on T2-weighted images; fatty tumors produce hyperintense signals on T1-weighted images	MR-guided stereotactic microsurgery for resection For unresectable tumors, surgical debulking followed by radiation therapy
Pineal tumor	Germ cell tumors of the pineal gland	MRI—sagittal scans demonstrate compression of midbrain; germinomas are isointense on T1- and T2-weighted images; teratomas produce a mixed signal intensity because of their cystic components and fat CT—germinomas hyperdense or isodense, displacing 3rd ventricle, and show intense contrast enhancement; teratomas are hypodense masses with internal calcifications	Surgery (first choice) followed by radiation therapy Chemotherapy with radiation therapy when surgery is not an option
Chordoma	Arises from the embryonic neural tube	Radiograph—ill-defined bone destruction or cortical expansion CT—base-of-skull mass is slightly denser than brain tissue and only moderately enhanced MRI—sagittal images best demonstrate clival area and surrounding structures	Clival region—surgical resection followed by radiation therapy Lumbar region—complete surgical resection
Metastatic carcinoma	Carcinoma reaching the brain by hematogenous spread	MRI—single or multiple masses of high signal intensity; additional lesions often seen with paramagnetic contrast agent CT—multiple enhancing lesions of various sizes with areas of low density surrounding edema	Single lesion—surgical resection Multiple lesions—whole brain radiation; chemotherapy if metastasis occurs after radiation therapy

hematoma. Emergency CT has virtually replaced all other radiographic investigations in patients with suspected neurologic dysfunction resulting from head injury. Because the presence or absence of a skull fracture does not correlate with intracranial abnormalities, plain radiographs of the skull are no longer indicated in the patient with head trauma.

Because of medicolegal reasons and the fear of missing a skull fracture, CT scans (and plain skull radiographs) are often overused. The following indications have been established for the use of radiographic procedures in the patient with head trauma:

1. Unexplained focal neurologic signs
2. Unconsciousness (including the unarousable alcoholic)
3. Documented decreasing level of consciousness or progressive mental deterioration

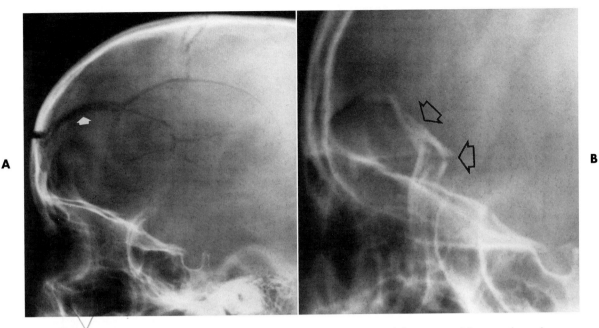

Figure 7-29 Skull fracture. **A,** Lateral projection of skull shows widely separated fracture *(arrow)* extending to star-shaped array of linear fractures. **B,** In another patient, lateral projection shows severely depressed skull fracture *(arrows).*

4. History of previous craniotomy with shunt tube in place
5. Skull depression or subcutaneous foreign body palpable or identified by a probe through a laceration or puncture wound
6. Hemotympanum or fluid discharge from the ear
7. Discharge of CSF from the nose
8. Ecchymosis over the mastoid process (Battle's sign)
9. Bilateral orbital ecchymoses (raccoon eyes)

Skull fracture

Radiographic appearance

A **linear skull fracture** appears on a plain radiograph as a sharp lucent line that is often irregular or jagged and occasionally branches (Figure 7-29). The fracture must be distinguished from suture lines, which generally have serrated edges and tend to be bilateral and symmetric, and vascular grooves, which usually have a smooth curving course and are not as sharp or distinct as a fracture line. The location of a linear skull fracture can indicate possible complications. A fracture that crosses a dural vascular groove may cause vessel laceration leading to an epidural hematoma. A fracture involving the sinuses or mastoid air cells may result in posttraumatic pneumocephalus, with air seen in the ventricles on plain radiographs. A **diastatic fracture** refers to a linear fracture that intersects a suture and courses along it, causing sutural separation.

More severe trauma, especially if localized to a small area of the skull, may force a fragment of bone to be separated and depressed into the cranial cavity (Figure 7-30). The underlying dura is frequently torn, and there is a relatively high incidence of cerebral parenchymal injury. **Depressed fractures** are often stellate (star shaped), with multiple fracture lines radiating outward from a central point. When the fracture is viewed en face, the overlap of fragments makes the fracture line appear denser than the normal bone. Tangential views are required to determine the amount of depression.

Fractures limited to the base of the skull are often hidden by the complex basal anatomy and may be very difficult to visualize on plain radiographs. A finding suggestive of a basilar skull fracture is an air–fluid level in the sphenoid sinus seen on an erect or cross-table lateral projection of the skull obtained with a horizontal x-ray beam. CT can demonstrate the presence of blood or fluid in the basilar cisterns and show some basilar skull fractures that are not visible on routine skull radiographs. Potential complications of basal skull fractures include leakage of CSF, meningitis, and damage to the facial nerve or auditory apparatus within the petrous bone.

It must be emphasized that the presence or absence of a skull fracture does not correlate with intracranial abnormalities. Indeed, serious treatable intracranial hematomas can be present without skull fractures.

Figure 7-30   Skull fracture. **A,** CT bone-window image demonstrates depressed temporal fracture *(long arrow).* Note the lateral orbital wall fracture *(short arrow),* the medial orbital wall fracture *(large arrowhead),* and the ethmoid opacification caused by hemorrhage. Also, air can be seen in the orbital soft tissues *(small arrowhead)* resulting from medial fracture into the ethmoids. **B,** Trauma resulted in a nondisplaced fracture in the supraorbital plate in this 24-year-old woman. (**A** From Pressman BD: In Eisenberg RL, editor: *Diagnostic imaging: an algorithmic approach,* Philadelphia, 1988, Lippincott.)

Figure 7-31   Acute epidural hematoma in a trauma patient. CT scan illustrates the characteristic lens-shaped epidural hematoma. Mass effect associated with the hematoma causes midline shift.

Treatment

The severity and location of the fracture and the complications resulting from the trauma determine the treatment.

Epidural hematoma

Epidural hematomas are caused by acute arterial bleeding and most commonly form over the parietotemporal convexity. Acute arterial bleeding is usually caused by laceration of the medial meningeal artery. Because of a high arterial pressure, epidural hematomas rapidly cause significant mass effect and acute neurologic symptoms.

Radiographic appearance

Because the dura is very adherent to the inner table of the skull, an epidural hematoma typically appears as a biconvex (lens-shaped), peripheral, high-density lesion (Figure 7-31). There is usually a shift of the midline structures toward the opposite side unless a contralateral balancing hematoma is present. If not promptly recognized, an epidural hematoma can lead to rapid progressive loss of consciousness, dilatation of the ipsilateral pupil, compression of the upper mid-

Figure 7-33 Bilateral subdural hematoma. Coronal MR image shows high signal intensity of bilateral subdural collections *(H)*.

Figure 7-32 Acute subdural hematoma. High-density, crescent-shaped lesion *(arrow)* adjacent to the inner table of the skull. Hematoma extends into interhemispheric fissure *(arrowhead)*.

brain, and eventually compression of the entire brainstem and death.

Treatment

To prevent death, emergency surgical decompression is required to relieve intracranial pressure.

Subdural hematoma

Subdural hematomas reflect venous bleeding, most commonly from ruptured veins between the dura and meninges. Symptoms may occur within the first few minutes; however, because of the low pressure of venous bleeding, patients with subdural hematomas tend to have a chronic course with symptoms of headache, agitation, confusion, drowsiness, and gradual neurologic deficits.

Radiographic appearance

An acute subdural hematoma typically appears on CT scans as a peripheral zone of increased density that follows the surface of the brain and has a crescentic shape adjacent to the inner table of the skull (Figure 7-32). On CT, the finding of isodense to hypodense areas within a hyperdense hematoma indicates rapid bleeding with an accumulation of

unclotted blood. There is usually an associated mass effect with displacement of midline structures and obliteration of sulci over the affected hemisphere. The absence of displacement away from the side of a lesion may indicate the not-infrequent presence of bilateral subdural hematomas. On MRI scans, a subdural hematoma is detectable within a few days as an extraaxial mass of high signal intensity representing the accumulation of methemoglobin (Figure 7-33).

Serial CT scans demonstrate a gradual decrease in the attenuation value of a subdural hematoma over a period of weeks. With absorption and lysis of the blood clot, the hematoma becomes isodense with normal brain tissue, and the lesion may be identified only because of its mass effect. At this stage, scanning after the administration of contrast material may be of value because of enhancement of the membrane around the subdural hematoma and identification of the cortical veins. MRI scanning of a lesion that is isodense by CT may show medial displacement of the superficial cerebral veins, an indication of an extracerebral mass, as well as the entire extent of the hematoma over the cerebral convexity. A chronic subdural hematoma has a density similar to that of spinal fluid (Figure 7-34). At times, the small bridging veins associated with a chronic subdural hematoma may bleed and produce the difficult problem of an acute subdural hematoma superimposed on a chronic one.

Treatment

In small subdural hematomas without any inclination to rebleed, the hemorrhage resorbs naturally, and no treatment is needed. Severe subdural hematomas

Figure 7-34 Chronic left subdural hematoma. Crescent-shaped high- and low-density regions in the left parietal area. The anterior is isodense (chronic hygroma); posteriorly, a hyperdense crescent shape resulting from acute bleeding can be seen. Midline shift and dilated right lateral ventricle are evident.

Figure 7-35 Cerebral contusion. CT scan shows small punctate hemorrhages (high density) within extensive areas of edema (low density). (From Pressman BD: In Eisenberg RL, editor: *Diagnostic imaging: an algorithmic approach*, Philadelphia, 1988, Lippincott.)

require surgical ligation and evacuation of the hematoma to prevent transtentorial herniation. Less-invasive methods of decreasing intracranial pressure include drug therapy or placement of an intraventricular catheter to remove CSF, which may prevent herniation.

Cerebral contusion

Cerebral contusion is an injury to brain tissue caused by movement of the brain within the calvaria after blunt trauma to the skull. Contusions occur when the brain contacts rough skull surfaces such as the superior orbital roof and petrous ridges. The patient loses consciousness and cannot remember the traumatic event.

Radiographic appearance

Cerebral contusions typically appear on CT scans as low-density areas of edema and tissue necrosis, with or without non–homogeneous density zones, reflecting multiple small areas of hemorrhage (Figure 7-35). The frontal and anterior temporal regions are the most common sites of injury. After the administration of intravenous contrast material, contusions generally enhance for several weeks after the injury because of a

breakdown of the blood–brain barrier. On MRI scans, the cerebral edema causes high signal intensity on T2-weighted images; associated areas of hemorrhage may produce high-signal-intensity regions on T1-weighted scans.

Treatment

The patient is hospitalized to allow observation of any changes in neurologic function. If the contusion causes swelling, medications to decrease intracranial pressure are prescribed. Surgery is usually not necessary.

Intracerebral hematoma

Traumatic hemorrhage into the brain parenchyma can result from shearing forces to intraparenchymal arteries, which tend to occur at the junction of the gray and white matter. Injury to the intima of intracranial vessels can cause the development of traumatic aneurysms, which can rupture.

Radiographic appearance

On CT scans, an intracerebral hematoma appears as a well-circumscribed, homogeneous, high-density region that is usually surrounded by areas of low-density edema (Figure 7-36). As the blood components within

Figure 7-36 Intracerebral hematoma. Note the large, homogeneous, high-density area *(H)* with acute bleeding into lateral ventricles *(V)*.

the hematoma disintegrate, the lesion eventually becomes isodense with normal brain (usually 2 to 4 weeks after injury). On MRI scans, the hematoma shows high signal intensity. A chronic hematoma filled with hemosiderin appears black on T2-weighted images.

Treatment

Although most intracerebral hematomas develop immediately after head injury, delayed hemorrhage is common. This is especially frequent after the evacuation of acute subdural hematomas that are compressing (tamponing) potential bleeding sites. Therefore a repeat CT (or MRI) scan is often performed within 48 hours in patients who have undergone decompressive surgery.

Subarachnoid hemorrhage

Injury to surface veins, cerebral parenchyma, or cortical arteries can produce bleeding into the ventricular system.

Radiographic appearance

On a CT scan, a subarachnoid hemorrhage appears as increased density within the basilar cisterns, cerebral fissures, and sulci. Identification of the falx cerebri, straight sinus, or superior sagittal sinus on non-

contrast CT scans is often considered an indication of subarachnoid blood in the interhemispheric fissure. However, with high-resolution scanners this appearance may be seen in patients with a normal or calcified falx. MRI does not demonstrate the acute subarachnoid hemorrhage well, but T1-weighted scans show subacute hemorrhage as a high signal intensity because of the conversion of fresh blood to methemoglobin.

Treatment

Subarachnoid hemorrhage may require surgical evacuation and vessel repair if bleeding continues. Less invasive methods of decreasing intracranial pressure include drug therapy and the placement of an intraventricular catheter to remove cerebrospinal fluid.

Carotid artery injury

The extracerebral carotid arteries can be injured by penetrating trauma to the neck, as from gunshot wounds or stabbing. The internal carotid artery is associated in 50% of traumatic fistulas.

Radiographic appearance

Angiography can demonstrate laceration of the artery or intimal damage, which may result in either dissection or thrombotic occlusion (Figure 7-37). Hyperextension injuries from motor vehicle accidents can cause intimal damage to the carotid or vertebral arteries, which may result in pseudoaneurysm formation. Traumatic arteriovenous fistulas usually arise between the internal carotid artery and the cavernous sinus. In this condition carotid arteriography demonstrates opacification of the cavernous sinus during the arterial phase. Reverse flow from the cavernous sinus may rapidly opacify a greatly dilated ophthalmic vein. The cavernous sinus and superior ophthalmic vein appear enlarged on a CT scan. MRI normally demonstrates strong enhancement of normal venous spaces (cavernous sinus). A fistula produces a signal void as a result of high flow.

Treatment

The placement of a detachable balloon catheter within the fistula using angiographic guidance may eliminate the need for surgical intervention.

Facial fractures

Although it is padded by overlying skin and fat and the muscles of expression, the face consists of thin and poorly supported bone that can easily break in response to a traumatic force. The purpose of radiographic imaging in the patient with a facial injury is

Figure 7-37 Posttraumatic caroticocavernous fistula. A lateral projection of an external carotid artery angiogram shows a pseudoaneurysm *(A)* and rapid filling of the cavernous sinus *(S)* and pterygoid plexus *(PP)*. There is total interruption of the external carotid artery trunk beyond the takeoff of the facial artery. (From Eisenberg RL: *Diagnostic imaging in surgery,* New York, 1987, McGraw-Hill.)

Figure 7-38 Depressed nasal fracture *(arrow)*.

to demonstrate major disruptions of the facial skeleton and displacement of fracture fragments that will affect the surgical reduction and stabilization of the fracture.

Radiographic appearance

Plain radiographs of the face are usually performed as an initial screening procedure, especially in a severely traumatized patient with substantial injuries to multiple organ systems. Whenever possible, films should be obtained with the patient in the erect position to show any air–fluid levels within the sinuses that could indicate recent hemorrhage and raise the suspicion of an underlying fracture. When erect films cannot be obtained, a cross-table lateral using a horizontal x-ray beam will demonstrate air–fluid levels. Complex-motion (pluridirectional) tomography can blur unrelated overlying structures and thus display details of injury that are obscure or only suspected on plain radiographs. CT can demonstrate soft-tissue abnormalities, such as intraorbital or retrobulbar hematomas, that are impossible to detect by conventional means. In addition, bone detail and displacement can be exquisitely demonstrated when CT window and level settings are adjusted to optimize bony structures.

Fractures of the **nasal bones** are the most common facial fractures. Isolated nasal fractures vary from simple, nondisplaced linear fractures to comminuted lesions with depression of the septum and lateral splaying of the fracture fragments (Figure 7-38). These fractures are best demonstrated on right and left (underexposed) soft-tissue lateral projections, which also can define interruption of the anterior nasal spine—the anterior projection of the maxilla at the base of the cartilaginous nasal septum. Most fractures are transverse and tend to depress the distal portion of the nasal bones.

A **blowout fracture** is caused by a direct blow to the front of the orbit that causes a rapid increase in intraorbital pressure. The fracture occurs in the thinnest, weakest portion of the orbit, which is the orbital floor just above the maxillary sinus. Plain radiographs (modified Waters method), the preferred screening study, and thin-section tomography can demonstrate most blowout fractures (Figure 7-39), although CT may be necessary for better visualization and for detecting entrapment of the extraocular muscles in the upper portion of the adjacent maxillary sinus (Figure 7-40). The fracture segment can be comminuted, with a sagging, hammocklike appearance, or be of the trapdoor variety, with a displaced segment hanging into the antrum by a periosteal hinge. Herniation of orbital fat and extraocular muscles into the fractured orbital

Figure 7-39 Blowout fracture. Conventional tomogram shows comminuted fracture of floor of left orbit with inferior displacement of fracture fragments *(solid arrows)*. Note characteristic soft-tissue shadow *(open arrow)* protruding through floor into superior portion of maxillary sinus.

Figure 7-41 Zygomatic arch fracture. Submentovertex projection demonstrates two fractures on the right with depression of the zygomatic arch.

Figure 7-40 CT of orbital floor fracture. Coronal CT scan using bone window shows fractured orbital floor as double-hinged trap door with separation in center *(open arrow)*. There is opacification of the right maxillary sinus. Note displacement of inferior rectus muscle *(solid arrow)* in this patient who had limited upward gaze. (Courtesy Kenneth D. Dolan, Iowa City, Ia.)

floor produces a characteristic soft-tissue shadow protruding through the floor into the superior portion of the maxillary sinus. Opacification of the sinus caused by hemorrhage and mucosal edema is an indirect sign of orbital floor fracture. The presence of air within the orbit (orbital emphysema) indicates that there is a communication with a paranasal sinus, usually the ethmoid, as a result of an associated fracture of the medial wall of the orbit through the lamina papyracea.

The zygomatic arch is vulnerable to a blow from the side of the face, which can produce a fracture with inward displacement of the fragments centrally and outward displacement of the fragments at the zygomatic and temporal ends of the arch (Figure 7-41). **Zygomatic arch fractures** are best demonstrated on underexposed films taken in the basal (submentovertex) projection ("jug handle" view).

A **tripod fracture** consists of fractures of the zygomatic arch and the orbital floor or rim combined with separation of the zygomaticofrontal suture (Figure 7-42). It is so named because it reflects separation of the zygoma from its three principal attachments. The resulting free-floating zygoma may cause facial disfigurement if not diagnosed and properly treated.

The mandible is a prominent, exposed segment of the facial skeleton and is thus a common site for both intentional and accidental trauma. Plain radiographs with oblique views, combined with panoramic tomography, can demonstrate most **mandibular fractures** (Figure 7-43). The angle of the mandible is the most frequent site of fracture, although fractures can involve any portion of the body and the condylar and coronoid processes. Because the mandible functions essentially as a bony ring, bilateral fractures are common.

Le Fort fractures are severe injuries in which separation at the fracture site results in the formation of a large, complex, detached fragment that is unstable

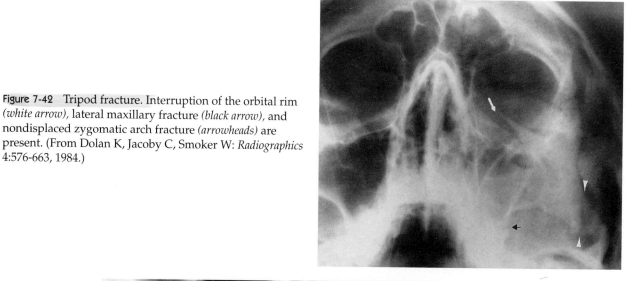

Figure 7-42 Tripod fracture. Interruption of the orbital rim *(white arrow)*, lateral maxillary fracture *(black arrow)*, and nondisplaced zygomatic arch fracture *(arrowheads)* are present. (From Dolan K, Jacoby C, Smoker W: *Radiographics* 4:576-663, 1984.)

Figure 7-43 Mandibular fracture. Panoramic examination in edentulous (without teeth) patient shows fractures of left angle and right body of mandible. (From Rogers LF: *Radiology of skeletal trauma*, New York, 1982, Churchill Livingstone.)

Summary of Findings for Traumatic Processes of the Brain and Skull

DISORDER	LOCATION	RADIOGRAPHIC APPEARANCE	TREATMENT
Skull fracture	Any cranial bone	Linear—sharp lucent line Depressed—stellate (star-shaped) fracture lines radiating outward CT—demonstrates fracture as well as associated intracranial complications	Treat associated complications
Epidural hematoma	Most commonly over parietotemporal convexity	CT—biconvex peripheral high-density lesion, showing midline shift	Emergency surgery to relieve increased intracranial pressure and to stop bleeding

Summary of Findings for Traumatic Processes of the Brain and Skull—cont'd

DISORDER	LOCATION	RADIOGRAPHIC APPEARANCE	TREATMENT
Subdural hematoma	Most commonly from ruptured veins between dura and meninges	CT—acute: crescent-shaped peripheral high-density lesion; chronic: isodense lesion MRI—extracerebral mass with high signal intensity	Resorption in small hematomas Surgical ligation and evacuation of hematoma Control intracranial pressure with drugs or intraventricular drainage catheter
Cranial contusion	Injury to brain tissue Frontal and anterior temporal most common	CT—low-density areas that usually enhance MRI—increased signal intensity on both T2-weighted (cerebral edema) and T1-weighted images (if hemorrhage)	Observation for neurologic change Surgery not usually required
Intracerebral hematoma	Hemorrhage into brain parenchyma	CT—well-circumscribed, homogeneous, high-density region surrounded by low-density regions of edema MRI—high-signal-intensity region; chronic hematoma is black on T2–weighted image	Surgical evacuation of hematoma
Subarachnoid hemorrhage	Injury to surface veins or cortical arteries	CT—increased density within the basilar cisterns, cerebral fissures, and sulci MRI—subacute hemorrhage shows high intensity on T1-weighted images	Surgical evacuation of the hemorrhage and vessel repair Drug therapy or an intraventricular catheter to decrease intracranial pressure
Carotid artery injury	Extracerebral carotid arteries	Angiography—demonstrates laceration of artery or intimal damage CT—large cavernous sinus and superior ophthalmic vein MRI—signal void caused by large cavernous vein resulting from high flow	Placement of detachable balloon within fistula Surgical intervention to eliminate fistula
Facial fracture	Nasal bone (most common) Blowout (orbit) Tripod (zygoma separation from other facial and cranial bones) Mandible Le Fort (bilateral and horizontal fracture of maxillae)	Plain films—cranial and facial bones (upright or horizontal beam image shows fluid levels in the sinuses) CT—soft-tissue abnormality and bone detail	Reduction of fracture Some require surgery to place internal or external fixation device

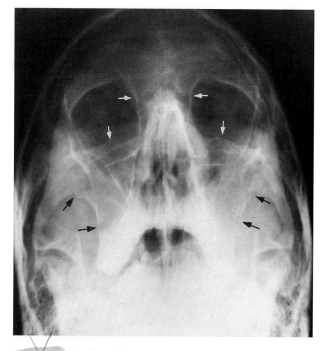

Figure 7-44 Le Fort II fracture. Waters projection shows large separated fragment produced by multiple fractures *(arrows)*. (From Dolan K, Jacoby C, Smoker W: *Radiographics* 4:576-663, 1984.)

and may have its position altered relative to its site of origin. Le Fort fractures involve bilateral and horizontal fractures of the maxillae and are classified as type I, II, or III, depending on the extent of injury (Figure 7-44).

Treatment

Treatment for nasal bone fractures varies depending on the amount of bony displacement. Reduction is required for fractures causing deviation of the nasal septum. More severe facial fractures require surgical reconstruction, possibly using internal or external fixation devices to prevent disfigurement.

■ Vascular Disease of the Central Nervous System

The term **cerebrovascular disease** refers to any process that is caused by an abnormality of the blood vessels or blood supply to the brain. Pathologic processes causing cerebrovascular disease include abnormalities of the vessel wall, occlusion by thrombus or emboli, rupture of blood vessels with subsequent hemorrhage, and decreased cerebral blood flow caused by lowered blood pressure or narrowed lumen caliber. Cerebrovascular diseases include arteriosclerosis, hypertensive hemorrhage, arteritis, aneurysms, and arteriovenous malformations.

Radiographic appearance

The radiographic evaluation of cerebrovascular disease depends on the presenting symptoms and the most likely diagnosis. For ease of classification, cerebrovascular disease can be divided into three categories: completed stroke, transient ischemic attacks (TIAs), and intracranial hemorrhage. Imaging modalities used today include duplex color-flow Doppler ultrasound, MRA, CTA, conventional angiography, and digital subtraction angiography.

Stroke syndrome

The term **stroke** denotes the sudden and dramatic development of a focal neurologic deficit, which may vary from dense hemiplegia (paralysis on one side of the body) and coma to only a trivial neurologic disorder. The specific neurologic defect depends on the arteries involved. A stroke, also known as an acute brain infarction, most commonly involves the circulation of the internal carotid arteries and is seen with symptoms that include acute hemiparesis (weakness of one side of the body) and dysarthria (difficulty speaking).

The purpose of radiographic evaluation in the acute stroke patient is not to confirm the diagnosis of a stroke but to exclude other processes that can simulate the clinical findings (e.g., parenchymal hemorrhage, subdural hematoma). Although the abrupt onset of a stroke may permit differentiation from other conditions that have a more gradual onset of symptoms, patients with focal neurologic deficits of various causes may initially be found comatose, so that the history of gradual onset is not elicited. Clearly it is essential to exclude an intracranial hemorrhage before considering the possibility of treating the stroke patient with anticoagulant therapy.

Radiographic appearance

Noncontrast CT (or MRI, if available) is the examination of choice for the evaluation of the stroke patient. Intravenous contrast material is contraindicated because it is a toxic substance that can cross the disrupted blood–brain barrier in the region of a cerebral infarct and lead to increased edema and a slower recovery for the patient. CT and MRI scans are normal in patients with small infarctions and in the early hours of large infarctions. The initial appearance (within 8 to 24 hours) of a cerebral infarction is a triangular or wedge-shaped area of hypodensity on CT (Figure 7-45) and high signal intensity on T2-weighted MRI sequences involving both the cortex and the underlying white matter down to the ventricular surface. The abnormality is confined to the vascular territory of the involved artery. Although little or no mass effect is evident during the

Figure 7-46   Chronic right middle cerebral artery infarct. Low-attenuation region *(arrows)* shows sharply defined borders and some midline shift.

Figure 7-45   Acute left middle cerebral artery infarct. CT scan obtained 20 hours after onset of acute hemiparesis and aphasia shows obliteration of normal sulci *(arrows)* in involved hemisphere. The gray and white matter in the distribution of the left middle cerebral artery demonstrate low density.

first day, progressive edema produces a mass effect that is maximal 7 to 10 days after the acute event (Figure 7-46). As an infarct ages, brain tissue atrophies, and the adjacent sulci and ventricular system enlarge (Figure 7-47). A combination of nonenhanced MRI and MRA is more sensitive than CT in detecting an infarct or ischemic edema, especially involving the brainstem. Occlusion or stenosis of an artery or vein can be demonstrated along with the associated hemorrhage due to ischemic infarction. A diffusion-weighted MRI scan usually demonstrates a positive hyperintense signal within 2 hours of the incident and plays a critical role in diagnosing and determining the age of the stroke. There is only a small window of 2 to 3 hours after the onset of a stroke in which fibrinolytic agents are effective in decreasing the amount of permanent neurologic deficits. A T2-weighted image detects edema sooner than CT and thus is considered more sensitive. In patients with classic stroke symptoms, follow-up CT or MRI scans are not indicated.

Figure 7-47   Chronic right middle cerebral artery infarct. Low-attenuation region shows sharply defined borders *(arrows)* and some dilatation of the adjacent ventricle.

Treatment

All stroke patients are placed on bed rest with reduced external stimuli to lower cerebral oxygen demands. Medications may be used to decrease intracranial pressure and intracranial edema. Patients with thrombotic strokes receive anticoagulants and possibly thrombolytic agents.

Transient ischemic attacks

TIAs present as focal neurologic deficits that completely resolve within 24 hours. They may result from emboli originating from the surface of an arteriosclerotic ulcerated plaque (embolic stroke), which causes temporary occlusion of cerebral vessels, or from stenosis of an extracerebral artery, which leads to a reduction in critical blood perfusion. Because almost two thirds of arteriosclerotic strokes are preceded by TIAs and the 5-year cumulative risk of stroke in patients with TIAs may be as high as 50%, accurate diagnosis and appropriate treatment are essential.

Radiographic appearance

The most common location of surgically treatable arteriosclerotic disease causing TIAs is the region of the carotid bifurcation in the neck. In patients with an asymptomatic bruit (a rumbling noise heard by a stethoscope) or an unclear history of a TIA, carotid duplex color-flow Doppler scanning is often the initial screening study (Figure 7-48). This technique combines high-resolution ultrasound imaging and Doppler ultrasound with spectral analysis into a "duplex" unit that avoids many of the problems associated with each of these modalities when used alone. In most cases, carotid duplex scanning when combined with MRA can reliably determine whether the extent of the disease is sufficient to warrant more invasive procedures (angiography). Patients with a normal or near-normal carotid duplex scan do not need to undergo more invasive diagnostic procedures for assessment of the carotid bifurcation. Limitations of the usefulness of carotid duplex scanning include its extreme operator dependence and the fact that 10% of patients cannot be successfully imaged with carotid duplex scanning because of anatomic factors (patients with extreme high carotid bifurcations and those with short, thick necks). High-resolution, real-time ultrasound techniques provide hemodynamic information about blood flow velocity. Using ultrasound techniques, it may be impossible to differentiate patients with a total occlusion of the internal carotid artery from those with a tiny residual lumen. This is an important clinical distinction because patients with even a small remaining lumen can undergo a successful carotid endarterectomy (surgical removal of atherosclerotic plaque).

Figure 7-48   Ultrasound of cervical arteriosclerotic occlusive disease. There is severe narrowing *(arrow)* of the origin of the internal carotid artery *(I)* by densely echogenic arteriosclerotic plaque *(asterisks). C,* Common carotid artery; *J,* jugular vein.

Noninvasive MRA provides accurate imaging of the carotid bifurcation and it demonstrates narrowing of the vertebral arteries (Figure 7-49). The reconstitution sign (flow gap) confirms a stenosis greater than 60%, indicating advanced disease requiring surgical intervention. Contrast-enhanced MRA also facilitates visualization of the aortic arch and the origins of the carotid and vertebral arteries.

Patients with a clear-cut episode of a TIA or a neurologic deficit usually are subjected to an angiographic study for evaluating the carotid arteries. Either intravenous or intraarterial digital subtraction angiography (DSA) or selective intraarterial carotid arteriography can be used to demonstrate TIA-producing stenotic or ulcerative lesions that may be amenable to surgical therapy (Figures 7-50 to 7-52). Angiographic evaluation of the aortic arch and vertebral arteries is infrequently indicated in the evaluation of patients with TIAs, because surgery on the origins of the great vessels and posterior circulation is both difficult and not commonly performed, and also because of the higher morbidity from arch and vertebral angiograms reported in some studies.

Treatment

Accurate diagnosis and appropriate treatment (antiplatelet therapy, anticoagulation therapy, or carotid

Figure 7-50 Normal carotid artery bifurcation. Common carotid arteriogram shows bulbous origin of the internal carotid artery *(solid arrow)* and multiple branches of the external carotid artery *(open arrows).*

Figure 7-49 Normal MRA carotid study. **A,** The anteroposterior perspective of the neck demonstrates from the subclavian arteries to the origin of the basilar artery, and the bifurcation of the common carotid arteries. **B,** The off-lateral perspective offers a second view of the vessels.

Figure 7-51 Ulceration of the internal carotid artery. Common carotid arteriogram shows ulcerated lesion *(arrowhead)* at the origin of the internal carotid artery, with severe stenosis of the internal carotid *(open arrow)* and external carotid *(black arrow)* arteries.

endarterectomy) are essential to prevent permanent deficits. Thrombolytic agents may also be used.

Intraparenchymal hemorrhage

Aside from head trauma, the principal cause of intraparenchymal hemorrhage (hemorrhagic stroke) is hypertensive vascular disease. Less frequent causes are rupture of a congenital berry aneurysm or an arteriovenous malformation. Hypertensive hemorrhages result in oval or circular collections that displace the surrounding brain and can cause a significant mass effect. Although they can occur at any location within the brain, hypertensive hemorrhages are most frequent in the basal ganglia, white matter, thalamus, cerebellar hemispheres, and pons. A frequent

Figure 7-52 Occluded internal carotid artery. Intravenous digital subtraction angiogram shows occlusion of the left internal carotid artery at its origin *(arrowhead).*

Figure 7-53   Intracerebral hematoma. Noncontrast CT scan shows homogeneous, high-density area in left thalamus. The low-density area *(arrowheads)* adjacent to the hematoma represents associated ischemia and edema. Hematoma has entered the ventricular system, and a prominent cerebrospinal fluid–blood level is seen in the dependent lateral ventricle *(arrow).* Such extension of blood into the ventricular system is an extremely poor prognostic sign. Mass effect caused by hematoma has compressed the third ventricle and the foramen of Monro and has resulted in obstructive enlargement of the lateral ventricles. (From Drayer BP: Neuroradiology. In Rosenberg RN, Heinz ER, editors: *The clinical neurosciences,* New York, 1984, Churchill Livingstone.)

complication is rupture of the hemorrhage into the ventricular system or subarachnoid space. Intraparenchymal hemorrhages resulting from congenital "berry" (saccular) aneurysms usually are associated with subarachnoid hemorrhage and tend to develop in regions where these congenital vascular anomalies most commonly occur. These include the sylvian fissure (middle cerebral artery) and the midline subfrontal area (anterior communicating artery). Arteriovenous malformations occur throughout the brain and tend to bleed into the white matter.

Radiographic appearance

Patients with a suspected intraparenchymal hemorrhage should be evaluated with MRI or a noncontrast CT scan. A fresh hematoma appears on CT as a homogeneously dense, well-defined lesion with a round to oval configuration (Figure 7-53). Hematomas produce ventricular compression and, when large, considerable midline shift and brain herniation. A hematoma that is not homogeneously dense is suggestive of hemorrhage occurring within a tumor, an inflammatory process, or an infarction. As the hematoma ages, its density changes. On CT, after passing through an isodense stage the hematoma becomes hypodense; by 6 months it appears as a well-defined, low-density region that is often considerably smaller than the original lesion. Contrast enhancement usually develops about the periphery of a hematoma after 7 to 10 days. On MRI, the preferred study, the high signal intensity within a hematoma (caused by the conversion of normal hemoglobin to

methemoglobin) arises after a few days and continues for several months (Figure 7-54). Once the methemoglobin is completely converted to paramagnetic hemosiderin, the hematoma demonstrates very low signal intensity on T2-weighted sequences.

Arteriography is not indicated in patients with classic hypertensive hematomas. However, arteriography remains the gold standard for those patients in whom an aneurysm or arteriovenous malformation is suspected as the underlying cause of the hematoma. In patients with a suspected aneurysm, it is important to determine the number of aneurysms, which aneurysm has ruptured, the location of the neck of the aneurysm, and the patency of the circle of Willis. Statistically, the largest of multiple aneurysms is the one that has ruptured; it is rare for an aneurysm less than 5 mm in diameter to rupture. Because an aneurysm

Figure 7-54   Intracerebral hematoma. Coronal T2-weighted MRI scan shows a large hematoma in the left thalamic region *(arrow)*. Hematoma consists of two portions: central area of increased signal intensity representing methemoglobin, and surrounding area of low signal intensity representing hemosiderin.

Figure 7-55   Arteriovenous malformation. Axial MRI scan shows large left parietal mass *(large arrowheads)* consisting of vascular structures of varying intensity, depending on whether there is rapid flow *(black)* or slow flow *(white)*. Note greatly dilated vessel *(small arrowhead)* that feeds the malformation.

generally ruptures at its apex, an irregular, multiloculated dome is suggestive of a prior rupture. Spasm in adjacent vessels and adjacent hematomas also assist in identifying which of several aneurysms has bled. Noncontrast CT demonstrates an aneurysm as a slightly hyperdense region. The intravenous injection of contrast material produces a strong uniform enhancement. On MRI, an aneurysm produces a flow void on both T1- and T2-weighted images. Imaging has improved to detect an aneurysm. CTA and MRA can visualize large and medium aneurysms, as well as feeding and draining vessels associated with an arteriovenous malformation. Angiography remains, however, the gold standard for demonstrating abnormalities involving small vessels.

In patients less than 20 years of age, arteriovenous malformation is the most common cause of nontraumatic intraparenchymal hemorrhage. On MRI (Figure 7-55), a cerebrovascular malformation appears as a mass of vascular structures of varying intensity, depending on whether there is rapid flow (black) or slow flow (white). On CT, the malformation consists of an irregular tangle of vessels (best seen after the intravenous injection of contrast material) and greatly dilated veins draining from the central tangle (Figure 7-56, *A*). Arteriography demonstrates an irregular, racemose tangle of abnormal vessels that are fed by

dilated cerebral or cerebellar arteries (Figure 7-56, *B*). There is rapid shunting of blood into dilated, tortuous draining veins. Because of the often multiple sources of blood flow to an arteriovenous malformation, the arteriographic evaluation should include selective injections of contrast material into both internal and external carotid arteries.

Treatment

Steroid therapy, especially in nontraumatic hematomas, usually controls the edema that produces much of the mass effect. In cases of hemorrhagic strokes, the first line of treatment consists of stopping the bleeding (i.e., correct any coagulopathy), and the second is to try to prevent a recurrence of bleeding (control blood pressure), and finally surgery is performed to correct pathology (aneurysm or arteriovenous malformation). For aneurysms, surgical placement of a clip at the neck of the lesion is required to close the pouch. Arteriovenous malformations require surgery or neurointerventional procedures.

Subarachnoid hemorrhage

A major cause of subarachnoid hemorrhage (hemorrhagic stroke) is rupture of a berry aneurysm (Figure 7-57). Patients with this condition usually have

A

Figure 7-57   Ruptured berry aneurysm. Left carotid arteriogram demonstrates left supraclinoid aneurysm of the internal carotid artery. Posterior bulge of the aneurysm *(arrow)* represents the site of rupture.

B

Figure 7-56   Arteriovenous malformation with hemorrhage. **A,** CT scan shows an irregular tangle of vessels in the parietal lobe, seen without a contrast injection. **B,** In another patient, carotid arteriogram shows dilated blood vessels constituting an arteriovenous malformation.

Figure 7-58   Berry aneurysm with subarachnoid hemorrhage. CT scan demonstrates subarachnoid bleed into the cisterns and ventricles (hyperdense) from a ruptured left middle cerebral aneurysm *(arrow).*

a generalized excruciating headache followed by unconsciousness.

Radiographic appearance

The radiographic procedure of choice is a noncontrast CT scan, which can demonstrate high-density blood in the subarachnoid spaces of the basal cisterns in more than 95% of cases (Figure 7-58). Bleeding may extend into the brain parenchyma adjacent to the aneurysm. Contrast-enhanced CT scans are not indicated in subarachnoid hemorrhage, because the sur-

geon will not operate for a suspected aneurysm without an angiogram and the patient would thus be exposed to the risk of an excessive load of contrast material. MRI is relatively insensitive for identifying acute subarachnoid bleeds but it does demonstrate

Summary of Findings for Vascular Disease of the Central Nervous System

DISORDER	LOCATION	RADIOGRAPHIC APPEARANCE	TREATMENT
Stroke syndrome	Neurologic deficit due to lack of circulation; internal carotid artery most common site	CT (initial exam)—a triangular or wedge-shaped hypodensity on noncontrast scan MRI—T2-weighted image produces high signal intensity of vascular territory involved Diffusion-weighted MRI—hyperintense signals within 2 hr of onset CT/MRI—mass effect seen 7-10 days after onset	Bed rest and reduced external stimuli for all stroke victims Medications to treat increased intracranial pressure if symptoms arise
Transient ischemic attack	Embolic stroke originating from arteriosclerotic ulcerated plaque	Duplex color-flow Doppler US—provides hemodynamic information including flow velocity (total occlusion vs. tiny residual flow) MRA—size and shape of diseased carotid and vertebral arteries; contrast-agent–enhanced scan shows aortic arch and origins of vessels DSA—invasive study provides the highest resolution of intraluminal vascular pathology	Anticoagulants and/or thrombolytic agents to treat cause Surgical endarterectomy
Intraparenchymal hemorrhage	Hemorrhage into brain tissue	CT—new hematoma appears as homogeneously dense, well-defined, round or oval lesion, becoming isodense over time; 6-month-old hematoma appears as a well-defined low-density lesion MRI—high signal intensity after a few days on T1- and T2-weighted images; with time, a low signal intensity is seen on T2-weighted images CTA/MRA—shows arteriovenous malformations in large and medium vessels and can detect an aneurysm Arteriography—utilized for small vessels	Steroid therapy Surgical clipping of aneurysm Surgery or neurointerventional procedures to correct arteriovenous malformation
Subarachnoid hemorrhage	Bleed beneath arachnoid layer of meninges	CT—noncontrast scan initally shows high attenuation of blood in the subarachnoid space MRI—best demonstrates chronic hemorrhages as hypointense areas on T2-weighted image CTA/MRA—shows large and medium vessels for detecting an aneurysm Arteriography—to localize and characterize small-vessel anatomy	Stop bleeding Prevent recurrence Surgical intervention to correct pathology

CTA, CT angiography; *DSA,* digital subtraction angiography; *MRA,* MR angiography; *US,* ultrasound.

chronic blood staining of the meninges by a marked hypointensity on T2-weighted images.

The timing of angiography in subarachnoid hemorrhage depends on the philosophy of the surgeon. Blood in the subarachnoid space is an irritant that causes vasospasm of the vessels of the circle of Willis and the middle cerebral artery. This vasospasm, which can lead to cerebral ischemia and frank infarction, is greatest 3 to 14 days after the acute episode.

Treatment

If emergency surgery within the first 72 hours after the hemorrhage is planned, emergency selective angiography is indicated. If surgical intervention is to be delayed, angiography should be postponed until just before surgery. The most common locations for berry aneurysms are the origins of the posterior cerebral and anterior communicating arteries and the trifurcation of the middle cerebral artery. Because of the 20% incidence of multiple aneurysms, the angiographic procedure should include evaluation of the internal carotid and vertebral arteries bilaterally.

■ Multiple Sclerosis

Multiple sclerosis is a the most common demyelinating disorder; it presents as recurrent attacks of focal neurologic deficits that primarily involve the spinal cord, optic nerves, and central white matter of the brain. The disease has a peak incidence between 20 and 40 years of age, a strong predominance in women, and a clinical course characterized by multiple relapses and remissions. Impairment of nerve conduction caused by the degeneration of myelin sheaths leads to such symptoms as double vision, nystagmus (involuntary, rapid movement of the eyeball in all directions), loss of balance and poor coordination, shaking tremor and muscular weakness, difficulty in speaking clearly, and bladder dysfunction.

Radiographic appearance

MRI is the modality of choice for demonstrating the scattered plaques of demyelination that are characteristic of multiple sclerosis. The plaques appear as multiple areas of increased signal intensity on T2-weighted images; these areas involve primarily the periventricular white matter, cerebellum, brainstem, and spinal cord (Figure 7-59). Lesions involving the optic nerve or chiasm require contrast enhancement and fat-suppression imaging (which increases the contrast difference between fat and water) to improve their detectability. On T1-weighted images, the plaques appear as isointense or hypointense lesions that may have a beveled edge. CT shows old inactive disease as well-defined areas of decreased attenuation in the deep white matter and periventricular regions. In the acute phase, CT performed after intravenous administration of contrast material demonstrates a mixture of nonenhancing focal areas of decreased density (representing old areas of demyelination) and enhancing regions that represent active foci.

Treatment

As the disease progresses and the symptoms increase in severity, immunosuppressive agents may help limit the autoimmune attack. Antiviral drugs may slow the progress of the disease. To reduce the number and severity of attacks, some patients receive subcutaneous injections of disease-modifying immunomodulatory agents (beta interferon). The treatments can only aid in slowing the progress of multiple sclerosis; there is no cure.

■ Epilepsy and Convulsive Disorders

Epilepsy is a condition in which brain impulses are temporarily disturbed, resulting in a spectrum of symptoms ranging from loss of consciousness for a few seconds to violent seizures (shaking and thrashing movements of all extremities). Although most cases of epilepsy are idiopathic, the disorder can be a result of injury (penetrating or nonpenetrating trauma, depressed skull fracture), birth trauma, or infection.

The mildest type of epilepsy, which occurs primarily in children, is called **petit mal.** This results in brief episodes of loss of consciousness, which may be associated with mild muscular twitching. Petit mal epilepsy usually disappears in young adulthood.

Grand mal epilepsy refers to generalized convulsions associated with the patient falling to the floor, hypersalivating (foaming at the mouth), and losing control of urine and sometimes feces. In many cases an approaching seizure is heralded by an aura, such as a ringing in the ears, a tingling sensation in the fingers, or spots before the eyes. After a seizure, the patient tends to be groggy and unaware of what has happened (i.e., in a postictal state).

Radiographic appearance

Whenever possible, the radiographic evaluation of a patient with a seizure disorder should be done when the patient is clinically stable. The appropriate procedure is an MRI scan to search for an unsuspected brain tumor, arteriovenous malformation, or hippocampal sclerosis (Figure 7-60). Hippocampal sclerosis (mesial temporal sclerosis) refers to neuronal loss and gliosis that occurs in the temporal region. High-resolution, thin-section, coronal T2-weighted images are the most specific. It is the most common cause of seizures that do not respond to medical therapy.

Figure 7-59 Multiple sclerosis. **A,** Axial T2-weighted MR image in a 35-year-old woman shows characteristic areas of increased signal intensity *(arrowheads)* in deep white matter. **B,** Sagittal image demonstrates periventricular plaques *(arrows).* **C,** Coronal plane image shows increased intensity of cervical cord plaque *(arrow).* (**B** and **C** courtesy Bartram J. Pierce, RT(R)(MR), Good Samaritan Regional Medical Center, Corvallis, Ore.)

Summary of Findings for Multiple Sclerosis

DISORDER	LOCATION	RADIOGRAPHIC APPEARANCE	TREATMENT
Multiple sclerosis	Most common demyelinating disorder of the CNS	MRI—plaques appear as a hyperintense signal on T2-weighted images and isointense to hypointense, possibly with beveled edges, on T1-weighted images MRI with contrast enhancement and fat suppression best demonstrates plaques involving the optic nerve and chiasm	Immunosuppressive agents Antiviral drugs Subcutaneous injections of beta-interferon

Figure 7-60   Seizure disorder caused by hippocampal sclerosis. **A,** Coronal T2-weighted MRI scan shows high-intensity signal in the left hippocampal region *(arrow).* **B,** Normal scan for comparison. (From Bronen RA: Epilepsy: the role of MR imaging, *AJR Am J Roentgenol* 159:1165-1174, 1992.)

Summary of Findings for Epilepsy and Convulsive Disorders

DISORDER	LOCATION	RADIOGRAPHIC APPEARANCE	TREATMENT
Epilepsy and convulsive disorders	Brain impulses temporarily disrupted	MRI—high-resolution, thin-section T2-weighted image is most specific PET—localizes seizure foci	Stabilize patient for safety Reverse chemical causes Medications to decrease number of seizures Surgical resection

PET, Positron emission tomography.

Since most seizure disorders are attributable to small areas of cortical brain injury resulting from trauma or infarction, CT or MRI scans are usually normal. If the MRI scan is normal, PET using ¹⁸F-fluorodeoxyglucose (FDG) may localize the seizure focus in a patient with hippocampal sclerosis. PET has a 70% to 80% sensitivity and a very low rate of false-positive results (Figure 7-61).

Treatment

For the patient who has an acute seizure, initial efforts are directed toward stabilization (securing adequate ventilation and perfusion) and stopping the seizure. Subsequently, a careful history, physical examination, and appropriate laboratory studies should be performed to exclude reversible chemical causes of seizures such as hypoglycemia, hyponatremia or hypernatremia,

and hypocalcemia or hypercalcemia. If the patient does not respond to routine anticonvulsive treatment, CT may be indicated to search for causes of an acute seizure disorder (e.g., subdural hematoma, intracerebral hematoma), which may be amenable to surgical intervention. These conditions can be adequately assessed with a noncontrast CT scan; plain skull radiographs are not required. Medications may help decrease the number of seizures a patient experiences. Surgical resection of the lesion is associated with a very good outcome.

■ Degenerative Diseases

Normal aging

During normal aging, a gradual loss of neurons results in enlargement of the ventricular system and sulci (Figure 7-62).

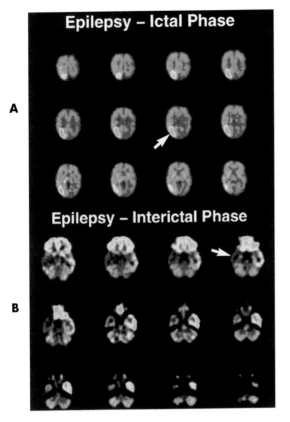

Figure 7-61 Epilepsy. In a patient with a history of epileptic seizures (ictal phase) **(A)**, FDG-PET brain images demonstrate an area of increased activity: the highlighted region in the posterior portion of the cerebrum *(arrow)*. **(B)**, The interictal phase (postseizure activity phase on the same patient) illustrates decreased activity in the temporal lobe *(arrow)* resulting from decreased blood flow during the seizure.

Figure 7-62 Normal aging. CT scan of 70-year-old man shows generalized ventricular dilatation with prominence of sulci over the surfaces of the cerebral hemisphere.

Radiographic appearance

Demyelination, which is also a part of normal aging, leads to the development of low density in the periventricular regions on CT and high signal intensity on T2-weighted MR images (Figure 7-63).

Alzheimer's disease

Alzheimer's disease (presenile dementia) is a diffuse form of progressive cerebral atrophy that develops at an earlier age than the senile period.

Radiographic appearance

CT and MRI demonstrate nonspecific findings of cerebral atrophy, including symmetrically enlarged ventricles with prominence of the cortical sulci (Figure 7-64). T2-weighted MR images demonstrate periventricular hyperintensities. FDG-PET metabolic brain imaging used in conjunction with automated brain mapping can help distinguish changes associated with progressive neurodegenerative processes such as

Figure 7-63 Degenerative changes of aging. Axial MRI scan demonstrates multiple areas of increased signal intensity around ventricles and in deep white matter, consistent with cerebral ischemia or infarction.

Figure 7-64 Alzheimer's disease. Noncontrast CT scan of a 56-year-old woman with progressive dementia shows generalized enlargement of ventricular system and sulci.

Alzheimer's dementia. When superimposed into an Alzheimer's data base, areas of significantly reduced glucose metabolism correspond with Alzheimer's regions (Figure 7-65).

Treatment

Diet, education, memory aids, and safety issues may slow the progression of dementia, but there is no cure at this time. Medications available today help to slow the progression of the disease and may reverse early symptoms to some degree.

Huntington's disease

Huntington's disease is an inherited (autosomal dominant) condition that predominantly involves men and presents in the early to middle adult years with dementia and typical choreiform movements (involuntary movements that are rapid, jerky, and continuous).

Radiographic appearance

The pathologic hallmark of Huntington's disease is atrophy of the caudate nucleus and putamen, which produces the typical CT appearance of focal dilatation of the frontal horns and a loss of their normal concave shape (Figure 7-66) as a result of caudate

Figure 7-65 Alzheimer's dementia. **A,** FDG-PET metabolic brain imaging demonstrates significantly reduced glucose metabolism in the left cerebrum on transverse images *(arrows).* **B,** When the brain map was superimposed, the area of reduced uptake (represented by the *dark gray area*) superimposed the Alzheimer's control data (represented by the *black area*). Significantly reduced glucose metabolism can be seen on the patient's left, which is consistent with a diagnosis of Alzheimer's dementia.

nucleus atrophy. Generalized enlargement of the ventricles and dilatation of the cortical sulci can also occur.

Treatment

At present there is no cure or treatment. Counseling is essential because of the hereditary genetic relationship.

Parkinson's disease

Parkinson's disease (shaking palsy) is a progressive degenerative disease characterized by stooped posture, stiffness and slowness of movement, fixed facial expression, and involuntary rhythmic tremor of the limbs that disappears with voluntary movement. A disorder of middle or later life, Parkinson's disease is very gradually progressive and exhibits a prolonged course.

The major degenerative changes in nerve cells in Parkinson's disease occur in the basal ganglia, especially the globus pallidus, the substantia nigra, and the fibers of the corpus striatum. The essence of the condition seems to be an enzyme defect that results in an inadequate production of the neuronal transmitter substance dopamine. The most recent method of treatment is the administration of L-dopa, a substance that is converted to dopamine in the brain. Although this drug therapy does not stop the neuronal degeneration, it dramatically improves both the appearance and behavior of the patient.

Radiographic appearance

CT scans in patients with Parkinson's disease often demonstrate cortical atrophy. However, because this condition is usually seen in older individuals, the ventricular enlargement and prominent cortical sulci found on CT scans may be indistinguishable from that caused by the normal aging process.

Treatment

Drug treatment is the first choice for controlling symptoms, as no cure currently exists. Stereotactic pallidotomy is a surgical option for some cases and may aid in long-term reduction of symptoms by creating lesions destroying the globus pallidus.

Cerebellar atrophy

Isolated atrophy of the cerebellum may represent an inherited disorder, a degenerative disease, or the toxic

Figure 7-66 Huntington's disease. **A,** CT scan in a normal patient shows the heads of the caudate nucleus *(black arrowheads)* producing a normal concavity of the frontal horns *(white arrowheads)*. **B,** In a patient with Huntington's disease, atrophy of the caudate nucleus causes a characteristic loss of the normal concavity *(white arrowheads)* of the frontal horns.

Summary of Findings for Degenerative Diseases of the Central Nervous System

DISORDER	LOCATION	RADIOGRAPHIC APPEARANCE	TREATMENT
Normal aging	Cerebral atrophy, enlarged ventricular system, demyelination	CT—low-density periventricular regions MRI—high signal intensity of periventricular regions on T2-weighted images	None in normal aging process
Alzheimer's disease	Cerebral atrophy before senile period	CT—cerebral atrophy with enlarged ventricles and prominent cortical sulci MRI—similar to CT; periventricular intensity on T2-weighted images PET—reduced glucose metabolism consistent with Alzheimer's regions	No cure Diet, education, and safety factors to slow progression Medications to slow progression
Huntington's disease	Atrophy of caudate nucleus and putamen	CT—focal ventricular dilation; loss of normal shape of frontal horns	No treatment at present Genetic counseling of families
Parkinson's disease	Degeneration of basal ganglia	CT appearance similar to that of normal aging process	Drug treatment No cure known Stereotactic pallidotomy
Cerebellar atrophy	Degeneration of cerebellum	MRI—size changes in cerebellum	Discontinue prolonged use of drugs (alcohol and phenytoin)
Amyotrophic lateral sclerosis	Upper and lower motor neurons	CT/MRI/myelography—inconclusive for diagnostic purposes; can demonstrate other causes of similar symptoms	Incurable Psychological support Education

Figure 7-67 Cerebellar atrophy. Sagittal MRI scan shows dramatic loss of substance of the vermis of the cerebellum *(arrows)* in a patient with severe alcoholism.

effect of prolonged use of such drugs as alcohol and phenytoin (Dilantin) (Figure 7-67).

Amyotrophic lateral sclerosis (Lou Gehrig's disease)

In this relentlessly progressive condition of unknown cause, there is widespread selective atrophy and loss of motor nerve cells leading to extensive paralysis and death from respiratory weakness or aspiration pneumonia.

Radiographic appearance

Although this disease cannot be diagnosed radiographically, CT, MRI, or myelography is often performed to exclude a spinal malignancy, which could produce a similar clinical appearance.

Treatment

Amyotrophic lateral sclerosis is uniformly fatal because there currently is no cure. Psychological support and education can be provided.

Figure 7-68 Hydrocephalus with obstruction at the level of the foramen of Monro. T1-weighted MRI scan shows a hyperintense colloid cyst causing bilateral enlargement of the frontal horns. (From Johnson CE, Zimmerman RD: *MRI Decisions* 3:2-16, 1989.)

Figure 7-69 Hydrocephalus caused by obstruction at the level of the aqueduct. Dilatation of the lateral *(L)* and third *(T)* ventricles can be seen in this patient with congenital hydrocephalus. Symptoms of headache and papilledema resolved after ventricular shunting.

▪ Hydrocephalus

Hydrocephalus refers to dilatation of the ventricular system that is usually associated with increased intracranial pressure. In **noncommunicating** (obstructive) hydrocephalus, there is an obstruction to the flow of CSF somewhere along the ventricular pathways from the lateral ventricles to the outlets of the fourth ventricle. Enlargement of the lateral ventricles with normal-size third and fourth ventricles indicates an obstruction at the level of the foramen of Monro. This is most commonly attributable to a colloid cyst (Figure 7-68) or a suprasellar tumor, especially craniopharyngioma. Enlargement of the lateral and third ventricles with a normal-size fourth ventricle indicates an obstruction at the level of the aqueduct of Sylvius (Figures 7-69 and 7-70). The most common causes of this appearance are congenital aqueduct stenosis or occlusion and neoplasm (pinealoma, teratoma). Enlargement of the entire ventricular system (with the fourth ventricle often dilated out of proportion [Dandy-Walker cyst]) indicates an obstruction at the level of the outlet of the fourth ventricle (Figure 7-71), a condition that may reflect congenital atresia,

infection, neoplasm, or downward herniation of the cerebellar tonsils through the foramen magnum.

In the much more common **communicating** hydrocephalus, the ventricular fluid passes freely into the extraventricular subarachnoid space. There is generalized ventricular enlargement with normal or absent sulci. Obstruction of the normal CSF pathway distal to the fourth ventricle usually involves the subarachnoid space at the basal cisterns, cerebral convexity, or foramen magnum. Causes include infection (meningitis, empyema), subarachnoid or subdural hemorrhage, congenital anomalies, neoplasm, and dural venous thrombosis. A similar radiographic pattern is seen in **"normal-pressure"** hydrocephalus, a syndrome of gait ataxia, urinary incontinence, and dementia associated with ventricular dilatation and relatively normal CSF pressure.

Radiographic appearance

CT clearly shows ventricular dilatation. MRI is more specific than CT in demonstrating the underlying cause of obstruction or excluding obstruction (communicating hydrocephalus). Contrast-enhanced MRI

Figure 7-70 Aqueductal stenosis. T1-weighted sagittal MRI scan shows pronounced narrowing of the inferior portion of the aqueduct *(arrow)*. There is flaring of the upper portion of the aqueduct and considerable enlargement of the third and lateral ventricles. Note that the fourth ventricle is of normal size. (From Stark DD, Bradley WG: *Magnetic resonance imaging,* ed 2, St Louis, 1991, Mosby.)

Figure 7-72 Choroid plexus papilloma. T1-weighted MRI scan shows a lobulated isointense mass *(arrows)* in a greatly dilated right lateral ventricle. (From Eisenberg RL: *Clinical imaging: an atlas of differential diagnosis,* Gaithersburg, Md, 1992, Aspen.)

Figure 7-71 Hydrocephalus caused by obstruction at the level of the outlet of the fourth ventricle. Huge low-density cyst (a Dandy-Walker cyst) occupies most of the enlarged posterior fossa and represents an extension of the dilated fourth ventricle.

may assist in distinguishing a congenital posterior fossa cyst from an enhancing cystic neoplasm. Ultrasound can show the ventricular dilatation either in utero or after birth as long as the sound waves can traverse the open fontanels.

Generalized enlargement of the ventricular system can also be attributable to the overproduction of CSF by a papilloma (Figure 7-72) or carcinoma arising in the choroid plexus (CSF-secreting vascular tissue in the ventricles). These rare tumors usually occur in the fourth ventricle in adults and the lateral ventricles in children.

Treatment

Hydrocephalus can often be treated by the placement of a shunt between the dilated ventricles and the heart or the peritoneal cavity. Successful shunting causes a decrease in the intracranial pressure and ventricular size; the latter can be monitored by CT or MRI.

■ Sinusitis

The paranasal sinuses (maxillary, ethmoid, frontal, and sphenoid) are paired, air-filled cavities that are lined with a mucous membrane that is directly con-

Figure 7-73 Chronic sinusitis. Mucosal thickening appears as soft-tissue density *(arrows)* lining the walls of the maxillary antra.

Figure 7-74 Acute sinusitis. There is mucosal thickening involving most of the paranasal sinuses, and air–fluid levels *(arrows)* in both maxillary antra.

tinuous with the nasal mucosa. The size and shape of the sinuses vary in different age periods, in different individuals, and on the two sides of the same individual. At birth, the maxillary sinus is only a slitlike space that later expands to fill the maxilla and is thus responsible for the growth of the face. The ethmoid sinuses can be seen radiographically by 6 years of age, whereas the frontal sinuses usually are not well demonstrated until about 10 years of age. The sphenoid sinuses begin to develop around 2 or 3 years of age and are fully developed by late adolescence.

Viral infection of the upper respiratory tract may lead to obstruction of drainage of the paranasal sinuses and the development of localized pain, tenderness, and fever.

Radiographic appearance

Radiographically, acute or chronic sinusitis causes mucosal thickening, which appears as a soft-tissue density lining the walls of the involved sinuses (Figure 7-73). The maxillary antra are most commonly affected and are best visualized on the Waters projection. An air–fluid level in a sinus is usually considered a manifestation of acute inflammatory disease (Figure 7-74). To demonstrate this finding, it is essential that all sinus films be obtained with the patient erect and with the use of a horizontal beam. The destruction of the bony wall of a sinus is an ominous sign indicating secondary osteomyelitis (Figure 7-75). CT, the proce-

Figure 7-75 Mucormycosis causing pansinusitis with osteomyelitis. Destruction of the roof of the right orbit and outer margins of the right frontal sinus can be seen.

dure of choice, demonstrates bony sinonasal anatomy; coronal images can show air–fluid levels (Figure 7-76). Coronal MRI provides the best method to detect suspected complications such as mucocele, osteomyelitis, or underlying intracranial disease.

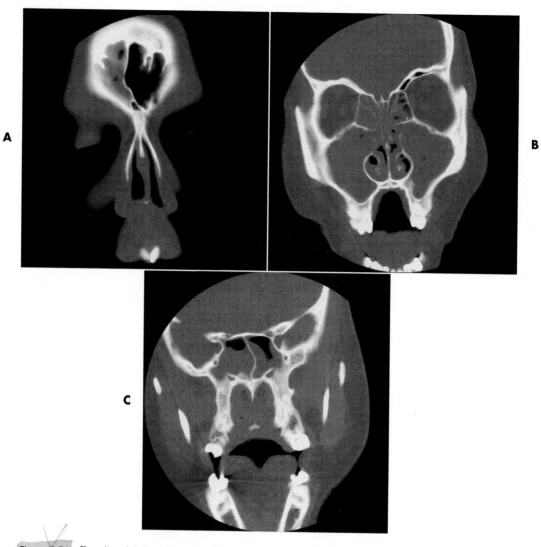

Figure 7-76 Pansinusitis in a 29-year-old woman with headache. The coronal CT scan shows fluid in the frontal sinus **(A)**, in the maxillary and ethmoid sinuses **(B)**, and in the sphenoid sinus **(C)**.

Summary of Findings for Other Diseases of the Central Nervous System

DISORDER	LOCATION	RADIOGRAPHIC APPEARANCE	TREATMENT
Hydrocephalus	Cerebral ventricular system	CT—demonstrates ventricular dilatation MRI—may also show underlying cause	Shunt placement
Sinusitis	Paranasal sinuses; maxillary most common	Sinus radiograph—mucosal thickening and fluid levels CT—demonstrates sinonasal anatomy and fluid levels on coronal imaging MRI—suspected complications	Antibiotics for bacterial infection Decongestants Surgery

Treatment

Sinusitis caused by bacteria is treated with antibiotics to eradicate the infection. Decongestants may be taken to relieve symptoms and aid in sinus drainage. Steroid nasal sprays help reduce mucosal inflammation. Chronic sinusitis may require surgery to clean and drain the sinus, as well as to repair a deviated septum or nasal obstruction that may be the cause of recurrent inflammation.

QUESTIONS

1. The imaging modality of choice to evaluate patients with suspected neurologic dysfunction caused by head trauma is _____.
   A. Ultrasound   C. CT
   B. MRI   D. Skull radiographs

2. Arterial bleeding sometimes associated with head trauma can cause _____ hematomas.
   A. Intracranial   C. Epidural
   B. Subdural   D. Acute

3. Venous bleeding sometimes associated with head trauma can cause _____ hematomas.
   A. Intracranial   C. Epidural
   B. Subdural   D. Acute

4. Movement of the brain within the calvaria following blunt trauma to the skull sometimes results in a cerebral _____.
   A. Subdural   C. Acute hematoma
      hematoma   D. Contusion
   B. Epidural
      hematoma

5. Bleeding into the ventricular system caused by injury to surface veins, cerebral parenchyma, or cortical arteries can cause _____ hemorrhage.
   A. Epidural   C. Epiarachnoid
   B. Subdural   D. Subarachnoid

6. Plain radiographs of the facial bones should always be made with the patient in the _____ position if possible.
   A. Supine   C. Lateral decubitus
   B. Erect   D. Anterior

7. The most common primary brain tumor is a _____.
   A. Glioma   C. Meningioma
   B. Glioblastoma   D. Neurinoma

8. A benign tumor that arises from arachnoid lining cells and is attached to the dura is named _____.
   A. Glioma   C. Meningioma
   B. Glioblastoma   D. Neurinoma

9. The most common neoplasms that metastasize to the brain arise in the _____ and _____.
   A. Lung, stomach C. Stomach, breast
   B. Lung, breast   D. Breast, prostate

10. A viral inflammation of the brain and meninges is called _____.
    A. Meningitis   C. Encephalitis
    B. Hydrocephalus D. Encephalomalacia

11. The best imaging modality to evaluate brain abscesses is _____.

12. The two imaging procedures of choice to evaluate the extent of a stroke in the brain are _____ and _____.

13. The initials *TIA* stands for _____.

14. The imaging modality of choice to demonstrate the plaques of demyelination that are characteristic of multiple sclerosis is _____.

15. A condition in which brain impulses are temporarily disturbed, the results of which range from loss of consciousness to violent seizures, is termed _____.

16. A diffuse form of progressive cerebral atrophy that develops at an earlier age than the senile period is called _____.

17. A progressive degenerative disease characterized by involuntary tremors of the extremities that disappear with voluntary movement is named _____.

18. Sinus radiographs should be taken using a _____ beam and with the patient in the _____ position.

19. The pathologic condition that refers to dilatation of the ventricular system and is usually associated with increased intracranial pressure is _____.

20. If a patient needing facial or sinus radiographs is unable to stand or sit erect, a(n) _____ using a(n) _____ beam may be performed to demonstrate any air–fluid levels that may be present.

Match the terms with the following definitions.

21. _____ Convolutions on the surface of the cerebrum

22. _____ The basic unit of the nervous system

23. _____ Combination of 12 pairs of cranial nerves, 31 pairs of spinal nerves, autonomic nerves, and ganglia

24. _____ Impulse conduction to and from the central nervous system

25. _____ Entity consisting of the brain and spinal cord

26. _____ Fatty covering that insulates axons

27. _____ Junction where impulses are passed from one neuron to another

28. _____ The part of the nervous system that supplies the striated skeletal muscles

29. _____ Projection leading from the nerve cell body

30. _____ The part of the nervous system that supplies smooth muscle, cardiac muscle, and glandular epithelial tissue

31. _____ Shallow grooves on the surface of the cerebrum

32. _____ Projection leading to a nerve cell body

33. _____ White matter connecting the two cerebral hemispheres

34. _____ Midbrain

35. _____ Transparent covering of the brain and spinal cord

36. _____ Projects down into the longitudinal fissure to separate the cerebral hemispheres

37. _____ Slitlike space between the right and left thalami

38. _____ Inflammation of the protective layers of the brain

39. _____ Covering over the cerebellum that separates it from the occipital lobe of the cerebrum

40. _____ Cobweb-like covering of the brain

41. _____ Diamond-shaped space in front of the cerebellum and behind the medulla and pons

42. _____ Outermost covering of the brain

43. _____ Canal connecting the third and fourth ventricles

44. _____ Result of an obstruction of cerebrospinal spinal fluid

45. _____ Foramen connecting the third and lateral ventricles

A. Dendrites
B. Dura mater
C. Axon
D. Gyri
E. Monro
F. Pia mater
G. Reflex arc
H. Corpus callosum
I. Synapse
J. Neuron
K. Hydrocephalus
L. Arachnoid
M. Somatic
N. Peripheral nervous system
O. Sulci
P. Myelin sheath
Q. Fourth ventricle
R. Autonomic
S. Falx cerebri
T. CNS
U. Meningitis
V. Mesencephalon
W. Third ventricle
X. Tentorium cerebelli
Y. Aqueduct of Sylvius

BIBLIOGRAPHY

Brant-Zawadzki M, Norman D: *Magnetic resonance imaging of the central nervous system,* New York, 1987, Raven Press.

Lee SH, Rao KCVG: *Cranial computed tomography and MRI,* New York, 1992, McGraw-Hill.

Osborn AG: *Handbook of neuroradiology,* St Louis, 1991, Mosby.

Ramsey RG: *Neuroradiology with computed tomography,* Philadelphia, 1987, Saunders.

Woodruff WW: *Fundamentals of neuroimaging,* Philadelphia, 1993, Saunders.

CHAPTER 8

Hematopoietic System

■ **Prerequisite Knowledge**

The student should have a basic knowledge of the physiology of the hematopoietic system.

■ **Goals**

To acquaint the student radiographer with the pathophysiology and radiographic manifestations of all the common and some of the unusual disorders of the hematopoietic system

■ **Objectives**

1. To understand and be able to define or describe all bold-faced terms in this chapter
2. To be able to describe the physiology of the hematopoietic system
3. To be able to identify the basic blood structures on diagrams
4. To be able to describe the various pathologic conditions affecting the hematopoietic system as well as their radiographic manifestations

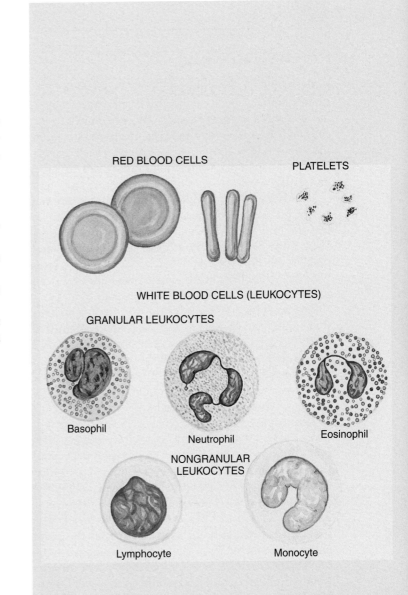

RED BLOOD CELLS   PLATELETS

WHITE BLOOD CELLS (LEUKOCYTES)

GRANULAR LEUKOCYTES

Basophil   Neutrophil   Eosinophil

NONGRANULAR LEUKOCYTES

Lymphocyte   Monocyte

■ ■ ■ ■ ■ ■ ■ ■ ■ **Radiographer Notes**

Although the hematopoietic system cannot be directly imaged, many blood disorders result in abnormalities that can be demonstrated radiographically. It may be necessary to increase or decrease exposure factors when imaging patients who manifest advanced stages of these diseases (see the Box in Chapter 1 labeled Relative Attenuation of X-rays in Advanced Stages of Diseases). The radiographer must be aware of the severe pain experienced by patients undergoing a sickle cell crisis. Patients with advanced leukemia or lymphoma who have an altered immune status may require protective isolation. Because many hematopoietic system diseases cause significant demineralization of bone, the radiographer must be alert to the possibility of pathologic fracture and thus exercise caution when moving and positioning these patients.

■ Physiology of the Blood

Blood and the cells within it are vital to life. An adequate blood supply to all body tissues is necessary to bring oxygen, nutrients, salts, and hormones to the cells and to carry away the waste products of cellular metabolism. The components of blood are also a major defense against infection, toxic substances, and foreign antigens.

Red bone marrow (found in vertebrae and flat bones such as the sternum, ribs, skull, and proximal femurs) and lymph nodes are the blood-forming tissues of the body. Red blood cells (erythrocytes) and platelets (thrombocytes) are made in red bone marrow, whereas white blood cells (leukocytes) are produced in both red marrow and lymphoid tissue.

Erythrocytes are biconcave disks without a nucleus that contain **hemoglobin,** an iron-based protein that carries oxygen from the respiratory tract to the body's tissues. In a normal person, there are 4.5 to 6 million red blood cells in each cubic millimeter of blood. The amount of hemoglobin per deciliter is approximately 14 g in women and 15 g in men.

Leukocytes, or white blood cells, normally number from 5000 to 10,000/mm^3 of blood. Unlike erythrocytes, there are several types of white blood cells. **Neutrophils (polymorphonuclear leukocytes),** which make up 55% to 75% of white blood cells, defend the body against bacteria by ingesting these foreign organisms and destroying them (phagocytosis). The number of polymorphonuclear leukocytes in the blood enormously increases in acute infections because the bone marrow rapidly releases into the bloodstream the large numbers of these cells kept in reserve. **Eosinophils** (1% to 4%) are red-staining cells whose number greatly increases in allergic and parasitic conditions. The third type of leukocyte is the **basophil** (0% to 1%), which contains granules that stain blue. These three types of cells are formed in the sinusoids of bone marrow, and they, like red blood cells, go through immature stages before reaching the adult form.

Lymphocytes represent about 25% to 40% of white blood cells. They play a major role in the immune system and aid in the synthesis of antibodies and the production of immunoglobulins.

The final type of white blood cell is the monocyte, which is actively phagocytic and plays an important part in the inflammatory process. **Monocytes** are formed in the bone marrow and represent about 2% to 8% of white blood cells.

Platelets, the smallest blood cells, are essential for blood clotting. Normally there are about 150,000 to 400,000 platelets in every cubic millimeter of blood.

■ Diseases of Red Blood Cells

Anemia

Anemia refers to a decrease in the amount of oxygen-carrying hemoglobin in the peripheral blood. This reduction can be attributable to improper formation of new red blood cells, an increased rate of red blood cell destruction, or a loss of red blood cells as a result of prolonged bleeding. Regardless of the cause, a hemoglobin deficiency causes the anemic person to appear pale. This is best appreciated in the mucous membranes of the mouth and conjunctiva, and in the nail beds. A decrease in the oxygen-carrying hemoglobin impairs the delivery of an adequate oxygen supply to the cells and tissues, leading to fatigue and muscular weakness, and often to shortness of breath on exertion (dyspnea). To meet the body's need for more oxygen, the respiratory rate increases and the heart beats more rapidly.

IRON DEFICIENCY ANEMIA

Iron deficiency is the most common cause of anemia. It most frequently results from chronic blood loss, as from an ulcer, a malignant tumor, or excessive bleeding during menstruation (menorrhagia). Other causes of iron deficiency anemia include inadequate dietary intake of iron and increased iron loss caused by intestinal parasites. Iron deficiency anemia also may develop during pregnancy because the mother's iron supply is depleted by red blood cell development in the fetus.

Treatment

If chronic blood loss causes the iron deficiency, the cause must be determined and treated. The first choice of treatment is for the patient to change dietary habits to include more foods rich in iron. The second option is on oral iron supplement, ferrous sulfate. When taking an iron supplement, it is important to remember that other products influence iron absorption. For example, increasing vitamin C intake enhances iron absorption. Iron deficiency can be treated successfully in most cases.

HEMOLYTIC ANEMIA

The underlying abnormality in hemolytic anemia is a shortened life span of the red blood cells with resulting hemolysis and the release of hemoglobin into the plasma. Most hemolytic anemias are caused by a hereditary defect that may produce abnormal red cells or abnormal hemoglobin. Less commonly, hemolytic anemia is acquired and related to circulating antibodies from autoimmune or allergic reactions (e.g., drugs such as sulfonamide) or the malarial parasite.

Spherocytosis, sickle cell anemia, and **thalassemia** are the major hereditary hemolytic anemias. In spherocytosis the erythrocytes have a circular rather than a biconcave shape, making them fragile and susceptible to rupture. In sickle cell anemia, which is generally confined to blacks, the hemoglobin molecule is abnormal and the red cells are crescentic or sickle shaped and tend to rupture. A defect in hemoglobin formation is also responsible for thalassemia, which predominantly occurs in persons living about the Mediterranean, especially those of Italian, Greek, or Sicilian descent.

The breakdown of hemoglobin produces bilirubin, a pigmented substance that is normally detoxified by the liver and converted into bile. The accumulation of large amounts of this orange pigment in the plasma causes the tissues to have a yellow appearance (jaundice).

Hemolytic anemia of the newborn (erythroblastosis fetalis) can result when the mother is Rh negative and the fetus has Rh-positive blood inherited from the father. Although the fetal and maternal circulations are separate, fetal blood can enter the mother's blood through ruptures in the placenta that occur at delivery. The mother thus becomes sensitized to the Rh factor of the fetus and makes antibodies against it. Any antibodies reaching the fetal blood through the placenta in future pregnancies cause hemolysis of the

Figure 8-1 Thalassemia. Pronounced widening of medullary spaces with thinning of cortical margins. Note the absence of normal modeling caused by the pressure of expanding marrow space. Localized radiolucencies simulating multiple osteolytic lesions represent tumorous collections of hypoplastic marrow.

fetal red blood cells. The severity of the disease ranges from mild anemia with jaundice to fetal death.

Radiographic appearance

The hemolytic anemias produce a variety of radiographic abnormalities. Although the radiographic findings are similar in the various types of hemolytic anemia, they tend to be most severe in thalassemia and least prominent in spherocytosis. Extensive marrow hyperplasia, the result of ineffective erythropoiesis and rapid destruction of newly formed red blood cells, causes generalized osteoporosis with pronounced widening of the medullary spaces and thinning of the cortices in long and tubular bones (Figure 8-1). As the fine secondary trabeculae are resorbed, new bone is laid down on the surviving trabeculae, thickening them and producing a coarsened pattern. Normal modeling of long bones does not occur because the expanding marrow flattens or even bulges the normally concave surfaces of the shafts.

In the skull, there is widening of the diploic space and thinning or complete obliteration of the outer

Figure 8-2 Thalassemia. Lateral projection of the skull demonstrates hair-on-end appearance. Note normal appearance of calvaria inferior to the internal occipital protuberance, an area in which there is no red marrow, and poor pneumatization of the visualized paranasal sinuses.

Figure 8-3 Extramedullary hematopoiesis in thalassemia. A lateral projection of the chest demonstrates lobulated posterior mediastinal masses of hematopoietic tissue *(arrows)* in the lower thoracic region. (From Leight TF: *Radiol Clin North Am* 1:377-393, 1963.)

table. When the hyperplastic marrow perforates or destroys the outer table, it proliferates under the invisible periosteum, and new bone spicules are laid down perpendicularly to the inner table. This produces the characteristic hair-on-end appearance of vertical striations in a radial pattern (Figure 8-2).

Extramedullary hematopoiesis is a compensatory mechanism of the reticuloendothelial system (liver, spleen, lymph nodes) in patients with prolonged erythrocyte deficiency resulting from the destruction of red blood cells or the inability of normal blood-forming organs to produce them. Paravertebral collections of hematopoietic tissue may appear on chest radiographs as single or multiple, smooth or lobulated, posterior mediastinal masses that are usually located at the lower thoracic levels (Figure 8-3).

In sickle cell anemia, expansile pressure of the adjacent intervertebral disks produces characteristic biconcave indentations on both the superior and inferior margins of the softened vertebral bodies, giving the appearance of fish vertebrae (Figure 8-4, *A*). Another typical appearance is the result of the development of localized steplike central depressions of multiple vertebral end plates (Figure 8-4, *B*). This is probably caused by circulatory stasis and ischemia, which retard growth in the central portion of the vertebral cartilaginous growth plate. The periphery of the growth plate, which has a different blood supply, continues to grow at a more normal rate.

Bulging of the abnormally shaped red blood cells in sickle cell anemia typically causes focal ischemia and infarction in multiple tissues. Bone infarcts commonly occur in infants and children. These most frequently involve the small bones of the hands and feet, producing an irregular area of bone destruction with overlying periosteal calcification, which may be indistinguishable from osteomyelitis. In older children and adults, bone infarction may initially appear as an ill-defined lucent area that becomes irregularly calcified.

A   B

Figure 8-4   Sickle cell anemia. **A,** Biconcave indentations on both superior and inferior margins of soft vertebral bodies produce characteristic fish vertebrae appearance. **B,** Localized steplike central depressions of multiple vertebral end plates.

Acute osteomyelitis, often caused by *Salmonella* infection, is a common complication in sickle cell disease. The resulting lytic destruction and periosteal reaction may be extensive, often involving the entire shaft and multiple bones (Figure 8-5). Radiographically, it may be impossible to distinguish between osteomyelitis and bone infarction without infection (Figure 8-6).

Throughout their lives, patients with sickle cell anemia are plagued by recurrent painful crises. These episodes are attributable to recurrent vasoocclusive phenomena and may appear with explosive suddenness and attack various parts of the body, especially the abdomen, chest, and joints. It is often difficult to distinguish between a painful sickle cell crisis and some other type of acute process such as biliary colic, appendicitis, or a perforated viscus. In the extremities, a sickle cell crisis may mimic osteomyelitis or an acute arthritis such as gout or rheumatoid arthritis.

The most common extraskeletal abnormality in the hemolytic anemias is cardiomegaly caused by severe anemia and increased cardiac output. The heart has a globular configuration reflecting enlargement of all chambers. Increased pulmonary blood flow produces engorgement of the pulmonary vessels,

Figure 8-5   Acute osteomyelitis in sickle cell anemia. Diffuse lytic destruction of the proximal humerus can be seen along with extensive periosteal reaction *(arrows).*

Figure 8-6 Aseptic necrosis of the femoral head in sickle cell anemia. Mottled areas of increased and decreased density reflect osteonecrosis without collapse. Trabeculae in neck and intertrochanteric region are thickened by apposition of new bone. Solid layer of new bone along the inner aspect of the cortex of the femoral shaft causes narrowing of the medullary canal. (From Moseley JE: *Semin Roentgenol* 9:169-184, 1984.)

giving a hypervascular appearance to the lungs. Pulmonary infarction, pulmonary edema and congestive failure, and pneumonia are frequent complications.

Renal abnormalities can be demonstrated by excretory urography in about two thirds of patients with sickle cell disease. A serious complication is renal papillary necrosis (see Figure 5-16), which is probably related to vessel obstruction within the papillae and may produce sinuses or cavity formation within one or more papillae.

Treatment

The cause and type of hemolytic anemia must be determined to successfully begin treatment. For spherocytosis, splenectomy is curative.

For sickle cell anemia, currently no cure exists. Therefore treatment consists of management and control of symptoms. The most invasive treatment, a bone marrow transplant, offers a possible cure. During a crisis, bed rest, maintenance of oxygen levels to prevent sickling, folic acid to aid in red blood cell pro-

duction, maintenance of fluids to keep electrolyte balance stable, and possible blood transfusion (of packed red cells) are appropriate. In some cases, prophylactic antibiotics are given.

If an Rh-negative mother delivers or aborts an Rh-positive infant, she is given a vaccine of Rh immunoglobulin within 24 hours to prevent the production of antibodies against the Rh factor. Blood testing to determine whether Rh incompatibility exists is now an essential part of prenatal care. An Rh-positive baby born to an Rh-negative mother receives a blood transfusion within 24 hours after birth.

MEGALOBLASTIC ANEMIA

A deficiency of vitamin B_{12} or of folic acid leads to defective DNA synthesis and an anemia in which there is a decreased number of red blood cells, although each cell contains the normal amount of hemoglobin. The most common cause of vitamin B_{12} deficiency is **pernicious anemia,** in which there is inadequate intrinsic factor secretion related to atrophy of the gastric mucosa. Intrinsic factor acts as a carrier in the small bowel absorption of vitamin B_{12}, which is essential for erythrocyte development.

A deficiency of folic acid (and vitamin B_{12}) may also be related to intestinal malabsorption. This in turn may be related to intestinal parasites or bacterial overproduction, especially in patients with stasis of bowel contents, as in blind loop syndrome and multiple jejunal diverticula. Other causes of megaloblastic anemia include a poor diet, such as strict vegetarianism, in which there are no sources of vitamin B_{12}, or long-term alcoholism, in which no folic acid is available.

Radiographic appearance

Gastric atrophy is seen radiographically as a tubular stomach with a bald appearance that reflects a decrease or absence of the usually prominent rugal folds (Figure 8-7). It must be emphasized, however, that radiographic findings of atrophic gastritis are often seen in older persons with no evidence of pernicious anemia.

Treatment

The treatment of megaloblastic anemia consists of correcting the deficiency of vitamin B_{12} or folic acid. Vitamin B_{12} deficiency requires an injection, because taking vitamin B_{12} orally does not reverse the process. Folic acid deficiency can be treated with an oral supplement. If needed, a blood transfusion is given.

APLASTIC ANEMIA

A generalized failure of the bone marrow to function (aplastic anemia) results in decreased levels of erythrocytes, leukocytes, and platelets. In addition to

Figure 8-7   Megaloblastic anemia in a patient with chronic atrophic gastritis, which is recognized by the tubular stomach with a striking decrease in the usually prominent rugal folds.

anemia, the patient cannot fight infection (a white blood cell function) and has a bleeding tendency (platelet depletion). Causes of aplastic anemia include exposure to chemical agents or drugs, infections, and invasion of the bone marrow by cancer.

Treatment

Patient prognosis depends on the severity and duration of the bone marrow aplasia. Regular blood transfusions are generally necessary for survival and to reduce symptoms. Because the patient has a suppressed immune response, preventative antibiotics are sometimes prescribed. Situations exposing the patient to an infection or a viral illness should be avoided. Some clinicians recommend medications to stimulate the bone marrow to produce more blood cells. Bone marrow transplantation is a new technique for treating these patients.

Myelophthisic anemia

Infiltration of bone marrow with nonhematopoietic cells such as tumor cells, or encroachment on marrow cavities caused by cortical thickening, can result in severe myelophthisic anemia and pancytopenia (decreased red and white blood cells and platelets). Tumors may arise from cells that are normally found in the bone marrow (leukemia, lymphoma, myeloma), or the marrow may be invaded by extensive metastases to bone (from carcinomas of the breast, prostate, lung, thyroid). Less common causes of marrow replacement include lipid storage disorders (Gaucher's disease), osteopetrosis (marble bones), and myelofibrosis.

Radiographic appearance

Skeletal films may demonstrate lytic or blastic lesions, depending on the progression of metastases. A radionuclide bone scan detects bone marrow abnormalities and skeletal metastases. MRI scans can demonstrate the extent of bone marrow infiltration.

Treatment

Treatment is focused on the underlying cause of the myelophthisic anemia. A packed red blood cell transfusion is used to treat the anemia and help stabilize the patient.

Polycythemia

Primary polycythemia (polycythemia vera)

Polycythemia vera is a hematologic disorder characterized by hyperplasia of the bone marrow (neoplastic) that results in increased production of erythrocytes, granulocytes, and platelets. The disease is slowly progressive and produces symptoms associated with increased blood volume and viscosity. Cerebrovascular and peripheral vascular insufficiencies are common, and many patients give a history of some thrombotic or hemorrhagic event during the course of their disease. There is an increased incidence of peptic ulcer disease, and the excessive cellular

Figure 8-8   Primary polycythemia. Severe hypoventilation caused by profound obesity causes engorgement of pulmonary vessels. Although cardiomegaly is uncommon in polycythemia, in this case it reflects pronounced elevation of the diaphragm as result of a huge abdominal girth and some underlying cardiac decompensation.

proliferation often results in increased levels of uric acid with secondary gout and the formation of urate stones. The spleen is often massively enlarged and may be seen as a left upper quadrant mass.

Radiographic appearance

Increased blood volume in polycythemia vera can lead to prominence of the pulmonary vascular shadows, usually without the cardiomegaly associated with the increased pulmonary vascularity that occurs in patients with congenital heart disease (Figure 8-8). Intravascular thrombosis may cause pulmonary infarctions that appear as focal areas of consolidation or as bands of fibrosis.

SECONDARY POLYCYTHEMIA

Secondary polycythemia may be the result of long-term inadequate oxygen supply in patients with severe chronic pulmonary disease or congenital cyanotic heart disease, or it may develop in persons living at high altitudes. An elevated hemoglobin concentration may also be caused by certain neoplasms (renal cell carcinoma, hepatoma, cerebellar hemangioblastoma) that result in an increased production of erythropoietin, which stimulates red blood cell formation.

Radiographic appearance

Because secondary polycythemia is a compensatory phenomenon, the pulmonary vasculature is normal in appearance and there is no evidence of the disease on chest radiographs. In children with severe secondary polycythemia caused by cyanotic heart

disease, the skull may show thickened tables and a hair-on-end appearance similar to the findings in congenital hemolytic anemias. CT may be used to investigate the kidneys and their function if a suspicion of tumor exists.

Treatment of polycythemias

Treatment for both primary and secondary polycythemias starts with bloodletting to remove excessive cellular elements. This improves circulation by lowering blood viscosity and is continued until the hemoglobin and hematocrit levels become normal. Chemotherapy helps to lower the platelet count, and it suppresses production of blood elements by the marrow. For primary polycythemia, clinicians may consider a splenectomy to alleviate painful enlargement of the organ, as well as for patients with repeated episodes of thrombosis causing splenic infarction. Patients who receive these treatments can expect to live about 15 to 20 years after their condition is diagnosed.

■ Diseases of White Blood Cells

Leukemia

Leukemia is a neoplastic proliferation of white blood cells. The two major types of leukemia are named for the site of malignancy. **Myelocytic leukemia** is a cancer of the bone marrow (myelocytes are the primitive white blood cells in bone marrow). In this condition, a huge increase in the number of circulating granulocytes occurs, and there is decreased production of red blood cells and platelets. **Lymphatic leukemia** is a malignancy of the lymph nodes; in lymphocytic leukemia, the only white blood cells that dramatically increase are lymphocytes.

Leukemia may be chronic or acute. Acute lymphocytic leukemia, which has an abrupt onset and progresses rapidly, is the most common form in children. Acute myelocytic leukemia is more common in adults. Chronic leukemias run a more prolonged course and may involve either cell type.

Because of the exuberant white cell production, there is generally a decrease in the number of circulating red blood cells and platelets. This results in a typical clinical appearance of weakness, shortness of breath, and cardiac palpitations. A decrease in the number of platelets interferes with the blood-clotting mechanism and results in a bleeding tendency. Even though there are more circulating white blood cells than normal, most are immature and thus the patient becomes highly susceptible to infection. Diffuse infiltration of white cells into the spleen and liver may cause massive enlargement of these organs (hepatosplenomegaly).

Summary of Findings for Diseases of Red Blood Cells

DISORDER	LOCATION	RADIOGRAPHIC APPEARANCE	TREATMENT
Hemolytic anemias	Shortened life span of red blood cells	Long bones—osteoporosis, widened medullary spaces with thinning of cortices; later stages: thickened, coarsened trabecular patterns Skull—thinning of outer table; vertical striation results from new bone formation	Spherocytosis—splenectomy Rh-negative mother and Rh-positive fetus—blood transfusion for baby and Rh immunoglobulin vaccine for mother
	Sickle cell anemia—hemoglobin molecule abnormal; red cells crescentic or sickle shaped	Spine—characteristic biconcave indentations superiorly and inferiorly on vertebral body Chest—cardiomegaly IVU—renal papillary necrosis	Sickle cell anemia—no cure exists Most invasive treatment—bone marrow transplant, offers possible cure Crisis—bed rest, maintenance of oxygen, folic acid, maintenance of fluids, possible blood transfusion
Megaloblastic anemia	Lack of small bowel absorption of vitamin B_{12} or folic acid	GI series—tubular stomach with bald appearance (decrease or absence of rugal folds)	Vitamin B_{12} deficiency requires an injection Folic acid deficiency can be treated with an oral supplement Possible blood transfusion
Polycythemia	Primary (neoplastic)—increased production of erythrocytes, granulocytes, and platelets	Chest film—prominent vascular markings without cardiomegaly	Bloodletting Chemotherapy Splenectomy
	Secondary (nonneoplastic)—elevated hemoglobin concentration	Chest film—normal Skull (of child)—thickened tables, hair-on-end appearance; similar to congenital hemolytic anemia	

IVU, IV urography.

Radiographic appearance

In childhood leukemia, radiographically detectable skeletal involvement is extremely common as a result of the infiltration of leukemic cells into the marrow. The earliest radiographic sign of disease is usually a transverse radiolucent band at the metaphyseal ends of the long bones, most commonly about the knees, ankles, and wrists (Figure 8-9). Although in infancy this appearance is nonspecific and it also oc-curs with malnutrition or systemic disease, the presence of these transverse lucent metaphyseal bands after 2 years of age is strongly suggestive of acute leukemia.

As the proliferation of neoplastic cells in the marrow becomes more extensive, actual destruction of bone may occur. This may cause patchy lytic lesions, a permeative moth-eaten appearance, or diffuse destruction with cortical erosion (Figure 8-10). A reac-

Figure 8-9   Acute leukemia. In addition to radiolucent metaphyseal bands, there is frank bone destruction with cortical erosion involving many metatarsals and proximal phalanges.

Figure 8-10   Acute leukemia. Proliferation of neoplastic cells in the marrow has caused extensive destruction of bone in both femurs.

tive response to proliferating leukemic cells can cause patchy or uniform osteosclerosis; subperiosteal proliferation incites the formation of periosteal new bone. Diffuse skeletal demineralization may result in vertebral compression fractures.

Enlargement of mediastinal and hilar lymph nodes is the most common abnormality on chest radiographs. Diffuse bilateral reticular changes may simulate lymphangitic spread of carcinoma. The nonspecific pulmonary infiltrates seen in patients with acute leukemia are usually attributable to hemorrhage or secondary infection.

The radiographic abnormalities in chronic leukemia are often similar to those in the acute disease, although their frequency and degree may vary. Skeletal changes are much less common and are usually limited to generalized demineralization in the flat bones, where active marrow persists in adulthood. The demonstration of focal areas of destruction, or periosteal new bone formation, indicates probable transformation into an acute phase of the disease.

Hilar and mediastinal adenopathy are common, especially in chronic lymphocytic leukemia. Congestive heart failure commonly results from the associated severe anemia.

Splenomegaly is an almost constant finding in patients with chronic leukemia (Figure 8-11). Leukemic infiltration of the gastrointestinal tract can produce single or multiple intraluminal filling defects, and the infiltrative process may be indistinguishable from carcinoma. Renal infiltration can cause bilateral enlargement of the kidneys. In chronic lymphocytic leukemia, enlargement of retroperitoneal or mesenteric lymph nodes can cause displacement or obstruction of structures in the genitourinary or gastrointestinal tracts.

Treatment

Leukemia treatment may require multidrug chemotherapy, bone marrow transplant, antibiotics to help prevent infections, or a transfusion to reverse the blood cell imbalance.

Figure 8-12   Lymphoma. **A,** Initial chest film demonstrates considerable widening of upper half of the mediastinum caused by pronounced lymphadenopathy. **B,** After chemotherapy, there is dramatic decrease in the width of the upper mediastinum.

Figure 8-11   Chronic leukemia. **A,** Massive splenomegaly causes downward displacement of splenic flexure of colon. *Arrows* point to inferior margin of spleen. **B,** Indium-111 whole-body scan. Indium-111 tagged to white blood cells illustrates a grossly enlarged spleen on images taken 27 hours after injection.

Lymphoma

Lymphomas are neoplasms of the lymphoreticular system, which includes the lymph nodes, the spleen, and the lymphoid tissues of parenchymal organs such as the gastrointestinal tract, lung, and skin. They are usually divided into two major types: Hodgkin's and non-Hodgkin's lymphomas. Ninety percent of cases of Hodgkin's disease originate in the lymph nodes; 10% are of extranodal origin. In contrast, parenchymal organs are more often involved in non-Hodgkin's lymphomas, about 40% of which are of extranodal origin.

Radiographic appearance

Mediastinal lymph node enlargement is the most common radiographic finding in lymphoma (Figure 8-12). It is seen on initial chest radiographs of about half the patients with Hodgkin's disease and about one third of those with non-Hodgkin's lymphoma. Mediastinal lymph node enlargement is usually bilateral but asymmetric.

Involvement of anterior mediastinal and retrosternal nodes is common, a major factor in differentiating lymphoma from sarcoidosis, which rarely produces radiographically visible enlargement of nodes in the anterior compartment. Calcification may develop in intrathoracic lymph nodes after mediastinal irradiation.

Involvement of the pulmonary parenchyma and pleura usually occurs by direct extension from mediastinal nodes along the lymphatic vessels of the bronchovascular sheaths. Radiographically, this may appear as a coarse interstitial pattern (Figure 8-13), as solitary or multiple ill-defined nodules, or as patchy areas of parenchymal infiltrate that may coalesce to form a large homogeneous mass. At times, it may be difficult to distinguish a superimposed infection after radiation therapy or chemotherapy from the contin-

ued spread of lymphomatous tissue. Pleural effusion occurs in up to one third of patients with thoracic lymphoma; extension of the tumor to the pericardium can cause pericardial effusion.

About 5% to 10% of patients with lymphoma have involvement of the gastrointestinal tract, primarily of the stomach and small bowel. Gastric lymphoma often is seen as a large, bulky polypoid mass, usually irregular and ulcerated, that may be indistinguishable from a carcinoma (Figure 8-14). A multiplicity of malignant ulcers or an aneurysmal appearance of a single huge ulcer (the diameter of which exceeds that of the adjacent gastric lumen) is characteristic of lymphoma. Additional findings suggestive of lymphoma include relative flexibility of the gastric wall, enlargement of the spleen, and associated prominence of retrogastric and other regional lymph nodes that cause extrinsic impressions on the barium-filled stomach. Other manifestations of gastric lymphoma include thickening, distortion, and nodularity of rugal folds (Figure 8-15) and generalized gastric narrowing caused by a severe fibrotic reaction.

Lymphoma can produce virtually any pattern of abnormality in the small bowel. The disease may be localized to a single intestinal segment, it may be multifocal, or it may cause diffuse involvement. The major radiographic appearances include irregular thickening of mucosal folds, large ulcerating masses, and multiple intraluminal or intramural filling defects simulating metastatic disease.

Skeletal involvement can be demonstrated in about 15% of patients with lymphoma. Direct extension from adjacent lymph nodes causes bone erosion, especially of the anterior surface of the upper lumbar

Figure 8-13 Lymphoma. Diffuse reticular and reticulonodular changes causing prominence of interstitial lung markings. Note enlargement of left hilar region.

Figure 8-14 Lymphoma presenting as a large mass almost filled by a huge ulcer *(arrows)*.

and lower thoracic spine. Paravertebral soft-tissue masses may occur. The hematogenous spread of lymphoma produces a mottled pattern of destruction and sclerosis, which may simulate metastatic disease. Dense vertebral sclerosis (ivory vertebra) may develop in Hodgkin's disease (Figure 8-16).

Figure 8-15 Lymphoma of the stomach. Note the diffuse thickening, distortion, and nodularity of the gastric folds.

Diffuse lymphomatous infiltration may cause renal enlargement, with distortion, elongation, and compression of the calyces (Figure 8-17). Single or multiple renal nodules or perirenal masses may displace or distort the kidney. Diffuse retroperitoneal lymphoma can displace the kidneys or ureters and obliterate one or both psoas margins.

Staging

Once the diagnosis of lymphoma is made, it is essential to determine the status of the abdominal and pelvic lymph nodes. This is necessary both for the initial staging and treatment planning and for assessing the efficacy of treatment and detecting tumor recurrence.

Although lymphography was the procedure of choice in the past, magnetic resonance imaging (MRI) and positron emission tomography (PET) are now the noninvasive techniques employed to demonstrate lymphomatous involvement of the abdominal and pelvic nodes. In practice, computed tomography (CT) of the chest, abdomen, and pelvis is generally the first imaging procedures used in staging lymphoma patients. This is especially true for those with non-Hodgkin's lymphoma, which tends to produce bulky masses in the mesenteric and high retrocrural areas. An abnormal CT scan may eliminate the need for more invasive procedures (Figure 8-18); a normal CT scan obtained at 2-cm intervals can exclude retroperitoneal adenopathy with a high degree of confidence. CT is usually used because of standardization and repeatability for patients. Malignant nodes appear round or oval and their transverse-to-longitudinal ratio is greater then 2. A narrow or absent hilus of the node also suggests malignancy.

Figure 8-16 Lymphoma. Ivory vertebra.

Figure 8-17 Lymphoma. Right kidney is completely replaced by a lymphomatous mass (L). Note the extensive involvement of lymph nodes (M).

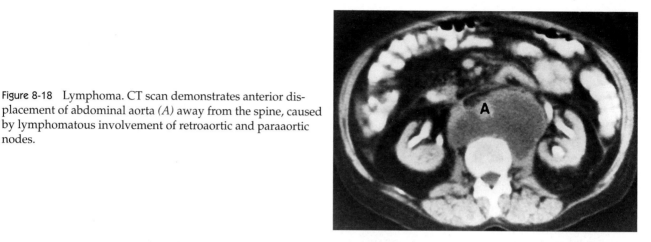

Figure 8-18 Lymphoma. CT scan demonstrates anterior displacement of abdominal aorta *(A)* away from the spine, caused by lymphomatous involvement of retroaortic and paraaortic nodes.

Figure 8-19 Lymphoma in a 16-year-old girl with a 3-week history of supraclavicular adenopathy. The PET body scan demonstrates FDG uptake in the supraclavicular fossae, the mediastinum, and the lungs; this indicates a metabolically active neoplasm, which is consistent with the clinically suspected lymphoma.

Figure 8-20 CT scan of patient with non-Hodgkin's lymphoma. The patient was diagnosed 8 months earlier with a pancreatic tumor measuring 4 × 6 × 4 cm. After chemotherapy, this scan shows a smaller tumor (3 × 5 × 3 cm) and no mass in the tail.

Ultrasound can detect enlarged retroperitoneal nodes, characterize them, and measure them accurately. For retroperitoneal adenopathy, ultrasound is 80% to 90% accurate, and it has the ability to detect extranodal disease, which typically produces discrete hyperechoic masses. MRI is considered the superior technique because it can detect subtle detail using multiple sequences.

Gallium scans may illustrate increased nodal uptake (indicating swelling or inflammation), and it can assess the response to treatment and detect early recurrence of tumor. PET imaging using fluorodeoxyglucose (FDG) uptake is considered superior to the gallium scan and CT because it can detect microscopic tumor foci and alterations in function within normal-size nodes. PET also has the ability to

Figure 8-21 Infectious mononucleosis. Frontal **(A)** and lateral **(B)** projections of chest demonstrate pronounced enlargement of hilar lymph nodes bilaterally *(arrows)*.

distinguish large nodes that contain tumor from those that have only benign reactive changes. PET can also be used to monitor the effectiveness of the therapy and identify tumor recurrence (Figure 8-19).

To ensure proper diagnosis and staging of both Hodgkin's and non-Hodgkin's lymphoma, biopsies are performed to extract cell and tissue samples. Freehand fine needle aspiration biopsy works best for superficial nodes, whereas CT-guided or ultrasound-guided biopsy is required for deep node evaluation. Patients unable to tolerate surgical procedures may undergo a large-needle core biopsy to determine the extent of the disease before beginning treatment.

Treatment

The best treatment available for Hodgkin's lymphoma is multidrug chemotherapy and radiation therapy. For non-Hodgkin's lymphoma, more aggressive chemotherapy is required if the disease process is diffuse (Figure 8-20), whereas conservative chemotherapy is utilized for low-level disease. Bone marrow transplant may be necessary.

Infectious mononucleosis

Mononucleosis is a self-limited viral disease of the lymphoreticular system characterized by vague symptoms of mild fever, fatigue, sore throat, and swollen lymph nodes caused by an intense increase of lymphoid cells. The Epstein-Barr virus may cause this disease process. It primarily infects young adults and, although often termed the "kissing disease," is not particularly contagious. Blood tests show an elevated white cell count with an abnormally high percentage of atypical lymphocytes, which resemble monocytes. The diagnosis is based on the presence of antibodies to the virus in the blood.

Radiographic appearance

Generalized lymphadenopathy and splenomegaly are characteristic clinical and radiographic findings in infectious mononucleosis. Hilar lymph node enlargement, usually bilateral, can be demonstrated in about 15% of cases (Figure 8-21). Pneumonia is a rare complication that can appear as a diffuse reticular pattern indicating interstitial disease, or as a patchy, nonspecific air-space consolidation.

Treatment

Because infectious mononucleosis is a self-limited disease, the usual treatment includes supportive therapy, adequate bed rest, and hydration.

Summary of Findings for Diseases of White Blood Cells

DISORDER	LOCATION	RADIOGRAPHIC APPEARANCE	TREATMENT
Leukemia	Neoplastic proliferation of white blood cells	Skeletal radiograph in child—radiolucent bands at metaphyses on long bones after 2 years of age, bone destruction (moth-eaten appearance with resulting osteosclerosis), possible pathologic fractures Chest film—enlarged mediastinal and hilar lymph nodes, bilateral reticular changes Chest film—congestive heart failure KUB/US—splenomegaly Organ infiltration—displacement or obstruction of GI or GU system	Multidrug chemotherapy Bone marrow transplant Antibiotics Blood transfusion
Lymphoma	Neoplasm of lymphoreticular system	Chest film—asymmetric, bilaterally enlarged mediastinal lymph nodes GI series—irregular and ulcerated polypoid mass (multiple ulcers or a huge single ulcer); thickening of rugal folds Skeletal radiograph—bone erosion of thoracolumbar spine with mottled pattern and sclerosis CT—detects increased node size PET—metabolically active neoplasm	Hodgkin's lymphoma—multidrug chemotherapy and radiation therapy Non-Hodgkin's lymphoma—aggressive chemotherapy for diffuse disease; conservative chemotherapy for low-level disease Bone marrow transplant
Infectious mononucleosis	Viral disease of lymphoreticular system	Generalized lymphadenopathy and splenomegaly	Self-limited—supportive treatment, bed rest, and hydration

GU, Genitourinary; *KUB*, kidney–ureter–bladder radiograph; *PET*, positron emission tomography; *US*, ultrasound.

■ Diseases of Platelets (Bleeding Disorders)

Blood coagulation (clotting) is a complicated mechanism requiring platelets, calcium, and 12 coenzymes and proteins called **coagulation factors.** A deficiency in quantity or activity of any of these elements may lead to an inability to control hemorrhage or may even lead to spontaneous bleeding.

Hemophilia

Hemophilia is an inherited (by a sex-linked recessive gene) anomaly of blood coagulation that appears clinically only in males. Patients with this disease have a decreased or absent serum concentration of antihemophilic globulin (factor VIII) and suffer a lifelong tendency to spontaneous hemorrhage or severe bleeding from even minor cuts or injuries.

Figure 8-22 Hemophilia. **A,** Large subchondral cysts about the elbow. **B,** Destructive, expansile lesion of the lower tibial shaft. (From Stoker DJ, Murray RO: Skeletal changes in hemophilia and other bleeding disorders, *Semin Roentgenol* 9:185-193, 1974.)

Radiographic appearance

The major radiographic changes in hemophilia are complications of recurrent bleeding into the joints, most commonly involving the knees, elbows, and ankles. Initially, the hemorrhage produces a generalized nonspecific soft-tissue prominence of the distended joint. Deposition of iron pigment may produce areas of cloudy, increased density in the periarticular soft tissues. Although complete resorption of intraarticular blood may leave no residual change, subsequent episodes of bleeding result in synovial hypertrophy. In chronic disease, the hyperplastic synovium causes cartilage destruction and joint space narrowing and

often leads to the development of multiple subchondral cysts of varying sizes in the immediate juxtaarticular bone (Figure 8-22, *A*). Destruction of articular cartilage and continued use of the damaged joint lead to subchondral sclerosis and collapse, extensive and bizarre spur formation, and often pronounced soft-tissue calcification. Hemorrhage extending into the adjacent bony structures may cause extensive destruction (pseudotumor of hemophilia), which can mimic a malignant tumor (Figure 8-22, *B*).

Repeated joint hemorrhages lead to increased blood flow in the region of the epiphysis and growth plate. These structures may ossify prematurely,

Figure 8-23   Hemophilia. Intercondylar notch is greatly widened, and coarse trabeculae, narrowing of joint space, and hypertrophic spurring can be seen.

Figure 8-24   Chronic idiopathic thrombocytopenic purpura. Hemorrhage into the wall of the small bowel causes regular thickening of the mucosal folds.

become abnormally large, or fuse prematurely with the metaphysis. The increased blood flow and atrophy of bone and muscle that may follow an episode of joint bleeding result in severe osteoporosis. Common signs suggestive of, though not pathognomonic for, hemophilia include widening and deepening of the intercondylar notch of the femur (Figure 8-23) and "squaring" of the inferior border of the patella. Asymmetric growth of the distal tibial epiphysis may result in "slanting" of the talotibial joint. Hemarthrosis can cause occlusion of epiphyseal vessels and result in avascular necrosis. This most commonly involves the femoral and radial heads, both of which have a totally intracapsular epiphysis and are therefore especially vulnerable to deprivation of their vascular supply from compression by a tense joint effusion.

As in the other bleeding disorders, submucosal bleeding into the wall of the gastrointestinal tract may develop in patients with hemophilia. This most commonly involves the small bowel and produces a short or long segment with regular thickening of folds. In the colon, bleeding may produce the thumbprint pattern of sharply defined, fingerlike, marginal indentations along the contours of the colon wall.

Treatment

Hemophilia is usually treated with transfusions and factor VIII replacement.

Purpura (thrombocytopenia)

Purpura refers to a deficiency in the number of platelets, and it results in spontaneous hemorrhages in the skin, mucous membranes of the mouth, and internal organs. The decreased number of platelets results from decreased production, increased destruction, or splenic sequestration of platelets. In the skin, purpura leads to the development of small, flat, red spots (petechiae) or larger hemorrhagic areas (ecchymoses).

Acute idiopathic thrombocytopenic purpura typically has the sudden onset of severe purpura 1 to 2 weeks after a sore throat or upper respiratory infection in an otherwise healthy child. In most patients the disorder is self-limited and clears spontaneously within a few weeks. Unlike the acute form, chronic idiopathic thrombocytopenic purpura occurs primarily in young women and has an insidious onset with a relatively long history of easy bruising and menorrhagia. This condition is generally considered to be an autoimmune disorder, since most patients have a circulating platelet autoantibody that develops without underlying disease or significant exposure to drugs.

Purpura can also be a complication of conditions that suppress the bone marrow (aplastic anemia) or infiltrate the bone marrow with tumor cells (leukemia, lymphoma, myeloma, metastases).

. . . .

Summary of Findings for Bleeding Disorders

DISORDER	LOCATION	RADIOGRAPHIC APPEARANCE	TREATMENT
Hemophilia	Anomaly of blood coagulation	Joint films—cloudy increased density in periarticular soft tissues Chronic—cartilage destruction with joint narrowing, multiple subchondral cysts; widening and deepening of intracondylar notch	Blood transfusion Factor VIII replacement
Purpura	Deficiency in number of platelets	Small bowel—uniform regular thickening of mucosal folds Splenomegaly	Self-limited—spontaneous recovery Drug-induced—discontinuation of drug Virus-induced—improves with cure of infection Splenectomy

. . . .

Radiographic appearance

The radiographic changes caused by either acute or chronic idiopathic thrombocytopenic purpura primarily involve the gastrointestinal tract. Hemorrhage into the small bowel produces characteristic uniform, regular thickening of mucosal folds in the affected intestinal segment (Figure 8-24). Splenomegaly is commonly present; splenectomy is often required to remove this important site of platelet destruction and major source of synthesis of platelet antibodies.

Treatment

Drug-induced thrombocytopenia responds well to discontinuing the offending drug. Virus-induced thrombocytopenia shows improvement following a cure of the infection.

QUESTIONS

1. When diseases of the hematopoietic system result in demineralization of bone, the radiographer must be alert to the possibility of _____.
   A. Patient infection C. Pathologic fracture
   B. Self-infection D. Syncope

2. Red blood cells are called _____.
   A. Erythrocytes C. Thrombocytes
   B. Leukocytes D. Hemoglobin

3. Platelets are called _____.
   A. Erythrocytes C. Thrombocytes
   B. Leukocytes D. Lymphocytes

4. White blood cells are called _____.
   A. Erythrocytes C. Thrombocytes
   B. Leukocytes D. Paracytes

5. The smallest blood cells, platelets, are essential for what process?
   A. Immunity C. Carrying oxygen
   B. Clotting D. Fighting infection

6. Lymphocytes play a major role in the _____ system.
   A. Endocrine C. Immune
   B. Hematopoietic D. Metabolic

7. Which term refers to a decrease in the amount of oxygen-carrying hemoglobin in the blood?
   A. Spherocytosis C. Anemia
   B. Thalassemia D. Hematopoiesis

8. What type of anemia can cause painful bone infarcts and is generally confined to the black race?
   A. Spherocytosis C. Sickle cell
   B. Thalassemia D. *Salmonella*

9. A hematologic disorder characterized by an increase in the production of erythrocytes, granulocytes, and platelets is _____.
   A. Polycythemia vera C. Sickle cell anemia
   B. Erythrocytosis D. Hemolytic anemia

10. A cancerous disease of the hematopoietic system characterized by an increase in white blood cells is _____.
    A. Anemia C. Leukemia
    B. Thrombocytopenia D. Hemophilia

11. What is the name of an inherited anomaly of blood coagulation?
    A. Sickle cell anemia   C. Leukemia
    B. Hemophilia   D. Leukocytosis

12. What pathologic condition refers to a deficiency in the number of platelets resulting in spontaneous hemorrhages in the skin, internal organs, and mucous membranes of the mouth?
    A. Hemophilia   C. Leukemia
    B. Purpura   D. Sickle cell anemia

BIBLIOGRAPHY

Estrada DA: Lymphoma, non-Hodgkin's, *eMedicine Journal* 2:9, 2001. http://www.emedicine.com/med/tomic1363.htm

Korsten J et al: Extramedullary hematopoiesis in patients with thalassemia anemia, *Radiology* 95:257-264, 1970.

Pear BL: Skeletal manifestations of the lymphomas and leukemias, *Semin Roentgenol* 9:229-240, 1974.

Reynolds J: Radiologic manifestations of sickle cell hemoglobulinopathy, *JAMA* 238:247-250, 1977.

Stoker DJ, Murray RO: Skeletal changes in hemophilia and other bleeding disorders, *Semin Roentgenol* 9:185-193, 1974.

CHAPTER 9

Endocrine System

Prerequisite Knowledge

The student should have a basic knowledge of the anatomy and physiology of the endocrine system. In addition, proper learning and understanding of the material will be facilitated if the student has some clinical experience in general radiography and film evaluation, including a concept of the newer imaging modalities used to study the various body systems affected by endocrine abnormalities. These modalities include ultrasound, computed tomography (CT), magnetic resonance imaging (MRI), and positron emission tomography (PET).

Goals

To acquaint the student radiographer with the pathophysiology and radiographic manifestations of all of the common and some of the unusual disorders of the endocrine system

Objectives

1. To understand and be able to define or describe all bold-faced terms in this chapter
2. To be able to describe the physiology of the endocrine system
3. To be able to identify anatomic structures on both diagrams and images of the endocrine system
4. To be able to describe the various pathologic conditions affecting the endocrine system as well as their radiographic manifestations

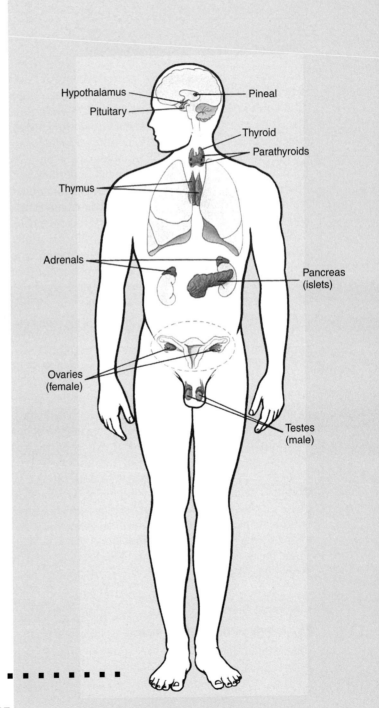

▪ Radiographer Notes

Imaging modalities are used to diagnose both the underlying endocrine disorder and the secondary changes that may occur in various areas of the body. Disorders of the endocrine glands themselves are usually evaluated by ultrasound, CT, MRI, and radionuclide scanning. Secondary pathologic manifestations elsewhere in the body are generally evaluated on plain radiographs, for which the routine exposure techniques may have to be al-

tered (see the Box in Chapter 1 labeled Relative Attenuation of X-rays in Advanced Stages of Diseases). For example, Cushing's syndrome causes extensive osteoporosis, which requires a decrease in kilovolts-peak for adequate visualization of the demineralized bones. It should also be noted that patients with this condition can easily sustain pathologic fractures and thus should always be handled with caution.

▪ Physiology of the Endocrine System

The endocrine system is a biochemical communication network through which several small glands control a broad range of vital body activities. The endocrine glands secrete chemical messengers called hormones, which circulate in the blood and may affect a single target organ or the entire body. Hormones may be proteins (growth hormone), steroids (cortisone), peptides (antidiuretic hormone), amino acids (thyroxine), or amines (epinephrine). They range from small to large molecules and have chemical structures of various complexities.

The major endocrine glands are the pituitary, adrenal, thyroid, and parathyroid glands. Inadequate **(hypoactive)** or excess **(hyperactive)** production of hormones from these endocrine glands can give rise to a wide variety of clinical symptoms and radiographic abnormalities.

Because hormones are powerful chemicals, it is essential that their circulating levels be carefully controlled. One type of control is called the negative feedback mechanism. In this system, an adequate level of a hormone in the blood automatically stops the release of additional hormone (somewhat like a thermostat). As the blood level of the hormone decreases, the gland is stimulated to secrete more of it. Another control mechanism is the production of two different hormones whose actions are opposite to each other. For example, insulin is secreted by the pancreas when the blood glucose level rises. When the blood glucose level falls below normal, a second hormone, glucagon, is secreted by the pancreas to raise the blood glucose level. Thus these two hormones are balanced so that a proper blood glucose level is continually maintained.

▪ Adrenal Glands

Physiology of the adrenal glands

The adrenal glands, which are situated at the top of each kidney, consist of an outer cortex and an inner medulla. The adrenal cortex secretes several different

types of steroid hormones, which can be divided into three general groups. The **mineralocorticoids** (primarily aldosterone) regulate salt and water balance by controlling sodium retention and potassium excretion by the kidneys. The production of aldosterone is primarily regulated by the secretion of renin from specialized cells (the juxtaglomerular apparatus) in the kidney. Reduced blood volume (as in hemorrhage) causes low blood pressure, which is detected by the juxtaglomerular apparatus and eventually results in increased aldosterone secretion from the adrenal cortex.

Glucocorticoids (especially cortisone) regulate carbohydrate metabolism and are under the regulation of adrenocorticotropic hormone (ACTH) from the anterior pituitary gland. Cortisone also depresses the inflammatory response to almost all forms of injury, thus leading to its use in the treatment of trauma, rheumatoid arthritis, bursitis, and asthma, and as an immunosuppressive agent to help limit rejection after organ transplantation.

Androgens are sex hormones that tend to masculinize the body, to retain amino acids, and to enhance protein synthesis. It is these hormones that are used both illegally and unwisely by athletes in an attempt to increase body strength.

The adrenal medulla secretes epinephrine (adrenaline) and norepinephrine. These fight-or-flight hormones are secreted in stress situations when additional energy and strength are needed. Epinephrine stimulates heart activity, raises blood pressure, and increases the level of blood glucose. By constricting some blood vessels and dilating others, epinephrine shunts blood to active muscles where oxygen and nutrients are urgently needed.

Diseases of the adrenal cortex

CUSHING'S SYNDROME

The excess production of glucocorticoid hormones in Cushing's syndrome may be attributable to generalized bilateral hyperplasia of the adrenal cortex, or it may be a result of a functioning adrenal or even non-adrenal tumor. It can also be the result of the exogenous administration of cortisone. Excess secretion of glucocorticoid hormones mobilizes lipids and increases their level in the blood. This produces a characteristic obesity that is confined to the trunk of the body and is associated with a round, moon-shaped face and a pathognomonic fat pad that forms behind the shoulders (buffalo hump). Retention of salt and water results in hypertension.

Radiographic appearance

Generalized enlargement of the adrenal glands is best demonstrated by CT, which shows thickening of the wings of the adrenal gland, which appear to have a stellate or Y-shaped configuration in cross section. Ultrasound can also show diffuse adrenal gland enlargement.

Benign and malignant tumors of the adrenal cortex are less common causes of Cushing's syndrome than is nontumorous adrenal hyperfunction. As a general rule, the larger the adrenocortical tumor and the more abrupt the onset of clinical symptoms and signs, the more likely the tumor is to be malignant (Figure 9-1). However, the differentiation between adenoma and carcinoma may be impossible at the time of histologic examination, and the nature of the tumor may have to be defined by the clinical course alone. Both CT and ultrasound can demonstrate an adrenal tumor (Figure 9-2), but CT is often more valuable because the abundance of retroperitoneal fat may prevent an optimal ultrasound examination. Adrenal venography has been widely used to demonstrate adrenal masses, and it also permits the aspiration of blood samples for assessment of the level of adrenal hormones.

Cushing's syndrome produces radiographic changes in multiple systems. Diffuse osteoporosis causes generalized skeletal demineralization, which may lead to the collapse of vertebral bodies, spontaneous fractures, and aseptic necrosis of the head of the femur or humerus. Widening of the mediastinum as a result of excessive fat deposition sometimes develops in Cushing's syndrome and can be confirmed by CT. Hypercalciuria caused by the elevated steroid levels can lead to renal calculi and nephrocalcinosis.

Imaging of the sella turcica by conventional tomography or CT is important in the routine assessment of the patient with Cushing's syndrome. Most patients with nontumorous adrenal hyperfunction are found at surgery to have an intrasellar lesion. It is important to emphasize, however, that small pituitary microadenomas may be present in asymptomatic patients. The modality of choice to detect a functioning microadenoma causing adrenal hyper-

Figure 9-1 Cushing's syndrome caused by large adrenal adenoma. Nephrotomogram demonstrates huge suprarenal mass *(arrows)* causing indentation and downward displacement of left kidney.

Figure 9-2 Cushing's syndrome caused by functioning cortical adenoma. A 4-cm mass in the left adrenal gland *(arrows)* is seen posterior to the tail of pancreas and anterior to the kidney *(K)*. Arrowhead points to the normal right adrenal gland. (From Lee JKT, Sagel SS, Stanley RJ, editors: *Computed body tomography*, New York, 1983, Raven Press.)

plasia is contrast-enhanced MRI. After adrenal surgery, a pituitary adenoma develops in up to one third of the patients and produces progressive sellar enlargement. For this reason, yearly follow-up sellar tomograms may be indicated after adrenalectomy.

Nonpituitary tumors producing ACTH may cause adrenal hyperfunction and Cushing's syndrome. The most common sites of origin are the lung, thymus, and pancreas; about half of these tumors can be demonstrated on chest radiographs. Octreotide scintigraphy (a nuclear medicine exam) detects ectopic ACTH tumors based on increased uptake of tumor cell surface receptors for somatostatin.

Treatment

Treatment for Cushing's syndrome depends on the cause of the excess production of glucocorticoid hormones. Surgical resection is the treatment of choice to eliminate the excessive hormone production. Medical suppression of abnormal endocrine stimulation and radiation therapy directed to the hyperfunctioning tumor are alternatives if the tumor is inoperable.

ALDOSTERONISM

An overproduction of mineralocorticoid hormones produced by the most superficial layer of the cortex causes retention of sodium and water and abnormal loss of potassium in the urine. This results in hypertension, muscular weakness or paralysis, and excessive thirst (polydipsia). Aldosteronism may be attributable to an adrenocortical adenoma (Conn's syndrome) or to bilateral hyperplasia of the superficial cortical layer. Aldosteronism may also be the result of renin-secreting tumors, renal artery stenosis, malignant hypertension, and bilateral chronic renal disease.

Radiographic appearance

The role of radiographic imaging is to demonstrate the location of adenomas that may otherwise be difficult to detect during exploratory surgery.

Noncontrast CT, the most widely used imaging modality, demonstrates the small adrenocortical adenoma as a contour abnormality of the gland (Figure 9-3). Adrenal venography with biochemical assay of a sample of adrenal blood is another important technique for localizing aldosteronomas and determining primary versus secondary hyperaldosteronism.

Treatment

Hypertension and other clinical manifestations of aldosteronism can be cured by the resection of an adenoma but are little affected by the removal of both adrenal glands in the patient with bilateral hyperplasia. Medical antihypertensive agents, especially long-acting calcium channel blockers, are available if the adenoma is inoperable.

ADRENOGENITAL SYNDROME

The adrenogenital syndrome (adrenal virilism) is caused by the excessive secretion of androgenically active substances by the adrenal gland. In the congenital form, a specific enzyme deficiency that prevents the formation of androgenic hormones causes continuous ACTH stimulation and bilateral hyperplasia. The elevated levels of androgens result in accelerated skeletal maturation along with premature epiphyseal fusion, which may lead to dwarfism.

In women, the tumor causes masculinization, with the development of hair on the face (hirsutism). The

Figure 9-3 Aldosteronoma. Note the small mass (*arrow*) anterior to the left kidney.

Figure 9-4 Adrenogenital syndrome caused by a functioning adrenocortical tumor (*arrow*).

breasts diminish, the clitoris enlarges, and ovulation and menstruation cease.

Radiographic appearance

Most cases of acquired adrenogenital syndrome are caused by adrenocortical tumors, which can be detected by CT (Figure 9-4), ultrasound, or adrenal venography. CT is currently the imaging modality of choice.

Treatment

Surgical resection of a hyperfunctioning tumor with replacement therapy allows normal development. Medical suppression of abnormal stimuli prevents the excessive release of ACTH, allowing female features to develop normally. If not treated, a masculinized woman may require reconstructive surgery.

Figure 9-5   Adrenocortical insufficiency caused by disseminated histoplasmosis. CT scan demonstrates bilateral adrenal enlargement *(arrows)*. (From Karstaedt N et al: Computed tomography of the adrenal gland, *Radiology* 129:723-730, 1978.)

HYPOADRENALISM

The clinical manifestations of adrenal insufficiency vary from those of a chronic insidious disorder (easy fatigability, anorexia, weakness, weight loss, increased melanin pigmentation) to those of an acute collapse with hypotension, rapid pulse, vomiting, and diarrhea.

The most common cause of adrenal insufficiency is the excessive administration of steroids. Primary adrenocortical insufficiency (Addison's disease) results from progressive cortical destruction, which must involve more than 90% of the glands before clinical signs of adrenal insufficiency appear. In the past, Addison's disease was usually attributed to tuberculosis; at present, most cases reflect idiopathic atrophy, probably on an autoimmune basis. In areas where the disease is endemic, histoplasmosis is an occasional cause of adrenal insufficiency.

Radiographic appearance

Acute inflammatory disease causes generalized enlargement of the adrenal glands, which can be demonstrated by a variety of imaging techniques (Figure 9-5). MRI can differentiate adrenal masses better than CT, but MRI cannot distinguish a tumor from an inflammatory process. Other radiographic findings occasionally seen in patients with adrenal insufficiency include a small heart and calcification of the cartilage of the ear.

Treatment

Corticosteroids produce a fast recovery and must be administered regularly for the patient's survival. Morbidity and mortality are high without treatment.

ADRENAL CARCINOMA

About half of adrenal carcinomas are functioning tumors that cause Cushing's syndrome, virilization, femi-

Figure 9-6   Adrenal carcinoma. **A,** Ultrasound identifies a heterogeneous lobulated mass (12 × 7 × 11 cm) involving the upper pole of the left kidney. **B,** CT scan 1 month later shows diffuse inhomogeneous enhancement with the appearance of some low-density areas suggesting necrosis.

nization, or aldosteronism. The tumors grow rapidly and are usually large necrotic masses at the time of clinical presentation.

Radiographic appearance

Ultrasound shows the tumor as a complex mass that may be difficult to separate from an upper pole renal tumor (Figure 9-6). CT demonstrates an adrenal carcinoma as a large unilateral mass with an irregular edge that often contains low-density areas resulting from central necrosis or prior hemorrhage (Figure 9-7). For adrenal exams, spiral CT with 3- to 5-cm-section reconstructions offers the best resolution and may identify tumors 1 cm or smaller.

Because lymphatic and hepatic metastases are common at the time of clinical presentation, CT scans at multiple abdominal levels are necessary to define the extent of the primary tumor and to detect metastases before surgical resection is attempted. Extension of the tumor into the renal vein and inferior vena cava

Figure 9-7 Adrenal carcinoma. Large soft-tissue tumor *(T)* invades the anteromedial aspect of the left kidney *(K)* and the left crus of the diaphragm *(arrow)*. (Courtesy Nolan Karstaedt and Neil Wolfman, Winston-Salem, N.C.)

Figure 9-8 Adrenal carcinoma. **A,** Axial MRI scan demonstrates a large left adrenal tumor invading the left renal vein and inferior vena cava *(arrow)*. **B,** In another patient, a coronal MRI scan shows an adrenal mass *(A)* above the kidney with a tumor thrombus of slightly higher signal intensity filling the inferior vena cava *(T)*. (From Stark DD, Bradley WG: *Magnetic resonance imaging,* ed 2, St Louis, 1991, Mosby.)

can also be detected by CT, especially after the injection of intravenous contrast material, or by MRI (Figure 9-8). On MRI scans, the higher signal intensity of the tumor in comparison to the liver on T2-weighted images (lower signal on T1-weighted images) may distinguish adrenal carcinoma from nonfunctioning adenomas and pheochromocytomas.

Treatment

The treatment management of choice is surgical resection by open laparotomy or laparoscopy. Chemotherapy using mitotane, an adrenocortical cytotoxin and adrenal inhibitor, may improve symptoms if resection is not an option.

METASTASES TO THE ADRENAL GLAND

The adrenal gland is one of the most common sites of metastatic disease. The primary tumors that most frequently metastasize to the adrenal gland are carcinomas of the lung, breast, kidney, ovary, and gastrointestinal tract, and melanomas.

Radiographic appearance

Metastatic enlargement of an adrenal gland can cause downward displacement of the kidney with flattening of the upper pole. Ultrasound and CT demonstrate adrenal metastases as solid, soft-tissue masses that vary considerably in size and are frequently bilateral (Figure 9-9). However, the ultrasound and CT patterns are indistinguishable from those of primary malignancies of the gland. Therefore, when a known primary tumor exists elsewhere, it is usually assumed that an adrenal mass is metastatic.

Figure 9-9 Adrenal metastases. Note huge irregular low-attenuation mass *(M)* representing adrenal metastasis from oat cell carcinoma of the lung. The left adrenal gland *(arrow)* is normal. *G,* Gallbladder; *L,* liver.

Summary of Findings for Diseases of the Adrenal Cortex

DISORDER	LOCATION	RADIOGRAPHIC APPEARANCE	TREATMENT
Cushing's syndrome	Bilateral adrenal hyperplasia	CT (noncontrast)—thickening of adrenal wings, which appear stellate or in a Y-shape US—diffuse adrenal gland enlargement	Surgical resection Medical suppression of endocrine stimulation if tumor is inoperable Radiation therapy if tumor is inoperable
	Adrenal tumor	CT—to evaluate sella turcica MRI—detects functioning pituitary microadenoma causing adrenal hyperplasia	
Aldosteronism	Overproduction of mineralocorticoid hormones	CT—locates small adrenocortical adenoma as a contour abnormality of the gland Venography (adrenal)—to acquire material for biochemical assay	Resection of altered adrenal gland Therapeutic option: antihypertensive drugs
Adrenogenital syndrome	Excessive secretion of androgenically active substances	CT/US—demonstrates underlying adrenal neoplasm or hyperplasia Venography (adrenal)—to acquire material for biochemical assay	Surgical resection Medical suppression Reconstructive surgery if necessary
Hypoadrenalism	Adrenal insufficiency	Abdominal film—calcification of adrenals CT—enlarged adrenal glands or atrophic adrenals	Corticosteroids Morbidity and mortality high without treatment
Adrenal carcinoma	Tumor of adrenal cortex	US—complex mass above upper pole of kidney; homogeneous when small; heterogeneous when large, with central necrosis or hemorrhage CT—mass containing low-density areas; metastasis also detected MRI—higher signal intensity than liver on T2-weighted images	Surgical resection Chemotherapy
Adrenal metastases	Adrenal gland	US/CT—demonstrates type of mass and whether bilateral MRI—high signal intensity on T2-weighted images; greater contrast enhancement with metastases than benign adenoma Chemical shift imaging—lipid-laden adenoma produces low signal intensity on an out-of-phase image US/CT—guided biopsy	Adrenalectomy with replacement therapy

US, Ultrasound.

On MR imaging, metastases typically have higher signal intensity on T2-weighted images than benign adenomas, and they also demonstrate increased contrast enhancement on T1-weighted, fat-suppressed images. In-phase and out-of-phase pulse sequences (also known as chemical shift imaging) are highly accurate for distinguishing between adrenal adenomas and metastases. Lipid-laden adenomas show low signal intensity on out-of-phase images and intermediate to high signal intensity on in-phase images.

If necessary, a needle biopsy using ultrasound or CT guidance may be of value to determine whether the adrenal lesion is primary or metastatic.

Treatment

The most common form of treatment is an adrenalectomy followed by replacement therapy; however, as metastasis has occurred, the prognosis is unfavorable.

Diseases of the adrenal medulla

PHEOCHROMOCYTOMA

A pheochromocytoma is a tumor that most commonly arises in the adrenal medulla and produces an excess of vasopressor substances (epinephrine and norepinephrine), which can cause an uncommon but curable form of hypertension. About 10% of pheochromocytomas are extraadrenal in origin. About 10% of patients have bilateral tumors, and a similar percentage of pheochromocytomas are malignant.

Because in almost all patients the diagnosis of a pheochromocytoma can be made with biochemical tests, radiographic imaging serves as a confirmatory study and as a means of localizing the tumor. Excretory urography, even with nephrotomography, may be of limited value because the kidney is often not displaced even when the adrenal pheochromocytoma is large.

Radiographic appearance

CT and ultrasound (Figure 9-10) are very useful in the localization of pheochromocytomas. The cross-sectional images not only detail the extent of the adrenal lesion but also define the status of adjacent structures and can demonstrate bilateral or multiple pheochromocytomas, extraadrenal tumors, and metastases. Pheochromocytomas generally appear as round, oval, or pear-shaped masses that are slightly less echogenic than liver and kidney parenchyma on ultrasound and have an attenuation value less than these organs on CT (Figure 9-11). Most extraadrenal pheochromocytomas arise in the abdomen (Figure 9-12); a few are found in the chest or neck. The tumor may be located anywhere along the sympathetic nervous system, in the organ of Zuckerkandl, and in chemoreceptor tissues such as the carotid body or the glomus jugulare, in the wall of the urinary bladder, or even in the kidney or ureter. Masses may displace the ureter or kidney or may appear as filling defects in the bladder.

MRI can demonstrate the relationship of the tumor to surrounding structures in the coronal plane (Figure 9-13) and has a higher sensitivity than CT. On T2-weighted scans, the extreme hyperintensity of the tumor (due to its water content) makes it stand out from the surrounding structures. When CT and MRI are inconclusive, a radionuclide scan using metaiodobenzylguanidine is highly sensitive for localizing ectopic pheochromocytomas, but this agent is not readily available.

In patients with pheochromocytomas, the arterial injection of contrast material causes a sharp elevation in blood pressure, which must be controlled by α-adrenergic blocking agents. Therefore arteriography is hazardous in these patients.

Treatment

Surgical removal of the tumor results in stabilizing the blood pressure and curing the hypertension. Most tumors are benign and well encapsulated, which makes removal successful.

NEUROBLASTOMA

Neuroblastoma, a tumor of adrenal medullary origin, is the second most common malignancy in children. About 10% of these tumors arise outside the adrenal gland, primarily in sympathetic ganglia in the neck, chest, abdomen, or pelvis. The tumor is highly malignant and tends to attain great size before detection.

Radiographic appearance

Calcification is common in neuroblastoma (occurring in about 50% of cases) in contrast to the relatively infrequent calcification in Wilms' tumor, from which neuroblastoma must be differentiated. Calcification in a neuroblastoma has a fine granular or stippled appearance (Figure 9-14, *A*). Occasionally there may be a single mass of amorphous calcification. Calcification can also develop in metastases of neuroblastoma in paravertebral lymph nodes and liver.

Excretory urography usually demonstrates downward and lateral renal displacement by the tumor mass (Figure 9-15). Neuroblastoma tends to cause the entire kidney and its collecting system to be displaced as a unit, unlike Wilms' tumor, which has an intrarenal origin and thus tends to distort and widen the pelvicalyceal system.

Because of its nonionizing character, ultrasound is a superb modality for evaluating abdominal masses in children. A neuroblastoma appears as a solid or

Figure 9-10 Pheochromocytoma. Longitudinal **(A)** and transverse **(B)** ultrasound images show a cystic and necrotic mass superior to the right kidney (note measuring markers). **C,** The mass *(M)* elevates the inferior vena cava *(arrows)*. The patient's history of increased heart rate (up to 200 beats per minute) and elevated blood pressure are consistent with a diagnosis of pheochromocytoma.

Figure 9-11 Pheochromocytoma. Large pear-shaped mass *(arrows)* is seen anterior to left kidney.

Figure 9-12   Ectopic pheochromocytoma. **A,** Soft-tissue mass *(arrow)* is seen adjacent to the aorta and in front of the left renal vein. **B,** CT scan taken at a higher level demonstrates that both right and left adrenal glands are normal *(arrows)*. *L,* Liver; *S,* spleen. (From Welch TJ et al: Pheochromocytoma: value of computed tomography, *Radiology* 148:501-503, 1983.)

Figure 9-13   Pheochromocytoma. Axial MRI scans (**A** and **B**) at two levels demonstrate bilateral low-intensity lesions *(arrows)*. Coronal MRI scan (**C**) in a different patient shows a left suprarenal mass. (From Stark DD, Bradley WG: *Magnetic resonance imaging,* ed 2, St. Louis, 1991, Mosby.)

Figure 9-14   Neuroblastoma metastatic to bone. **A,** Plain film of the upper abdomen shows diffuse granular calcification within a large primary tumor. **B,** Lateral projection of the skull shows similar calcified deposits within a metastatic lesion in the calvaria. Note sutural widening *(arrowhead)* consistent with increased intracranial pressure. (From Eisenberg RL: *Diagnostic imaging in surgery,* New York, 1987, McGraw-Hill.)

Figure 9-15   Neuroblastoma. Nephrotomogram demonstrates downward and lateral displacement of the upper pole of the left kidney.

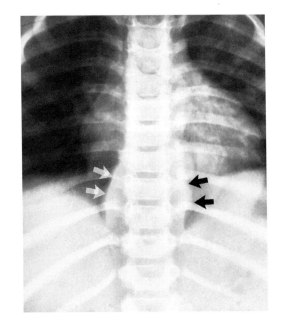

Figure 9-16   Neuroblastoma. Bilateral widening of the paravertebral stripes *(arrows)* represents metastatic deposits. (From Friedland GW et al: *Uroradiology: an integrated approach,* New York, 1983, Churchill Livingstone.)

semisolid mass that is separate from the kidney. It appears as a poorly defined heterogenic mass, unlike the well-defined and relatively homogeneous Wilms' tumor. The tumor is often diffusely hyperechogenic, probably because of necrosis, calcification, and hemorrhage. CT can show evidence of tumor spread to lymph nodes and the sympathetic chain, widening of the paravertebral stripe (also seen on plain films) (Figure 9-16), and metastases to the liver and chest. This modality can also be used to assess the response to treatment.

Metastases to bone, liver, and lungs are common in neuroblastoma. Metastases to the skull typically cause spreading of cranial sutures because of plaques of tumor tissue growing along the surface of the brain (Figure 9-17). Bone destruction leads to a granular pattern of osteoporosis that is often associated with thin, whiskerlike calcifications coursing outward and inward from the tables of the skull (see Figure 9-14, *B*). Metastases in long tubular bones are often multiple and relatively symmetric and present a permeative destructive pattern.

Neuroblastomas arising in the chest appear as posterior mediastinal masses. Metastases to the chest most commonly cause asymmetric enlargement of mediastinal nodes; metastases to the pulmonary parenchyma are infrequent.

Treatment

Combining surgery, chemotherapy, and radiation therapy has dramatically improved the prognosis to about a 90% cure rate.

Figure 9-17   Neuroblastoma. Bone scan performed in a 1-year-old baby boy with left adrenal neuroblastoma to evaluate for osseous involvement. Temporal bones and orbital zygomatic region demonstrate increased uptake appearing as "raccoon eyes."

■ Pituitary Gland

Physiology of the pituitary gland

The pituitary gland is often called the master gland because the many hormones it secretes control the level of most glandular activity throughout the body. The hormone secretion of the pituitary gland itself is controlled by the hypothalamus.

■ ■

Summary of Findings for Diseases of the Adrenal Medulla

DISORDER	LOCATION	RADIOGRAPHIC APPEARANCE	TREATMENT
Pheochromocytoma	Adrenal medulla—excessive epinephrine and norepinephrine	CT—round, oval, or pear-shaped mass with lower attenuation than liver or kidney parenchyma US—mass shows lower echogenicity than normal liver and kidney parenchyma MRI—T2-weighted hyperintense signal NM metaiodobenzylguanidine scan—supersensitive for localizing when ectopic	Surgical resection
Neuroblastoma	Adrenal medullary origin	Radiograph—calcification of tumor; destructive metastatic bone lesions IVU—inferior and lateral kidney displacement US—solid to semisolid mass separate from kidney; poorly defined, heterogeneous mass with irregular hyperechoic areas	Combination treatment: surgical resection, chemotherapy, and radiation therapy

■ ■

IVU, Intravenous urography; *NM,* nuclear medicine; *US,* ultrasound.

The pituitary is a tiny gland, about the size of a pea, that is suspended from the base of the brain by a slender stalk (infundibulum) and sits in the bony depression of the sella turcica. It is divided into anterior and posterior portions, each of which secretes different hormones.

The anterior lobe of the pituitary gland secretes growth hormone, thyroid-stimulating hormone (TSH), ACTH, and a group of hormones that affect the sex organs, or gonads. These gonadotropins include follicle-stimulating hormone (FSH) and luteinizing hormone (LH), which regulate the menstrual cycle and secretion of male and female sex hormones, and prolactin, which stimulates the production of milk during pregnancy and after delivery.

Growth hormone affects all parts of the body by promoting the growth and development of the tissues. Before puberty, it stimulates the growth of long bones (increasing the child's height) and the size of such organs as the liver, heart, and kidneys. After adolescence, growth hormone is secreted in lesser amounts but continues to function in promoting tissue replacement and repair. TSH controls the secretion of thyroid hormone, which regulates the body's metabolism (production and use of energy). ACTH controls the level of activity of the adrenal cortex.

The posterior lobe of the pituitary gland (neurohypophysis) produces two hormones: vasopressin (antidiuretic hormone) and oxytocin. Antidiuretic hormone (ADH) increases the rate of reabsorption of water and electrolytes by the renal tubules, thus decreasing the output of urine and protecting the individual from excessive water loss. Oxytocin causes contraction of smooth muscle, especially in the uterus, and thus strengthens contractions during labor and helps to prevent hemorrhage after delivery.

Diseases of the pituitary gland

HYPERPITUITARISM

Hyperpituitarism results from an excess of growth hormone produced by a tumor (see Figures 7-17 and 7-18) or generalized hyperplasia of the anterior lobe of the pituitary gland. The development of this condition before enchondral bone growth has ceased results in **gigantism;** hyperpituitarism beginning after bone growth has stopped produces **acromegaly.**

Generalized overgrowth of all the body tissues is the underlying abnormality in acromegaly. Although the long bones can no longer grow because the epiphyses are closed, the bones of the hands, feet, and face enlarge, and there is excessive growth of soft tissues. Proliferation of cartilage may cause joint space

Figure 9-18   Acromegaly. Prominent thickening of the heel pad measuring 32 mm, which is highly suggestive of acromegaly.

Figure 9-19   Pituitary adenoma causing acromegaly. Ballooning of the sella turcica with downward displacement of the floor is demonstrated.

widening, especially of the metacarpophalangeal and hip joints. The slight increase in length of each of the seven articular cartilages for each digit leads to perceptible lengthening of the fingers. Overgrowth of the tips of the distal phalanges produces thick bony tufts with pointed lateral margins. The associated hypertrophy of the soft tissues produces the characteristic square, spade-shaped hand of acromegaly. Degenerative changes develop early and are associated with prominent hypertrophic spurring. Unlike typical osteoarthritis, acromegaly results in joint spaces that remain normal or are even widened.

Radiographic appearance

Thickening of the heel pads (the soft tissue inferior to the plantar aspect of the calcaneus) to greater than 23 mm is highly suggestive of acromegaly (Figure 9-18). However, a similar appearance may also be seen in patients with obesity, myxedema, or generalized edema.

The bones of the skull become thickened and have increased density, often with obliteration of the diploic space. This bone thickening is especially prominent in the frontal and occipital regions, leading to characteristic frontal bossing and enlargement of the occipital protuberance. The paranasal sinuses (especially the frontal) become enlarged, and the mastoid processes are usually overpneumatized. Lengthening of the mandible and an increased mandibular angle produce prognathism, one of the typical clinical features of acromegaly. Thickening of the tongue may lead to slurred speech. Pituitary enlargement causes expansion and erosion of the sella turcica (Figure 9-19).

Figure 9-20   Acromegaly. Posterior scalloping *(arrows)* associated with enlargement of vertebral bodies (especially in anteroposterior dimension).

In the spine, hypertrophy of cartilage causes an increased width of the intervertebral disk spaces. An increase in the size of the vertebral bodies is best seen on lateral projections. Hypertrophy of soft tissues may produce an increased concavity of the posterior aspect of the vertebral bodies (scalloping) that is most prominent in the lumbar spine (Figure 9-20).

Extraskeletal manifestations of acromegaly include visceral enlargement, especially of the heart and kidney, enlargement of the tongue, and calcification of cartilage in the pinna of the ear.

Gigantism is manifested as an excessively large skeleton. If hypersecretion of growth hormone continues after epiphyseal closure, the soft tissue and bony changes of acromegaly are superimposed.

To diagnose the pituitary tumor causing the excessive growth, MRI provides the most exact definition of the sella turcica and tissue contained within. Its superior sensitivity and multiplanar capabilities make MRI the modality of choice. Thin-section coronal and sagittal T1-weighted images permit clear distinction of the sphenoid sinus and carotid artery for surgical planning.

Treatment

Surgical resection of the tumor remains the treatment of choice. Even with treatment, any changes or damage in the skeleton will remain unchanged. Radiation therapy or medications to decrease growth hormone levels may provide some relief if resection is not a viable option for the patient.

HYPOPITUITARISM

Because the pituitary gland controls the level of secretion of gonadal and thyroid hormones and the production of growth hormone, decreased function of the pituitary gland causes profound generalized disturbances in bone growth and maturation. In children, hypopituitarism typically leads to a type of dwarfism in which the delayed appearance of epiphyseal centers causes the failure of bones to grow normally in length or width. This results in a person who is small in stature and sexually immature, although well proportioned and of normal mentality. In many patients there is a delay in the eruption of the teeth, which tend to become impacted because their size is not affected. The arrest in the growth of the skeleton occurs during childhood, when the cranial vault is proportionally greater in relation to the facial bones than in the adult. Because this discrepancy remains into adulthood in hypopituitary dwarfism, the relatively large skull may be mistakenly believed to result from hydrocephaly.

Hypopituitarism occurring after adolescence results in hypofunction of the thyroid gland, adrenal glands, and gonads but usually causes few radiologic findings. The heart and kidneys are often small, and calcification or ossification may develop in the articular cartilages.

Radiographic appearance

MRI is the preferred imaging modality as it has superb sensitivity and can directly image the sella and parasellar regions in multiple planes. The use of contrast enhancement may help define a microadenoma,

Summary of Findings for Diseases of the Pituitary Gland

DISORDER	LOCATION	RADIOGRAPHIC APPEARANCE	TREATMENT
Hyperpituitarism	Excessive growth hormone—anterior pituitary	Radiograph—widened joints, thickened heel pad, thickened skull tables with frontal bossing, paranasal sinus enlargement, mandibular changes, vertebral enlargement with scalloping, hypertrophy of cartilage MRI—superior sensitivity and multiplanar imaging to evaluate the pituitary gland	Surgical resection of pituitary tumor
Hypopituitarism	Loss of secretion of any anterior pituitary hormone	Radiograph—skeletal changes in size; dwarfism MRI—detects pituitary tumor by multiplanar imaging	Children—subcutaneous injection of growth hormone
Diabetes insipidus	Deficient release of hormones from the posterior lobe of the pituitary	MRI—detection of pituitary tumor by multiplanar imaging	Drugs to mimic antidiuretic hormone

or detect sarcoidosis in an older patient with Addison's disease.

Treatment

For children, a subcutaneous injection of recombinant growth hormone several times per week during puberty and earlier is recommended to prevent the arrest in growth. In adults, usually no treatment is required.

DIABETES INSIPIDUS

The impaired ability of the kidneys to conserve water in diabetes insipidus results from low blood levels of ADH, reflecting deficient vasopressin release by the posterior lobe of the pituitary gland in response to normal physiologic stimuli. In response to excessive water loss in the urine (polyuria), the body compensates by developing an insatiable thirst (polydipsia). Another type of diabetes insipidus occurs when the kidneys fail to respond to circulating ADH; this is known as nephrogenic diabetes insipidus. It must be stressed that diabetes insipidus is completely unrelated to diabetes mellitus.

Radiographic appearance

Severe polyuria can lead to massive dilatation of the renal pelves, calyces, and ureters. This probably represents a compensatory alteration to accommodate the huge volume of excreted urine.

Treatment

Treatment for diabetes insipidus consists of taking drugs that mimic antidiuretic hormone, delivered most commonly in a nasal spray. For the nephrogenic type, treatment with thiazide diuretics allows the kidney to resorb an increased amount of fluid.

▪ Thyroid Gland

Physiology of the thyroid gland

The thyroid is a butterfly-shaped gland located in the neck at the level of the larynx. It consists of two lobes, one on each side of the trachea, and a connecting strip (the isthmus) that runs anterior to the trachea and connects the lower portions of the two lobes. The thyroid lies just below the Adam's apple, the protrusion formed by the cricoid cartilage of the larynx. Microscopically, the thyroid gland consists of innumerable follicles surrounding a central core of colloid, the storage form of the active material known as thyroxine, which is the only natural iodine-containing substance in the body.

The thyroid gland picks up iodine from the bloodstream and combines it with the amino acid tyrosine to synthesize thyroid hormones, which are stored in the gland until released into the bloodstream when stimulated by TSH from the anterior lobe of the pituitary gland. The active hormone, **thyroxine,** is a small molecule that may contain either three iodine molecules (T_3) or four iodine molecules (T_4). These substances stimulate cellular metabolism in response to the body's need for increased energy production. The increased cellular metabolism requires that additional oxygen be circulated to the cells and that more waste materials be removed, which in turn requires increased blood flow and greater cardiac output. The increased demand for oxygen stimulates the respiratory center and results in a faster rate and greater depth of breathing. Increased cellular metabolism produces heat, which is dissipated by perspiration and by increased blood flow through dilated vessels in the skin, giving the person a flushed appearance. Thyroid hormone also increases the secretion of digestive juices and the movement of ingested material through the intestinal tract.

The release of thyroid hormone is controlled by TSH, which is secreted by the anterior lobe of the pituitary gland. This process is a negative feedback mechanism, in which a high blood level of thyroxine inhibits the anterior pituitary and TSH release, whereas a low level of thyroxine forces the anterior pituitary to release TSH again.

Diseases of the thyroid gland

RADIOACTIVE IODINE SCANNING

Scanning after the administration of radioactive iodine is the superior imaging modality for demonstrating both functioning and nonfunctioning thyroid tissue. This technique is used to localize palpable nodules, to determine the function of nodules, to detect nonpalpable lesions (especially in patients with a history of neck irradiation), and to evaluate the extent of residual tissue after surgical or radioisotopic thyroid ablation. Radionuclide scanning may be combined with uptake, stimulation, or suppression techniques to better characterize the thyroid lesions.

Radiographic appearance

The distribution of radioactivity is uniform throughout the normal thyroid gland (Figure 9-21). Diffuse thyroid enlargement without hyperthyroidism most frequently represents a multinodular goiter of Hashimoto's thyroiditis. In a patient with hyperthyroidism, diffuse thyroid enlargement is suggestive of Graves' disease.

Masses within the thyroid gland appear as hyperfunctioning ("hot") or poorly functioning ("cold") nodules. A hot nodule demonstrates increased radionuclide uptake compared with surrounding thyroid tissue (Figure 9-22). These hot nodules usually represent autonomously functioning thyroid tissue and are rarely malignant, although malignancy is sometimes reported elsewhere in the same gland. Large

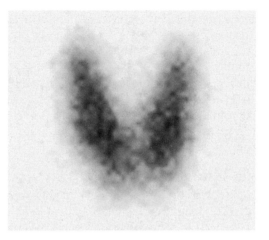

Figure 9-21   Normal radioactive iodine scan. There is uniform distribution of nuclide activity throughout the thyroid gland.

Figure 9-22   Hyperfunctioning (hot) nodules in two patients. Notice the variable amount of suppression in the remainder of the thyroid gland. (From Palmer EL, Scott JA, Strauss HW: *Practical nuclear medicine,* Philadelphia, 1992, Saunders.)

Figure 9-23   Nonfunctioning (cold) nodules in two patients. **A,** Uptake within the gland is normal. A cold nodule in the left lobe of the thyroid corresponds to the nodule seen on the ultrasound. The upper marker is at the thyroid cartilage; the inferior marker is at the suprasternal notch *(SSN).* **B,** Inhomogeneous right and left lobes demonstrate multiple cold nodules. There is a dominant cold nodule in the inferior left pole.

Figure 9-24 Hyperthyroidism. Radionuclide scans in two patients with Graves' disease show symmetrically enlarged thyroid glands with homogeneous increased iodine uptake.

hyperfunctioning nodules may completely suppress the remaining thyroid tissue so that only the nodule itself is visualized. An autonomous nodule may eventually develop central hemorrhage or cystic change and evolve into a nonfunctioning (cold) nodule.

Cold thyroid nodules contain less radionuclide per unit tissue mass than adjacent normal thyroid tissue (Figure 9-23). Most cold nodules represent poorly functioning adenomas. Thyroid cysts, carcinoma, and thyroiditis can also produce this appearance. In a young patient, the absence of uptake in the region of a solitary cold thyroid nodule is associated with a 10% to 25% probability that the nodule is malignant. Ultrasound can establish the precise location of the palpable mass and determine whether it is within the thyroid or in adjacent tissue. In patients who are at risk because of irradiation of the neck during their youth or a family history, but who have no palpable lesion, ultrasound may detect an occult thyroid nodule. Although ultrasound can distinguish a thyroid cyst from the other causes of cold nodules, this modality is of little value in further characterizing noncystic thyroid masses.

HYPERTHYROIDISM

Hyperthyroidism results from the excessive production of thyroid hormone, either from the entire gland (Graves' disease) or from one or more functioning adenomas. Graves' disease is a relatively common disorder that most often develops in the third and fourth decades and has a strong female predominance. The major clinical symptoms include nervousness, emotional lability, an inability to sleep, tremors, rapid pulse rate (tachycardia), palpitations, excessive sweating, and heat intolerance. Weight loss is frequent, usually despite an increased appetite. A characteristic physical finding is exophthalmos, outward protrusion of the eyeball caused by edema in the tissue behind the eyes.

Figure 9-25 Thyroid goiter. Ultrasound image shows thickened isthmus *(arrows)* and enlarged bilateral lobes. *T,* Trachea.

Radiographic appearance

Radioactive iodine scans in patients with Graves' disease typically demonstrate diffuse enlargement of the thyroid gland with increased radioiodine uptake (Figure 9-24), which rules out a single toxic adenoma. The degree of increased uptake on the scan helps to determine the dose of radioactive iodine for treatment.

In severe disease, high-output cardiac failure may develop along with generalized cardiomegaly and pulmonary congestion. Unilateral or bilateral exophthalmos as a result of Graves' disease can be demonstrated by CT as thickening of the extraocular muscles. Ultrasound imaging helps determine the size and location of the thyroid (Figure 9-25), and the image can be correlated with the radioactive scans.

Treatment

Antithyroid drugs are used to decrease thyroid response. Destruction of thyroid cells by radioactive iodine (^{131}I) or total thyroidectomy results in hypothyroidism.

HYPOTHYROIDISM

Hypothyroidism can result from any structural or functional abnormality that leads to an insufficient synthesis of thyroid hormone. Hypothyroidism dating from birth (cretinism) results in multiple developmental abnormalities. Children with cretinism typically have a short stature; coarse features with a protruding tongue, a broad, flattened nose, and widely set eyes; sparse hair; dry skin; and a protuberant abdomen with an umbilical hernia.

Adult hypothyroidism has an insidious onset with nonspecific symptoms including lethargy, somnolence (sleeping up to 16 hours a day), constipation, cold intolerance, slowing of intellectual and motor activity, and weight gain despite a decreased appetite. Dry skin, stiff aching muscles, and a deepening voice with hoarseness often occur. The facial features are thickened, and there is a doughy thickening of the skin (myxedema).

Radiographic appearance

The major radiographic abnormalities in children include a delay in the appearance and subsequent growth of ossification centers and retarded bone age. Skull changes are common and include an increase in the thickness of the cranial vault, underpneumatization of the sinuses and mastoid air cells, widened sutures with delayed closure, and a delay in the development and eruption of the teeth (Figure 9-26).

Radiographically, the heart in adults is typically enlarged because of pericardial effusion. Soft-tissue thickening is often seen on films of the extremities, and adynamic ileus is a common finding on abdominal radiographs.

Treatment

If a tumor is the cause of hypothyroidism, surgery, chemotherapy, and radiation therapy is the treatment of choice. For functional hypothyroidism, the thyroid hormone is replaced with a synthetic product (thyroxine).

GOITER

A goiter is an enlargement of the thyroid gland that does not result from an inflammatory or neoplastic process and is not initially associated with hyperthyroidism or myxedema. A simple (nontoxic) goiter results when one or more factors impair the capacity of the thyroid gland in the basal state to secrete the

Figure 9-26   Cretinism. Lateral projection of skull shows increased density at the base, small underdeveloped sinuses, and hypoplasia of teeth with delayed eruption. Retardation of facial maturation makes face appear small relative to size of calvaria.

quantities of active hormones necessary to meet the needs of the body. Because the blood level of thyroid hormone is low, there is nothing to inhibit the anterior pituitary, which continues to secrete thyroid-stimulating hormone, causing the thyroid gland to enlarge. In most cases, there is a sufficient increase in both the functioning thyroid mass and the cellular activity to overcome the mild or moderate impairment of hormone synthesis, permitting the patient to remain metabolically normal although goitrous.

Although goiters were once endemic in areas where there was insufficient iodine in the diet, this situation is now rare because iodine is added commercially to salt and bread.

Radiographic appearance

On a radioactive iodine scan, a nontoxic goiter usually appears as a symmetric or an asymmetric enlargement of the thyroid gland. Plain radiographs and esophagrams often show the enlarged thyroid gland impressing or displacing the trachea and esophagus (Figure 9-27).

A toxic multinodular goiter may be a consequence of a long-standing nontoxic goiter. In this condition, one or more areas of the gland become independent of TSH stimulation. Radioactive iodine scans most commonly show accumulation of iodine

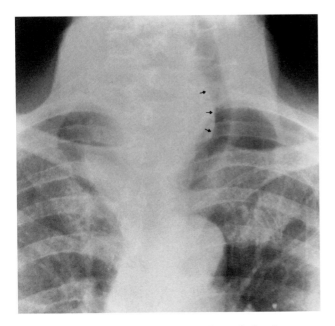

Figure 9-27   Goiter. Greatly enlarged thyroid gland appears as a soft-tissue mass impressing the trachea *(arrows)* and displacing it to the left.

Figure 9-28   Multinodular goiter. Radioactive iodine scan shows patchy uptake of the nuclide caused by increased and decreased uptake by the thyroid.

in diffuse but patchy foci throughout the gland (Figure 9-28). Another pattern consists of iodine accumulation in one or more discrete nodules within the gland, with the remainder of the gland being essentially nonfunctional.

Ultrasound is indicated to determine if a nonfunctioning mass detected on a radioactive iodine scan is cystic or solid (Figure 9-29). CT or MRI is employed only when there is a substernal thyroid that cannot be seen with ultrasound.

Treatment

The first-line treatment of small goiters is to control the nodule size with oral thyroxine. If the goiter continues to enlarge, the thyroid is surgically resected to relieve the compression of anatomic structures in the neck (trachea, esophagus).

BENIGN THYROID ADENOMAS

Benign thyroid adenomas are encapsulated tumors that vary greatly in size and usually compress adjacent tissue. They may be located within the neck, where they tend to cause deviation or compression of the trachea, or they may extend substernally and appear as masses in the superior portion of the anterior mediastinum.

Radiographic appearance of thyroid adenomas

Calcification may develop within the mass (Figure 9-30). Thyroid adenomas can appear as hot or cold nodules, depending on their functional capacity. Ultrasound usually demonstrates an adenoma as a

A

B

Figure 9-29   Multinodular goiter. **A,** Ultrasound image demonstrates solid nodular lesions (8 × 15 mm) in both lobes of the thyroid (left lobe shown here). **B,** The Doppler image demonstrates increased vascularity.

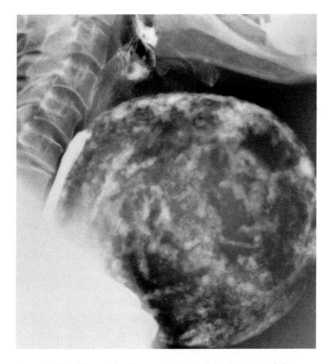

Figure 9-30 Thyroid adenoma. Lateral projection of the neck shows a huge calcified thyroid mass.

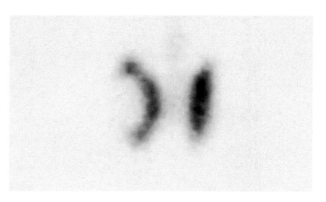

Figure 9-31 Thyroid carcinoma. Radioactive iodine scan shows a solitary cold nodule that corresponds to the patient's palpable mass.

solid mass with a consistent echogenicity. There is often a thick and smooth peripheral hypoechoic halo caused by the fibrous capsule and blood vessels.

THYROID CARCINOMAS

The three major types of thyroid carcinomas are papillary, follicular, and medullary. **Papillary carcinoma,** the most common type, has peaks of incidence occurring in adolescence and young adulthood and again in later life during the third to fifth decade. The tumor is usually slow-growing and cystic, and it typically spreads to regional lymph nodes, where it may remain silent for many years. Distant metastases to the lungs are rare and often cause only mild, nonspecific thickening of bronchovascular markings, although the metastases may also appear as miliary and nodular densities that predominantly involve the lower lobes.

Follicular carcinoma has a histologic appearance that closely mimics normal thyroid tissue. Typically (in about 75% of cases), this tumor occurs in women over 40 years of age. The tumor usually undergoes early hematogenous spread, especially to the lung and bone. Skeletal metastases, which may be the initial presentation, tend to produce entirely lytic, expansile destruction that extends into the soft tissues and is associated with little or no periosteal reaction.

Medullary carcinoma is the least common type of thyroid malignancy. At least 10% of the cases are familial, most often appearing as a component of a syn-

drome in which there are multiple endocrine tumors. Dense, amorphous calcifications can often be seen within the tumor. Medullary carcinomas readily metastasize via the lymphatic channels.

There is a substantially increased risk of thyroid cancer in persons with a history of therapeutic neck irradiation in childhood. In the past such radiation was used for benign disease such as enlargement of the tonsils, adenoids, and thymus; middle ear disease; and a variety of skin disorders, including acne.

Radiographic appearance of thyroid carcinomas

On radioactive iodine scans, thyroid carcinoma usually appears as a solitary cold nodule that corresponds to a palpable mass (Figure 9-31). A nodule that is functioning (hot) can essentially be excluded from a diagnosis of thyroid carcinoma.

On ultrasound, 90% of papillary carcinomas appear as solid hypoechoic masses that may contain microcalcifications, which appear as tiny hyperechoic foci (Figure 9-32). Follicular carcinomas, which have similar tissue consistency, cannot be distinguished from adenomas unless they demonstrate irregular tumor margins and a thick irregular halo (Figure 9-33). On color Doppler, tortuous or disordered blood vessel arrangement is common. Medullary carcinomas appear similar to papillary carcinomas, with bright echogenic foci caused by calcifications.

MRI and CT demonstrate substernal thyroids that ultrasound cannot detect because of bone interference. MRI may aid in defining the extent of the neoplasm.

Treatment of Thyroid Tumors

Thyroid adenoma treatment may be as simple as observation or as complex as a surgical lobectomy. Drug therapy options include TSH suppression or radioactive iodine. Appropriate treatment will depend on the size and location of the thyroid adenoma.

Figure 9-32 Ultrasound images of a complex thyroid mass. **A,** The mass has solid components and intercystic septations of various thicknesses. **B,** Echogenic foci with shadowing are evident *(arrows).* Together with the radioactive iodine scan, which showed a cold nodule, this suggests a malignant lesion.

Figure 9-33 Degenerative follicular adenoma. **A,** Radioactive iodine scan shows a prominent cold nodule. **B,** Ultrasound illustrates a lesion that is not smooth (note papillary projections, *arrow*) and that lacks back wall enhancement. These features most often indicate a degenerative follicular adenoma.

Summary of Findings for Diseases of the Thyroid Gland

DISORDER	LOCATION	RADIOGRAPHIC APPEARANCE	TREATMENT
Hyperthyroidism	Excessive hormone production	NM radionuclides—diffuse enlarged thyroid with increased uptake	Antithyroidal drugs Radioactive iodine Partial or total resection of thyroid
Hypothyroidism	Insufficient synthesis of thyroid hormone	Imaging not used for diagnosis Radiograph—retarded bone age; increased skull thickness with widened sutures and delayed suture closure Chest film (in adult)—enlarged heart with pericardial effusion	Replacement therapy If caused by tumor— surgery, radiation, and chemotherapy

NM, Nuclear medicine; *US,* ultrasound.

Continued

● ●

Summary of Findings for Diseases of the Thyroid Gland—cont'd

DISORDER	LOCATION	RADIOGRAPHIC APPEARANCE	TREATMENT
Goiter	Enlarged thyroid gland	NM radionuclides—enlargement of thyroid gland Esophagram—thyroid gland impresses or displaces trachea and esophagus	Thyroxin to manage goiter size Resection of enlarged portion of thyroid
Benign thyroid adenomas	Encapsulated tumor	X-ray calcification NM radionuclides—hot or cold nodule US—solid homogenetic mass with peripheral hypoechoic halo	Observation Lobectomy Drug therapy
Thyroid carcinomas	Papillary, follicular, or medullary	NM radionuclides—solitary cold nodule US—papillary carcinoma appears as a solid hypoechoic mass with hyperechoic foci; follicular carcinoma has irregular tumor margins and a thick irregular halo Color Doppler—tortuous or disordered blood vessel arrangement; medullary carcinomas appear similar to papillary carcinomas with bright echogenic foci MRI/CT—demonstrates substernal thyroid and may aid in defining the extent of the neoplasm	Thyroidectomy Suppressive drugs Chemotherapy with radioactive iodine Radiation therapy

● ●

NM, Nuclear medicine; *US,* ultrasound.

Thyroidectomy is the first choice of treatment, especially for papillary carcinomas. About 80% of patients survive longer than 10 years. If the patient cannot undergo surgery, alternative choices are suppressive drugs and chemotherapy with radioactive iodine, which may result in hypothyroidism. For patients with follicular carcinoma and widespread metastases, radioactive iodine treatment is the best treatment.

■ Parathyroid Glands

Physiology of the parathyroid glands

The parathyroids are four tiny glands, two on each side, that lie behind the upper and lower poles of the thyroid gland. They secrete **parathormone,** which is responsible for regulating the blood levels of calcium and phosphate. Parathormone raises a low serum calcium level by three mechanisms. First, it increases the amount of calcium absorbed from the intestinal tract by interaction with ingested vitamin D. Second, the hormone prevents a loss of calcium through the kidneys and releases calcium from bones by stimulating osteoclastic activity. Third, the parathyroid glands also secrete calcitonin, which decreases the serum calcium level and appears to play a role analogous to that of glucagon in the pancreas.

Diseases of the parathyroid glands

HYPERPARATHYROIDISM

Excessive secretion of parathormone leads to a generalized disorder of calcium, phosphate, and bone metabolism that results in elevated serum levels of calcium and phosphate. **Primary hyperparathyroidism** may be caused by a discrete adenoma (80%) or carcinoma (2%) or by generalized hyperplasia (18%) of all glands. Other causes include nonparathyroid tumors that secrete a parathormone-like substance and the familial syndrome of multiple endocrine neoplasia. **Secondary hyperparathyroidism** occurs more frequently than the primary form and is most often attributable to chronic renal failure. **Tertiary hyperparathyroidism** refers to the development of autonomous functioning parathyroid glands in patients who demonstrate progressive bone disease in the presence of biochemical and clinically controlled renal disease.

Figure 9-34 Hyperparathyroidism. Subperiosteal bone resorption can be seen that predominantly involves the radial margins of the middle phalanges of the second, third, and fourth digits *(arrows)*. Notice also resorption of terminal tufts.

Figure 9-35 Hyperparathyroidism. Characteristic erosion of the distal clavicle *(arrow)* is shown. Metaphyseal subperiosteal resorption beneath the proximal humeral head has led to a pathologic fracture with slippage of the humeral head.

Radiographic appearance

The radiographic findings of primary and secondary hyperparathyroidism are similar, except that in the secondary form brown tumors (focal areas of bone destruction) are rare and osteosclerosis is more common. The earliest change is subperiosteal bone resorption, which particularly involves the radial margins of the middle phalanges (Figure 9-34), the distal clavicles (Figure 9-35), and the medial aspect of the upper third of the tibias. Loss of normal cortical definition is followed by an irregularly lacy resorption, with the endosteal margin initially remaining intact. Erosions of the terminal tufts of the fingers and loss of the lamina dura of the teeth often occur, although these are nonspecific findings that also are seen in other conditions.

Generalized loss of bone density may produce a ground-glass appearance. So-called brown tumors may become large and expansile and even simulate a malignant process (Figure 9-36). Pathologic fractures may lead to bizarre deformities. Irregular demineral-ization of the calvaria produces the characteristic salt-and-pepper skull (Figure 9-37).

A generalized increase in bone density (osteosclerosis) may develop in patients with hyperparathyroidism, especially when it is a result of renal failure. Thick bands of increased density adjacent to the superior and inferior margins of vertebral bodies produce the characteristic "rugger-jersey" spine (Figure 9-38).

Soft-tissue calcification is common, especially in secondary hyperparathyroidism. Calcific deposits may develop in vessels, articular cartilages, menisci, joint capsules, and periarticular tissues (Figure 9-39). Elevated serum calcium and decreased excretion of calcium in the urine may result in nephrocalcinosis and urinary tract stones. Increased incidences of pancreatic calculi and pancreatitis, peptic ulcer, and gallstones have also been reported in patients with hyperparathyroidism.

The preoperative localization of a functioning parathyroid adenoma has long been a difficult imaging problem. Ultrasound can detect 80% to 85% of the

Figure 9-36 Hyperparathyroidism. Brown tumors have produced multiple lytic lesions about the knee.

parathyroid abnormalities. Parathyroid carcinomas usually have a more heterogeneous internal structure than adenomas. Preoperative parathyroid localization is not required unless the patient has had a previous neck surgery. Plain radiographs and barium studies are of virtually no value unless the tumor is huge.

The major role of sophisticated imaging modalities in the localization of functioning parathyroid adenomas is in patients who remain hypercalcemic, or in whom hypercalcemia recurs (Figure 9-40), after neck surgery for hyperparathyroidism. In these patients, normal anatomic relationships are disturbed, landmarks may be absent, and scarring and adhesions distort the field and complicate the surgical technique. Also, the elusive parathyroid tumor is more likely to be situated in an ectopic position (Figure 9-41). Indeed, the success rate for parathyroid reexploration without help from imaging is less than 65%.

Thus CT and MRI are required to detect ectopic parathyroid tissue location (such as in the thymus). Radionuclide subtraction imaging using technetium-99m (Figure 9-42, *A*) and thallium can detect parathyroid adenomas with a fairly high sensitivity and specificity. An adenoma takes up only the thallium (Figure 9-42, *B*) and a residual focus of activity appears when the technetium is subtracted from the initial image (Figure 9-42, *C*). The normal thyroid can be distinguished from the tumor because it concentrates both radionuclides.

Using ultrasound or CT guidance for preoperative fine-needle aspiration biopsy can increase the specificity of localizing and confirming the exact site of a parathyroid adenoma, especially in patients who have

Figure 9-37 Hyperparathyroidism. Characteristic salt-and-pepper skull.

The union of an ovum and a spermatozoon (fertilization) normally occurs in the fallopian tubes. About 1 day later, the resulting embryo reaches the uterus, where it begins to implant itself in the endometrium. Occasionally, implantation occurs in the fallopian tube or pelvic cavity instead of in the uterus, resulting in an **ectopic pregnancy.** Within 10 days, there is the earliest development of the placenta, which is derived in part from both the developing embryo and the maternal tissues and serves to nourish the fetus and anchor it to the uterus. Although they are closely related, maternal and fetal blood do not mix, and the exchange of nutrients occurs across the important fetal membrane termed the **chorion.**

The menstrual cycle refers to the changes in the endometrium of the uterus that occur in women throughout the childbearing years. Each cycle lasts about 28 days and is divided into three phases: proliferative, secretory, and menstrual. Although the first day of menstruation is normally considered as the first day of the cycle, for ease of description the menstrual phase will be described last.

The **proliferative,** or **postmenstrual,** phase occurs between the end of the menses and ovulation. Production of estrogen by ovarian follicular cells under the influence of FSH causes proliferation of the endometrium of the uterus. In a typical 28-day cycle, the proliferative phase usually includes cycle days 6 to 13 or 14. However, there is far more variability in the length of this phase than in the others.

The **secretory,** or **postovulatory,** phase occurs between ovulation and the onset of the menses. The high level of estrogen in the blood after ovulation inhibits the secretion of FSH, and the anterior lobe of the pituitary gland begins to secrete LH. This stimulates the corpus luteum to produce the hormone progesterone, which stimulates a further increase in the thickness of the endometrium and prepares the uterus for implantation of the ovum should fertilization occur. The length of the secretory phase is fairly constant and usually lasts 14 days.

If fertilization of the ovum does not occur, the high level of progesterone in the blood inhibits the secretion of LH so that the corpus luteum begins to degenerate and ceases to produce progesterone. As the superficial layers of the hypertrophied endometrium begin to break down, denuded bleeding areas are exposed. The flow of blood, mucus, and sloughed endometrium from the uterus is called the menstrual flow. This **menstrual** phase of the cycle lasts about 4 to 6 days, until the low level of progesterone causes the pituitary gland to again secrete FSH and a new menstrual cycle begins. Of course, if the ovum is fertilized, the corpus luteum does not degenerate and the endometrium remains intact throughout pregnancy.

The reproductive years terminate with the cessation of menstrual periods **(menopause),** which usually begins when a woman is in her late 40s or early 50s.

■ Pelvic Inflammatory Disease

Inflammation of the pelvic reproductive organs is usually the result of venereal disease (especially gonorrhea) in women of childbearing age. It can also develop from an unsterile abortion or delivery, or it may be a complication of intrauterine devices. If pelvic inflammatory disease is not promptly and adequately treated, spread of infection to the fallopian tubes may cause fibrous adhesions that obstruct the inner portion near the uterus. If the outer ends of the tubes remain open, the spill of purulent material can lead to peritonitis and the formation of a pelvic abscess. More commonly, the outer ends close and the fallopian tubes fill with pus **(pyosalpinx).** After antibiotic therapy, the infection subsides and the tubes may remain filled with a watery fluid **(hydrosalpinx).** Obstruction of the fallopian tubes can result in infertility or ectopic pregnancy. Spread of infection to involve the ovaries can produce tuboovarian abscesses, which are usually bilateral.

Radiographic appearance

Ultrasound is the imaging procedure of choice for detecting pelvic inflammatory disease and pelvic abscesses. The transabdominal approach best demonstrates the extent of the disease process, whereas the endovaginal approach is most sensitive for detecting dilated tubes, inflammatory changes, and abscesses. The fluid-filled urinary bladder provides an excellent acoustic window and permits confusing loops of small bowel to be displaced out of the pelvis. Endometritis may occur after childbirth or in association with pelvic inflammatory disease. Ultrasound demonstrates a thickened endometrium, possibly with irregularity that may contain fluid (Figure 10-26). Pyosalpinx and tuboovarian abscesses typically are seen as tubular adnexal masses that are sonolucent and compatible with fluid collections (Figure 10-27). However, abscesses may also have thick and irregular (or "shaggy") walls or may contain echoes or fluid levels representing the layering of purulent debris (Figure 10-28). In severe cases, CT may aid in assessing the full extent of the disease. MRI is unnecessary unless the patient has an iodine allergy.

The status of the fallopian tubes can be assessed radiographically by hysterosalpingography, in which the uterine cavity and fallopian tubes are opacified after the injection of contrast material into the uterus. In the woman with normal patent fallopian tubes, contrast material extravasating into the pelvic peritoneal

Figure 10-26   Endometritis. Ultrasound illustrates an enlarged endometrial cavity with a heterogeneous echogenicity (between *cursors*) associated with a therapeutic abortion.

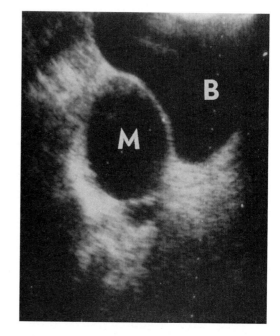

Figure 10-27   Tuboovarian abscess. Ultrasound scan demonstrates a large sonolucent mass *(M)* posterior to the bladder *(B)*.

Figure 10-28   Chronic pelvic inflammatory disease. Transverse sonogram demonstrates large, complex cystic and echogenic masses *(arrows)* posterior to the echo-free bladder. (From Callen PW, editor: *Ultrasonography in obstetrics and gynecology,* Philadelphia, 1983, Saunders.)

Figure 10-29   Normal hysterosalpingogram. Arrows point to a bilateral spill of contrast material into the peritoneal cavity. *Cx,* internal cervical os; *c,* cornua of the uterus; *f,* fimbriated portion of fallopian tube; *Rt* and *Lt,* right and left fallopian tubes. (From Yune HY et al: Hysterosalpingography in infertility, *Am J Roentgenol Radium Ther Nucl Med* 122:642-651, 1974.)

Figure 10-30   Hydrosalpinx. Unilateral **(A)** and bilateral **(B)** gross dilatation of fallopian tubes without evidence of free spill of contrast material into peritoneal cavity.

cavity outlines the peritoneal surfaces and often loops of bowel within the pelvis (Figure 10-29). If the fallopian tubes are occluded by fibrosis from pelvic inflammatory disease or developmental anomalies, there is no evidence of the contrast material reaching the peritoneal cavity (Figure 10-30).

Plain abdominal or pelvic radiographs are of little value in detecting pelvic inflammatory disease and pelvic abscesses. Abnormal gas collections can be masked by fecal material in the rectum and in loops of small bowel.

Treatment

Antibiotic therapy and abstaining from sexual intercourse until the inflammation subsides are the usual treatments. In more complex instances, ultrasound-guided aspiration and drainage may be required. Thick purulent materials require catheter drainage; most nonpurulent abscesses need only aspiration. The healing phase may leave the fallopian tubes scarred and obstructed.

▪ Cysts and Tumors

Ovarian cysts and tumors

Physiologic ovarian cysts are most common in the female infant and in women of childbearing age. They include follicular cysts (unruptured, enlarged follicles) and corpus luteum cysts, which occur after continued hemorrhage or lack of resolution of the corpus luteum.

The most common malignancies involving the ovaries are metastatic tumors, which primarily arise from carcinomas of the breast, colon, and stomach. They are frequently bilateral and often asymptomatic.

Radiographic appearance

On ultrasound, cysts appear as rounded, anechoic adnexal masses (Figure 10-31). **Primary cystadenocarcinoma** of the ovary often contains psammomatous bodies, depositions of calcium carbonate located in the fibrous stroma of the tumor that can be detected on plain abdominal radiographs. These psammomatous calcifications appear as scattered, fine amorphous shadows that are barely denser than the normal soft tissues and can therefore be easily missed unless they are extensive (Figure 10-32). On ultrasound examination, cystadenocarcinoma typically appears as a large cystic mass with internal septa. It may be difficult to distinguish cystadenocarcinoma (Figure 10-33) from **cystadenoma** (Figure 10-34), its benign counterpart. The more solid and irregular the areas within the mass on ultrasound images, the more likely it is that it represents a malignant tumor. In addition, the association of ascites with an ovarian mass is strongly suggestive of underlying malignancy. MRI is a more definitive study to determine whether the tumor has benign or malignant characteristics.

Ovarian carcinomas usually spread by implanting widely on the omental and peritoneal surfaces. This can produce the characteristic CT appearance of an "omental cake," an irregular sheet of soft-tissue densities beneath the anterior abdominal wall (Figure 10-35). CT is also of value in detecting tumor adherence to bowel, ureteral involvement, and retroperitoneal adenopathy. This makes CT the modality of choice for staging and surgical planning. Positron emission tomography (PET) may be used in determining recurrence of ovarian carcinoma (Figure 10-36).

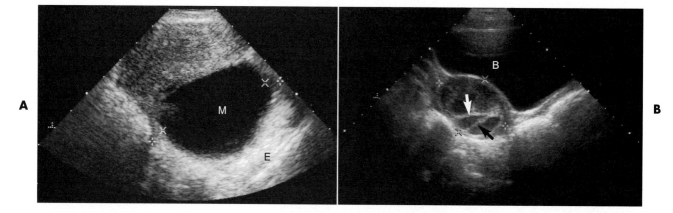

Figure 10-31 Ovarian cysts. **A,** Ultrasound scan demonstrates a large (5 × 6 cm) sonolucent mass *(m)* with backwall enhancement *(E)* involving the right ovary. **B,** In another patient, the longitudinal scan of the right ovary demonstrates a septated *(arrows)* mass (between *cursors*) with homogeneous sonolucent components measuring 5 × 6.7 cm located posterior to the bladder *(B).*

Figure 10-32 Psammomatous calcifications. Diffuse, ill-defined collections of granular amorphous calcification are visible within this cystadenocarcinoma of ovary. (From Eisenberg RL: *Diagnostic imaging in surgery,* New York, 1987, McGraw-Hill.)

Figure 10-33 Endovaginal sonogram of a cystadenocarcinoma. **A,** The transverse image demonstrates a thickened wall and septations within the ovary the left measuring 9 × 7 × 10 cm. **B,** The longitudinal image illustrates an enlarged uterus with a large, complex mass. The CT scan had demonstrated posterior wall thickening in the cyst and irregular densities within the liver—highly suggestive of cystadenocarcinoma.

Figure 10-34   Cystadenoma. Longitudinal **(A)** and transverse **(B)** sonograms demonstrate a complex, predominantly cystic mass (sonolucent) containing several thin and well-defined septations *(arrows)*, which suggest a benign lesion—a mucinous cystadenoma.

Figure 10-35   Omental cake. Metastases *(M)* resulting from cystadenocarcinoma of the ovary cause an irregular sheet of soft-tissue densities beneath the anterior abdominal wall that posteriorly displaces the adjacent contrast-filled bowel loops. (From Lee JKT, Sagel SS, Stanley RJ, editors: *Computed body tomography*, New York, 1983, Raven Press.)

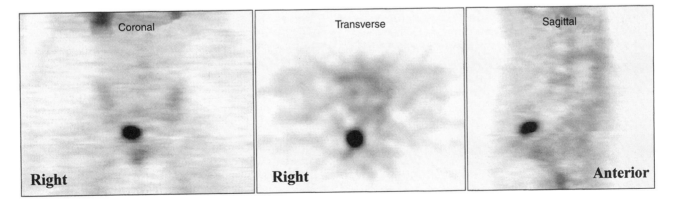

Figure 10-36   Recurrence of ovarian carcinoma. PET scan revealed a solitary focus of intense fluorodeoxyglucose (FDG) uptake in the right paramidline retrocystic location, suggestive of an active neoplasm and consistent with regional recurrence of the patient's ovarian carcinoma. The finding resulted in a change in treatment: the tumor focus, identified by PET-FDG to be in the right posterior pelvis, was successfully resected.

Figure 10-37 Dermoid cyst containing multiple well-formed teeth. Notice the relative lucency of the mass *(arrows)*, which is composed largely of fatty tissue.

Figure 10-39 Dermoid cyst. **A,** Kidney–ureter–bladder study demonstrates two tooth-like densities *(arrow)* beside the coccyx. **B,** A transverse sonogram has a heterogeneous mass (between *cursors*) with a high-amplitude echogenic focus *(arrows)* due to the tooth-like densities.

Figure 10-38 Dermoid cyst. Sagittal sonogram demonstrates only the near wall of the dermoid because of acoustic shadowing from a hairball *(arrows)*, producing the so-called tip of the iceberg sign. (From Eisenberg R: *Atlas of signs in radiology,* Philadelphia, 1984, Lippincott.)

Treatment

With surgical treatment, there is currently a 25% to 30% survival rate.

Dermoid cyst (teratoma)

A dermoid cyst, the most common type of germ cell tumor, contains skin, hair, teeth, and fatty elements, all of which typically derive from ectodermal tissue. These cysts are of no clinical significance unless they grow so large that they produce symptoms by com-

pressing adjacent structures. About half of all ovarian dermoid cysts contain some calcification. This is usually in the form of a partially or completely formed tooth (Figure 10-37); less frequently, the wall of the cyst is partially calcified.

Radiographic appearance

The characteristic calcification combined with the relative radiolucency of the lipid material within the lesion is pathognomonic of an ovarian dermoid cyst.

The most common ultrasound appearance of a dermoid cyst is a complex, primarily solid mass containing high-level echoes arising from hair or calcification within the mass (Figures 10-38 and 10-39). The highly echogenic nature of these masses may make it difficult to delineate the lesion completely or to distinguish it from surrounding gas-containing loops of bowel.

Treatment

Surgical removal is recommended since the cyst may undergo transformation and become malignant.

Uterine fibroids

Fibroids (leiomyomas) of the uterus are benign smooth-muscle tumors that are very common; they are often multiple and vary greatly in size. Growth of fibroid tumors is stimulated by estrogen. They develop only during the reproductive years and tend to shrink after menopause. Abnormal bleeding between periods or excessively heavy menstrual flow is the most common symptom. Large tumors may project from the uterus, causing pressure on surrounding organs, resulting in pelvic pain. They can also interfere with delivery or, if on a stalk (pedunculated), protrude into the vagina.

Radiographic appearance

Uterine fibroids are by far the most common calcified lesions of the female genital tract. They have a characteristic mottled, mulberry, or popcorn type of calcification and appear on plain abdominal radiographs as smooth or lobulated nodules with a stippled or whorled appearance. A very large calcified fibroid occasionally occupies the entire pelvis or even extends out of the pelvis to lie in the lower abdomen (Figure 10-40).

During excretory urography, persistent uterine opacification is often seen in patients with an underlying uterine fibroid tumor (Figure 10-41). The tumor typically presses on the fundus of the bladder, causing a lobulated extrinsic impression that differs from the smooth impression usually seen with ovarian cysts. Extension of a fibroid into the adjacent tissues (parametrium) may cause medial displacement of the pelvic ureter or ureteral compression leading to hydronephrosis.

The classic ultrasound appearance of a uterine fibroid is a hypoechoic, solid, contour-deforming mass in an enlarged, inhomogeneous uterus (Figure 10-42). Fatty degeneration and calcification cause focal increased echogenicity; the calcification may result in acoustic shadowing. A subserosal fibroid projecting from the uterus but attached to it by a large stalk may occasionally simulate an adnexal mass or an ovarian tumor.

Endovaginal ultrasound is the best modality to demonstrate small and submucosal uterine fibroids (Figure 10-43). MRI is more sensitive than CT or ultrasound, but it is indicated only when ultrasound is inconclusive in differentiating between uterine and adnexal masses or between leiomyoma and adenomyosis, and when searching for submucosal fibroids in the patient with unexplained bleeding.

Treatment

In many cases, no treatment is required. Medications can induce a temporary chemical menopause that causes a temporary shrinkage of the fibroid. If bleed-

Figure 10-40 Calcified uterine fibroid. Calcified mass extends well beyond the confines of the pelvis.

Figure 10-41 Uterine fibroid. Excretory urogram demonstrates persistent dense opacification of a huge uterine leiomyoma *(arrows)*.

ing and fibroid size cannot be controlled with medications, surgery is performed. In younger women and for superficial fibroids, a myomectomy (removal of the leiomyoma) is performed to preserve the uterus. Large or multiple tumors usually require hysterectomy, especially if childbearing is complete.

Figure 10-42 Uterine fibroid. Longitudinal sonogram demonstrates a pedunculated leiomyoma as a hypoechoic mass *(M)* projecting from the fundus of the uterus *(U)*. Decreased sound transmission through the mass indicates its solid nature. (From Callen PW, editor: *Ultrasonography in obstetrics and gynecology,* Philadelphia, 1983, Saunders.)

Figure 10-44 Endometrial carcinoma. Endovaginal scan localizing irregular endometrial thickening *(arrows)* with echogenic polypoid projections into the fluid-filled endometrial canal *(F)*. (From Rumack CM, Wilson SR, Charboneau JW: *Diagnostic ultrasound,* St Louis, 1998, Mosby.)

Figure 10-43 Submucosal uterine fibroid. Endovaginal ultrasound of the uterus in the sagittal plane demonstrates a fibroid filling the superior endometrial cavity *(arrow)*.

Many new techniques are becoming available: multilaser technique, myolysis (electrical coagulation of the myoma), uterine artery embolization, and medications, but they are not yet proven.

Endometrial carcinoma

Adenocarcinoma of the endometrium is the predominant neoplasm of the uterine body and is the most common invasive gynecologic neoplasm. It usually occurs in postmenopausal women, especially those who have never had children. Most patients are seen clinically with postmenopausal bleeding.

Radiographic appearance

Excretory urography may demonstrate an enlarged uterus impressing or invading the posterior wall and fundus of the bladder. The typical ultrasound appearance of endometrial carcinoma is an enlarged uterus with irregular areas of low-level echoes and bizarre clusters of high-intensity echoes (Figure 10-44). Unless evidence of local invasion can be demonstrated, the ultrasound findings are indistinguishable from those of fibroid tumors, which often occur in patients with endometrial carcinoma. The endovaginal approach is generally preferred to measure endometrial thickness and to determine whether dilation and curettage (D & C—dilation of the cervix to allow scraping of the uterine wall) is required for histologic examination.

CT demonstrates focal or diffuse enlargement of the body of the uterus (Figure 10-45). This modality is especially useful for detecting clinically unsuspected omental and nodal metastases in patients with advanced disease, as well as for evaluating patients with suspected neoplastic recurrence and for checking the response to chemotherapy or radiation treatment.

MRI allows differentiation of the endometrium (the inner lining) from the myometrium (the muscle layer) of the uterus and has been shown to be useful for demonstrating focal or diffuse endometrial tumors (Figure 10-46). The excellent contrast resolution of this technique may allow determination of the depth of myometrial invasion. For staging purposes, MRI is superior to CT for demonstrating extension of the tumor into the cervix, broad ligaments, and

Figure 10-45   Bladder invasion by endometrial carcinoma. CT scan shows a mass *(M)* obliterating the fat planes between the bladder *(b)* and the uterus. Urine within the bladder outlines thickening of the posterior bladder wall. Nodular extension into the ischiorectal fossa indicates local extension of the tumor.

Figure 10-46   Endometrial carcinoma. Sagittal T2-weighted MR scan shows extensive tumor of mixed signal intensity *(1)* that has invaded the endocervix and permits identification only of the ectocervix *(2)*. Tumor has extended interiorly along the serosal surface of the uterus into the vesicovaginal septum *(3)* and bladder wall *(4)*. Low-intensity foci in the vagina represent radiotherapy implants *(5)*. Note the normal urinary bladder wall superiorly *(6)*. (From Lupetin AR: In Stark DD, Bradley WG, editors: *Magnetic resonance imaging*, St Louis, 1988, Mosby.)

ovaries. Lymphatic involvement of the pelvis and retroperitoneal lymph nodes can also be visualized; the use of a contrast agent makes the resolution even greater.

Treatment

The first option for treatment is a hysterectomy with resection of the enlarged lymph nodes. Radiation therapy may follow surgery, especially in cases of advanced disease or an incomplete resection. For inoperable cancers, the preferred choice is chemotherapy.

Endometriosis

Endometriosis is the presence of normal-appearing endometrium in sites other than their normal location inside the uterus. Although tissues next to the uterus (ovaries, uterine ligaments, rectovaginal septum, pelvic peritoneum) are most frequently involved in endometriosis, the gastrointestinal and urinary tracts can also be affected. Current theories of the cause of endometriosis include (1) reflux of endometrial fragments backward through the fallopian tubes during menstruation, with implantation into the pelvis; (2) transformation of multipotential cells in the abdomen and pelvis; (3) implantation of endometrial fragments during surgery or delivery; and (4) spread of endometrial tissue by way of the bloodstream or lymphatic system.

Radiographic appearance

Even though the endometrial tissue lies outside the uterus, it still responds to hormonal changes and undergoes a proliferative and secretory phase along with sloughing and subsequent bleeding. Thus an endometrial implant within a closed space can continue to grow with each menstrual cycle (Figure 10-47). Clinical symptoms include abnormal bleeding, painful menstruation (dysmenorrhea), and pain during sexual intercourse (dyspareunia). Because endometriosis is usually clinically apparent only when ovarian function is active, most women who are symptomatic for endometriosis are between 20 and 45 years of age. Ultrasound may demonstrate cystic masses filled with old blood. However, differentiation of endometriosis from other adnexal masses requires MRI.

Endometriosis involving the urinary tract most commonly produces ureteral obstruction below the level of the pelvic brim. The condition mimics a ureteral tumor and may appear as an intraluminal mass or stricture or as a smooth, rounded, or multilobular filling defect in the bladder. In the gastrointestinal tract, endometriosis primarily affects those segments that are situated in the pelvis (especially the

Figure 10-47   Endometrioma. Endovaginal scan demonstrating diffuse, homogeneous, low-level echoes throughout the cystic mass *(arrows)*. (From Rumack CM, Wilson SR, Charboneau JW: *Diagnostic ultrasound,* St Louis, 1998, Mosby.)

Figure 10-48   Endometriosis. Three separate endometrial implants *(arrows* and *arrowheads)* are seen in the sigmoid colon. The most distal lesion has a smooth interface with the bowel wall, indicating no intramural invasion. The two more-proximal lesions have irregular borders, indicating intramural or submucosal invasion. (From Gedgaudas RK, et al: The value of the preoperative barium-enema examination in the assessment of pelvic masses, *Radiology* 146:609-616, 1983.)

rectosigmoid colon). It typically causes abdominal cramps and diarrhea during the menstrual period and may appear as single or multiple masses in the colon (Figure 10-48). Repeated shedding of endometrial tissue and blood into the peritoneal cavity can lead to the development of dense adhesive bands causing small bowel obstruction.

A rare complication of endometriosis with intrathoracic implants of endometrial tissue is recurrent catamenial pneumothorax, which is usually right sided and occurs during menstrual flow.

Treatment

The main functions of treatment include pain management, reduction of disease progression, and prevention or reversal of infertility. To manage pain and reduce disease progression, drugs can be used to interrupt the menstrual cycle by stopping proliferation and secretion of extrauterine cells. A conservative surgical treatment, laser surgery, is used to remove visible endometrial implants that obstruct the fallopian tubes. When pain is unbearable, the radical surgical treatment is a complete hysterectomy.

Carcinoma of the cervix

Carcinoma of the cervix is the second most common form of cancer in women. Development of the tumor appears to be related to chronic irritation, infection, and poor hygiene. A higher incidence occurs in women who have begun sexual activity at an early age and have had multiple sexual partners. The development of the Pap smear examination has permitted detection of cervical carcinoma at a very early stage (carcinoma in situ—confined to the site of origin), when it has not yet invaded the underlying tissues and is surgically curable. Widespread cervical cancer becomes inoperable, and radiation therapy is the usual treatment.

Radiographic appearance

At the time of the initial staging, one third of patients have unilateral or bilateral hydronephrosis that can be demonstrated by excretory urography or ultrasound. Indeed, the most common cause of death in patients with carcinoma of the cervix is impairment of renal function caused by ureteral obstruction. Extension of the tumor to the bladder may cause an irregular filling defect; direct infiltration of the perirectal tissues may produce irregular narrowing of the rectosigmoid colon and widening of the retrorectal space. Distant metastases to the skeleton or lungs are uncommon, even in patients with advanced disease.

Ultrasound usually demonstrates a cervical carcinoma as a solid mass behind the bladder (Figure 10-49). CT is more accurate in detecting pelvic sidewall invasion and therefore is usually the initial staging procedure in patients in whom there is a clinical suspicion of advanced disease (Figures 10-50 and 10-51). This modality is also the procedure of choice for monitoring tumor response to treatment and for assessing suspected recurrence.

MRI is superior to CT and is the preferred study to distinguish the cervix from the uterus and vagina. Thus MRI is of value in detecting and staging cervical carcinoma (Figures 10-52 and 10-53). CT cannot always differentiate tumor from adjacent normal tissue.

After radiation therapy for carcinoma of the cervix (and other types of pelvic carcinoma), it may be difficult to distinguish chronic rectal narrowing and widening of the retrorectal space caused by radiation effects from that caused by recurrence of

Figure 10-49   Carcinoma of cervix. Sonogram demonstrates a solid, echogenic mass *(asterisk)* lying behind the bladder *(Bl)* that is indistinguishable from a benign cervical myoma. (From Callen PW, editor: *Ultrasonography in obstetrics and gynecology,* Philadelphia, 1983, Saunders.)

Figure 10-50   Carcinoma of cervix. CT scan demonstrates the inhomogeneity of an enlarged cervix *(Cx)* without evidence of bladder invasion. (From Gross BH et al: Computed tomography of gynecologic diseases, *AJR Am J Roentgenol* 141:765-773, 1983.)

tumor. Radiation therapy can also lead to the development of fibrous inflammatory adhesions between loops of bowel and the bladder, resulting in the development of fistulas between bowel loops (enteric–enteric) and between a bowel loop and the urinary bladder (enteric–vesicular).

Treatment

A hysterectomy with resection of the involved nodes and surrounding tissues and followed by radiation is

Figure 10-51 Bladder invasion by carcinoma of the cervix. CT scan shows irregularity *(arrow)* of the posterior margin of a contrast-filled urinary bladder *(Bl)* and the adjacent inhomogeneous cervical mass *(M)*. (From Callen PW, editor: *Ultrasonography in obstetrics and gynecology,* Philadelphia, 1983, Saunders.)

Figure 10-52 Cervical carcinoma. On this sagittal T1-weighted MR scan, posterior cervical lobulation *(1)* is the only primary sign of infiltrating cervical neoplasm. Note the considerable widening of the central uterine high-intensity zone *(2)* caused by an accumulation of menstrual products in the endometrial canal resulting from tumor occlusion of the endocervical canal. Urine *(3)* within the vagina produces low signal intensity on this imaging sequence. (From Lupetin AR: In Stark DD, Bradley WG, editors: *Magnetic resonance imaging,* St Louis, 1988, Mosby.)

recommended for stage I and II cervical cancers. Advanced lesions require surgery with a combination of radiation and chemotherapy. A pelvic exenteration (removal of all the pelvic organs to debulk the tumor) is used as a last resort.

Figure 10-53 Carcinoma of the cervix. Sagittal T2-weighted MR image shows a bulky cervical neoplasm *(1)* with mottled high signal intensity. The lesion has invaded the upper third of the vaginal stroma *(2)* anteriorly and posteriorly but has spared the uterus *(3)*. The urethra *(4)* and urinary bladder *(5)* are anteriorly displaced by the tumor. (From Lupetin AR: In Stark DD, Bradley WG, editors: *Magnetic resonance imaging,* St Louis, 1988, Mosby.)

■ Breast Cancer

Breast cancer is the most common malignancy among women. Most tumors are classified as infiltrating duct carcinomas, which occur most frequently in the upper lateral quadrant. Current surgical and radiation therapy techniques provide highly effective treatment but only if the cancers are detected when localized to the breast itself. Today many breast tumors are diagnosed prior to their being palpable because routine screening is available (especially in the United States). In these instances, the prognosis is considerably better because the mass has not extended into surrounding tissue or beyond the breast. Unfortunately, most breast tumors are discovered accidentally rather than in the course of regular survey examinations. By this time, the majority have spread either to regional lymph nodes or systemically, accounting for the current high mortality (about 50%) that makes breast cancer the leading cause of cancer death in women.

Periodic careful physical examination of the breast, done either by a trained health professional or by the patient herself, will discover cancers that are small and more likely to be localized. Even smaller, nonpalpable, and potentially more curable lesions can be

Summary of Findings for Diseases of the Female Reproductive System

DISORDER	LOCATION	RADIOGRAPHIC APPEARANCE	TREATMENT
Pelvic inflammatory disease	Infection of uterus and fallopian tubes	US—fallopian tubes appear as adnexal masses that are sonolucent; multiloculated, irregular mass with scattered internal echoes CT—shows full extent of severe disease Hysterosalpingography—for nonvisualized fallopian tubes	Antibiotics Aspiration and drainage
Ovarian cysts	Follicular or corpus luteum	US—round, anechoic adnexal masses	Surgery
Ovarian tumors		KUB—scattered tumor calcifications US—solid irregular mass with associated ascites	Surgery
	Ovarian metastasis	CT—irregular sheet of soft-tissue densities beneath the anterior abdominal wall—omental cake	
Dermoid cyst (teratoma)	Germ cell tumor of ovary	Radiograph—calcifications US—complex, primarily solid mass containing high-level echoes	Surgery
Uterine fibroids (leiomyomas)	Uterus	IVU—lobulated extrinsic impressions of fundus of bladder US—hypoechoic, solid, contour-deforming mass in an enlarged inhomogeneous uterus (when endovaginal, small and submucosal fibroids) MRI—to differentiate anatomy and distinguish fibroid from adenomyosis	Medications Myomectomy Hysterectomy
Endometrial carcinoma	Uterine body	IVU—cancer invading posterior wall of bladder US—enlarged uterus with irregular hypoechoic areas and bizarre clusters of high-signal-intensity echoes CT—diffuse enlargement of the uterine body; omental and nodal metastases MRI—to determine depth of myometrial invasion	Hysterectomy Radiation therapy for incomplete resection Chemotherapy for inoperable tumors
Endometriosis	Endometrium outside normal location	US—sonolucent masses MRI—differentiates endometriosis from other adnexal masses	Medications to interrupt menstrual cycle Conservative surgery—laser technique Radical surgery—hysterectomy
Carcinoma of the cervix	Cervix	US—solid mass posterior to bladder CT—demonstrates pelvic side-wall invasion MRI—differentiates uterus from vagina; used for staging	Stage I and II—hysterectomy followed by radiation Advanced stages—surgery with radiation and chemotherapy

IVU, Intravenous urography; *KUB,* kidney–ureter–bladder image; *US,* ultrasound.

A

B

Figure 10-54   Breast cancer. Full **(A)** and magnified coned **(B)** views of the breast demonstrate an ill-defined, irregular mass with radiating spicules *(arrowheads).*

Figure 10-55   Benign breast mass. Screen-film mammogram demonstrates smooth, round fibroadenoma with clearly defined margins.

origin) and approximately 75% are negative for nodal involvement.

Radiographic appearance

The two major radiographic techniques for diagnosing breast cancer are screen-film mammography and the digital direct-capture system. Screen-film imaging uses a specially designed x-ray screen that permits the proper exposure of film by many fewer x-rays than would otherwise be necessary. This produces a conventional black-and-white image at a very low radiation dose. A direct-capture system relies on radiation captured by multiple cells that convert the radiation energy to electrical energy to produce a numerical value (i.e., a digitized image).

Almost all breast cancers are seen mammographically as a tumor mass, clustered calcifications, or both. Either feature, when clearly demonstrated, is so indicative of malignancy that prompt biopsy is required whether the lesion is palpable or not. Secondary changes of breast carcinoma include skin thickening and nipple retraction. Magnification imaging and compression techniques greatly improve the diagnostic value of the image.

The typical malignant tumor mass is poorly defined, has irregular margins, and demonstrates numerous fine linear strands or spicules radiating out from the mass (Figure 10-54). This appearance is characteristic but not diagnostic of malignancy and is in stark contrast to the typical mammographic picture of a benign mass, which has well-defined, smooth margins and a round, oval, or gently lobulated contour (Figure 10-55).

Clustered calcifications in breast cancer are typically numerous, very small, and localized to one segment

detected by mammography, a radiographic examination that is by far the most effective breast diagnostic procedure. Indeed, routine mammography combined with physical examination is the only approach currently available that promises to significantly reduce breast cancer mortality.

From screening mammography, 7% to 10% of the patients are recalled for more extensive imaging. Of these, 15% to 20% will require a biopsy, and 5% to 7% will have cancer detected. On screening examinations, 40% of the cancers detected are in situ (at the

Figure 10-56 Malignant calcifications in breast cancer. Numerous tiny calcific particles with linear *(straight arrows)*, curvilinear *(solid arrowhead)*, and branching *(open arrowhead)* forms characteristic of malignancy. Note the benign calcification in the arterial wall, which is easily recognized by its large size and tubular distribution *(curved arrow)*.

of the breast. They demonstrate a wide variety of shapes, including fine linear, curvilinear, and branching forms (Figure 10-56). Although only about half of breast cancers present mammographically as clusters of calcifications, typical calcifications are seen in many of the nonpalpable intraductal cancers that often do not form mass lesions and may otherwise escape detection.

Ultrasound provides a secondary diagnostic tool that can differentiate a benign cyst from a solid mass, and thus it substantially reduces the number of biopsies performed for benign cysts (Figures 10-57 and 10-58) and normal fibroglandular tissue. However, ultrasound is of limited value in detecting nonpalpable cancers, particularly those that present with calcifications alone, and thus it cannot substitute for mammography as a screening examination. In cases of ruptured silicone implants, an inflammatory process causes the development of silicone granulomas. These produce a "snowstorm" appearance (Figure 10-59) causing shadowing posteriorly that obscures the posterior border.

MRI with multiple sequences and contrast enhancement now has the ability to help differentiate between benign adenomas and carcinomas. The use of image subtraction (noncontrast image subtracted from the enhanced image) assists in highlighting the contrast-enhanced regions. Benign masses tend to have smooth borders, whereas malignancies appear as high-signal-intensity lesions with spiculation. Using longer sequences, carcinomas produce high signal intensity, whereas adenomas assume a lower signal intensity (and are not apparent). Fat suppression using water excitation best demonstrates the functional

Figure 10-57 Sonography for breast disease. **A,** Mammogram shows several rounded masses *(m)* that could be solid or cystic in a breast that is very dense anteriorly. **B,** Sonogram clearly shows that the largest mass *(M)* is cystic, as it contains no internal echoes and shows considerable posterior enhancement *(arrows)*.

parenchyma, and this technique helps differentiate among various lesions. For patients with breast implants, MRI may best demonstrate the surrounding breast tissue (Figure 10-60). This modality also demonstrates implant twisting or rupture, which may not be visible on other imaging techniques. Single photon emission computed tomography (SPECT) fusion imaging aids in determining lymphatic involvement for breast malignancies (Figure 10-61).

Figure 10-58   Spiculated lesion. **A,** Mammography using magnification-spot compression demonstrates microcalcifications and a spiculated lesion. **B,** Breast sonography demonstrates fingerlike projections emanating from the lesion measuring 1.8 × 1.25 cm.

Figure 10-59   Ruptured silicone breast implants. **A,** Mammogram shows retroglandular implant with extracapsular silicone *(arrows)*. **B,** Ultrasound image of the same patient shows typical "snowstorm" appearance of free extracapsular silicone *(arrowheads)*. (From Hagen-Ansert S: *Textbook of diagnostic ultrasound,* St Louis, 2001, Mosby.)

Figure 10-60   Breast implants. MRI distinguishes between breast tissue and the implant. A fold in the implant is also visualized *(arrow).*

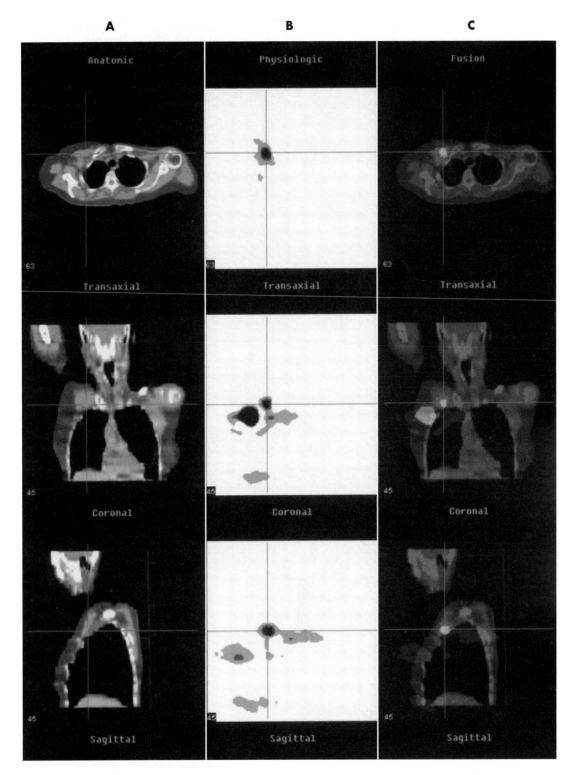

Figure 10-61   Right sentinel lymph node studied with single photon emission computed tomography (SPECT) and CT fusion imaging. **A,** A tri-planar anatomic CT image. **B,** A tri-planar SPECT physiologic image. **C,** A tri-planar fusion image. One sentinel node is located and marked for intraoperative removal.

Figure 10-62 Stereotaxic needle biopsy. **(A),** Stereotaxic scout images of breast lesion. **(B),** Stereotaxic images showing needle localization. **(C),** Postbiopsy images of lesion with needle pulled back to demonstrate lesion removal.

Although relatively infrequent (1 in 100), breast cancer also can develop in men. Breast cancer in men usually has a poor prognosis because it is often diagnosed in a later stage.

Treatment

Imaging also plays a role in surgical planning by providing guidance (by ultrasound or mammography) for needle localization (Figure 10-62). A conservative surgical approach is lumpectomy, which is used for isolated lesions. Mastectomy, a more aggressive surgical approach, includes the removal of all breast tissue and a dissection of the lymph nodes. If the lymph nodes are positive for cancerous cells, the axillary nodes are removed (radical mastectomy). Chemotherapy and radiation therapy are used in more advanced cases, depending on the type of cancer cells and whether the axillary nodes are involved. Hormonal chemotherapy with synthetic antiestrogens may be used if the tumor is positive for estrogen receptors.

- -

Summary of Findings for Breast Lesions

DISORDER	LOCATION	RADIOGRAPHIC APPEARANCE	TREATMENT
Breast carcinoma	Breast tissue	Mammography—poorly defined, irregular margins with numerous fine linear strands or spicules radiating from the mass US—differentiates benign cysts from a solid mass; ruptured silicone implants produce "snowstorm" appearance MRI (subtraction imaging)—benign masses tend to have smooth borders, whereas malignancies demonstrate high signal intensity with spiculation; fat suppression best demonstrates the functional parenchyma and helps differentiate lesions; best demonstrates the surrounding breast tissue in patients with implants	Lumpectomy Mastectomy Radical mastectomy Chemotherapy or hormonal therapy
Benign breast disease	Fibrocystic breast or single cysts	Mammography—smooth, well-circumscribed mass without invasion of surrounding tissue US—simple cyst appears as an anechoic center with a thin echogenic capsule	Pain management through diet Hormonal therapy Surgery for single cysts

- -

US, Ultrasound.

Benign breast disease

Fibrocystic disease of the breast is a common benign condition that occurs in about 20% of premenopausal women. It is usually bilateral, with cysts of various sizes distributed throughout the breasts that also contain an increased amount of fibrous tissue. The size of the cyst usually changes with the menstrual cycle, as does the amount or type of fluid in it.

Radiographic appearance

A fibroadenoma is the most common benign breast tumor. It generally appears as a smooth, well-circumscribed mass with no invasion of surrounding tissue (see Figure 10-55). Ultrasound permits differentiation of a solid fibroadenoma from a fluid-filled breast cyst. Sonographically, a simple cyst has an anechoic center with a thin echogenic capsule (see Figure 10-57). High-risk patients require monitoring of the cystic lesions for possible conversion to a cancerous process. Equivocal lesions may require imaging with other modalities.

Treatment

The most conservative treatment addresses pain management, usually by dietary modifications and re-ducing caffeine intake. If dietary changes do not reduce pain to a tolerable level, drainage of the cyst may be performed. Hormonal therapy with synthetic antiestrogens that block estrogen and progesterone is used in cases of cyclical pain. However, these drugs may produce intolerable side effects. Surgery is not the most effective treatment unless there is only a single cyst (and most patients have multiple cysts).

■ Imaging in Pregnancy

Because of its noninvasive and nonionizing character, ultrasound is the modality of choice in the evaluation of possible complications of pregnancy. A major role of ultrasound is to assess the gestational age, a measurement that is often highly inaccurate when based on the date of the last menstrual period. A knowledge of the true gestational age may be critically important for obstetric decisions, as the length of pregnancy is a major factor in interpreting the graphs that indicate the status of the fetus.

Measurements of fetal age by ultrasound include the longest biparietal diameter (BPD), the crown-to-rump length, and the length of the fetal femur. The

A

B

Figure 10-63 Biparietal diameter (BPD) in 27-week fetus. **A,** Cursor width indicates BPD, which is measured from outer margin of skull on one side to inner margin on other side. Arrows point to midline falx. **B,** Dotted line indicates head circumference.

Figure 10-64   Crown-to-rump length measurement. Cursors delineate the length of the fetus from the top of the head to the bottom of the torso. (From Rumack CM, Wilson SR, Charboneau JW: *Diagnostic ultrasound,* St Louis, 1998, Mosby.)

Figure 10-65   Fetal femur. Cursor measures a femur length of 3.96 cm and cartilage is not demonstrated indicating a fetal age earlier than 33 weeks.

BPD is measured from the outer margin of the skull on one side to the inner margin on the other side at the level of the thalami (Figure 10-63). A single measurement of the biparietal diameter has its greatest accuracy between 12 and 26 weeks; after this time, the size of the head and thus the BPD may be affected by a growth disturbance. The crown-to-rump length refers to the distance between the tip of the head and the bottom of the fetal trunk (Figure 10-64). This measurement is highly accurate for assessing gestational age in early pregnancy (less than 11 weeks). Fetal femoral length (Figure 10-65) aids in determining fetal age in the second and third trimester by identifying epiphyseal cartilage at the knee, which indicates a gestational age beyond 33 to 35 weeks.

An early diagnosis of multiple pregnancies can be made by ultrasound (Figure 10-66). This is essential so that therapeutic measures can be taken to reduce the high complication rate associated with twin (or more) fetuses.

Ultrasound can be used to detect an abnormal volume of amniotic fluid, which is often associated with underlying fetal anomalies. **Polyhydramnios** refers to an excessive accumulation of amniotic fluid that may be caused by maternal disorders such as diabetes mel-

Figure 10-67   Polyhydramnios. Excessive accumulation of amniotic fluid (hypoechoic area) surrounds the fetus in the mother of advanced maternal age.

Figure 10-66   Multiple pregnancies. **A,** Endovaginal sonogram shows two gestational sacs surrounded by the echogenic chorionic ring *(c)* composed of the decidua capsularis and the chorion laeve within the deciduas vera *(d)*. A yolk sac *(small arrow)* and live embryo *(arrowhead)* are present within each gestational sac. The crown-to-rump lengths measure 5.4 mm and 4.7 mm, corresponding to a gestational age of 6.5 weeks. **B,** Lateral abdominal radiograph of a woman with quadruplets clearly shows four separate fetal skulls and spines. (**A** from Rumack CM, Wilson SR, Charboneau JW: *Diagnostic ultrasound,* St Louis, 1998, Mosby.)

litus and Rh isoimmunization (Figure 10-67). Polyhydramnios is also caused by fetal abnormalities, especially those related to the central nervous system, the gastrointestinal tract, the circulatory system, and dwarfism. **Oligohydramnios** refers to a very small volume of amniotic fluid. This condition results primarily from fetal urinary tract disorders such as renal aplasia, renal dysplasia, and urethral obstruction. Oligohydramnios is also associated with intrauterine growth retardation.

Clinically significant errors of morphologic development occur in up to 5% of all children. The in utero

detection of these anomalies by ultrasound may permit in utero medical or surgical therapy, may provide an indication for termination of the pregnancy, or may influence the mode of delivery. Although a detailed description of the rapidly expanding field of prenatal sonography is beyond the scope of this book, some of the abnormalities that can be detected, and often treated, in utero are osseous (bony) and neural anomalies of the fetal cranium (Figures 10-68 and 10-69) and spine, gastrointestinal atresias and developmental cysts, cystic and obstructive lesions of the genitourinary tract, and congenital cardiac diseases and skeletal anomalies (Figure 10-70).

Because ultrasound examinations can demonstrate the fetus and placenta with no apparent risk to the mother or unborn child, ultrasonography is unquestionably the imaging study of choice for evaluating the gravid (pregnant) woman. In extremely rare instances, there may be justification for performing radiographic pelvimetry to demonstrate the architecture of the maternal pelvis and to compare the size of the fetal head with the size of the maternal bony pelvic outlet to determine whether the pelvic diameters are adequate for normal delivery or a cesarean section will be required. In almost all cases, however, the combination of careful clinical evaluation and ultrasonography is sufficient to make these decisions without the need to resort to radiographic pelvimetry with its high radiation dose. There is absolutely no indication ever to perform fetography, the radiographic demonstration of the fetus in utero. Ultrasound can provide far better diagnostic information and is not

Figure 10-68   Anencephaly. Long-axis image of third-trimester fetus shows that the head *(H)* is irregularly shaped, echogenic, and much smaller than the body *(arrowheads)*. *B,* Maternal bladder. (From Pasto ME, Kurtz AM: *Semin Ultrasound CT MR* 5:170-193, 1984.)

Figure 10-69   Ventriculomegaly. Cranial axial ultrasound image at 27 menstrual weeks shows obvious ventricular enlargement with convex surface of the lateral ventricle wall that parallels the bony calvaria. Note the dangling choroids *(c)*. (From Rumack CM, Wilson SR, Charboneau JW: *Diagnostic ultrasound*, St Louis, 1998, Mosby.)

Figure 10-70   Clubfoot. Prenatal ultrasound scan shows the feet with the foot at a right angle to the leg.

Figure 10-71   Ectopic pregnancy with live embryo in the adnexa. Endovaginal sonography shows tubal ring (*arrowheads*) and gestational sac, containing yolk sac and live embryo (*e*). Asterisk indicates free fluid. *U,* Uterus. (From Rumack CM, Wilson SR, Charboneau JW: *Diagnostic ultrasound,* St Louis, 1998, Mosby.)

Summary of Findings for Pregnancy

TYPE OF PREGNANCY	LOCATION	RADIOGRAPHIC APPEARANCE	TREATMENT
Uterine pregnancy	Fetus within the uterus	US—demonstrates the fetus and placenta	Normal birth
Ectopic Pregnancy	Fertilization outside the uterus	US—enlarged uterus without gestational sac and an appearance of an irregular adnexal mass	Surgical intervention

US, Ultrasound.

associated with the danger of producing radiation-induced fetal malformations.

Ectopic pregnancy

Although ectopic pregnancy is a life-threatening condition, responsible for up to one fourth of maternal deaths, the diagnosis is missed by the initial examining physician in up to three fourths of cases. More than 95% of ectopic pregnancies occur within the fallopian tubes, and more than half the patients with this complication of pregnancy have a history or pathologic evidence of pelvic inflammatory disease. Ectopic pregnancies are often associated with urine or plasma levels of human chorionic gonadotropin (HCG) that are substantially lower for the expected date of gestation than those in patients with normal intrauterine pregnancies.

Radiographic appearance

Ultrasound is the major imaging modality for diagnosing ectopic pregnancy. The classic appearance consists of an enlarged uterus that does not contain a gestational sac and is associated with an irregular adnexal mass, an "ectopic fetal head," or fluid in the cul-de-sac (Figure 10-71). The unequivocal demonstration of an intrauterine pregnancy virtually excludes an ectopic pregnancy, because the incidence of coexisting ectopic and intrauterine pregnancies is only one in 30,000.

Treatment

Emergency surgical intervention before a fatal hemorrhage occurs is required.

▪ Trophoblastic Disease

Trophoblastic disease refers to a spectrum of pregnancy-related disorders ranging from benign hydatidiform mole to the more malignant and frequently metastatic choriocarcinoma. A hydatidiform mole results from abnormal fertilization when there is an absence of the female chromosome. About half of choriocarcinomas follow pregnancies complicated by hydatidiform mole. The remainder occur after spontaneous abortion, ectopic pregnancy, or normal deliveries.

Figure 10-72 Hydatidiform mole. Longitudinal sonogram in a patient in her second trimester of pregnancy demonstrates large, moderately echogenic mass filling the central uterine cavity. Note the numerous small cystic spaces *(arrows)* that represent greatly hydropic chorionic villi. (From Callen PW, editor: *Ultrasonography in obstetrics and gynecology*, Philadelphia, 1983, Saunders.)

Figure 10-73 Uterine agenesis. Ultrasound on a 16-year-old girl who has never had a menstrual cycle. Midline sagittal view **(A)** demonstrates the bladder *(dark area)* with no uterus found posteriorly. Normal left **(B)** and right **(C)** ovaries are shown in the parasagittal plane.

Radiographic appearance

A hydatidiform mole typically appears on an ultrasound image as a large, soft-tissue mass of placental (trophoblastic) tissue filling the uterine cavity and containing echoes of low to moderate amplitude ("bunch of grapes") (Figure 10-72) without any signs of fetal movement. Endovaginal sonography confirms that there is no evidence of a developing fetus. On ultrasound images, choriocarcinoma resembles benign hydatidiform mole and usually appears as a large complex mass of central hemorrhage, with necrosis found in the expected position of the uterus. Choriocarcinoma tends to metastasize to the lungs, where it typically produces multiple large masses that rapidly regress once appropriate chemotherapy is instituted.

Treatment

Hydatidiform moles are treated by removal of all placental tissue by suction curettage of the uterus. If suction curettage does not lower the patient's HCG, the disease progresses and the patient requires chemotherapy. For choriocarcinoma, folic acid antagonists have a cure rate of approximately 80% if treatment begins before brain metastasis occurs.

■ Female Infertility

The causes of infertility in young women include anomalies in the reproductive organs, such as an abnormal uterus that cannot hold a fetus (Figure 10-73), obstructed fallopian tubes, ovaries that are unable to produce mature ova, and disruption of the path the ova normally follows en route to the uterus.

Radiographic appearance

The major radiographic procedure for evaluating infertile women is hysterosalpingography, in which the uterine cavity and fallopian tubes are opacified after the injection of contrast material into the uterus. In a woman with normal patent fallopian tubes, contrast material extravasating into the pelvic peritoneal cavity outlines the peritoneal surfaces and often loops of bowel within the pelvis (see Figure 10-29). Developmental anomalies or fibrosis from pelvic inflammatory disease may cause occlusion of one or both of the fallopian tubes; in such cases, there is no evidence of the contrast material reaching the peritoneal cavity (see Figure 10-30). In addition to assessing tubal patency, hysterosalpingography can also demonstrate uterine abnormalities that contribute to infertility, such as intrauterine fibroids, severe uterine flexion or retroversion, and other congenital and acquired malformations.

Summary of Findings for Trophoblastic Disease

DISORDER	LOCATION	RADIOGRAPHIC APPEARANCE	TREATMENT
Hydatidiform mole	Abnormal fertilization	US—large soft-tissue mass with "bunch of grapes" appearance	Suction curettage
Choriocarcinoma	Malignant transformation of hydatidiform mole	US—large complex mass	Chemotherapy of folic acid antagonist

US, Ultrasound.

Summary of Findings for Infertility

DISORDER	LOCATION	RADIOGRAPHIC APPEARANCE	TREATMENT
Female infertility	Lack of fertilization or implantation	Radiograph—hysterosalpingography to demonstrate the ovaries, fallopian tubes, and uterus US—screening for congenital anomalies, and to monitor treatment	Ovulation-induction agents

US, Ultrasound.

Treatment

For women who receive ovulation-induction agents as treatment for infertility, ultrasound can be used to monitor the maturation of ovarian follicles. Low-level internal echoes in mature ovarian follicles appear to be a prognostic indicator of fertility. They may represent a periovulatory state, which is an appropriate time for artificial insemination or in vitro fertilization. Ultrasound can also demonstrate the characteristic bilateral multicystic ovarian enlargement in the ovarian hyperstimulation syndrome, which may develop in women receiving menotropin (Pergonal) therapy for infertility.

QUESTIONS

1. Why has ultrasound become the major imaging modality for both the male and the female reproductive systems?

2. In addition to ultrasound, what are the main radiographic studies currently used for the female reproductive system?

3. The formation of sperm is known as _____.

4. What male hormone helps to regulate metabolism by promoting growth of skeletal muscles and is considered responsible for the greater degree of muscle development in men?

5. Severing of the vas deferens to create sterility is termed _____.

6. The second most common cause of malignancy in men is _____.

7. What imaging modality for demonstrating the prostate gland uses a probe inserted into the rectum?

8. Ultrasound studies of the prostate gland *cannot* always determine the malignant or benign status of prostatic disease. Is this TRUE or FALSE?

9. Prostatic carcinoma can often spread through the bloodstream to the bone and can sometimes cause sclerosis of an entire vertebra. This pathologic condition is termed _____.

10. What screening technique is usually employed to identify the location of an undescended testicle?

11. What is the term used to describe the twisting of the male gonad on its pedicle?

12. The most common neoplasms in men between 20 and 35 years of age are tumors that tend to metastasize through the _____ system.

13. The rupture and expulsion of the mature ovum into the pelvic cavity is termed _____.

14. A pregnancy that occurs in a fallopian tube or in the pelvic cavity is termed _____.

15. What is the name of the radiographic procedure used to demonstrate the patency or status of the fallopian tubes?

16. Untreated _____ can lead to cerebral cortical lesions causing mental disorders and involvement of the skeletal system and affects infants born to infected mothers.

17. The most common type of germ cell tumor, often containing teeth, hair, and fatty material, is called a(n) _____.

18. Leiomyomas, more commonly referred to as _____, are benign smooth-muscle tumors of the uterus.

19. The most common malignancy among women occurs in the _____.

20. The second most common form of cancer in women is _____.

BIBLIOGRAPHY

Callen PW: *Ultrasonography in obstetrics and gynecology,* Philadelphia, 1992, Saunders.

de Paredes ES: *Atlas of film-screen mammogram,* Baltimore, 1992, Williams & Wilkins.

Eisenberg RL, Margulis AR: *What to order when,* ed 2, Philadelphia, 2000, Lippincott Williams & Wilkins.

Rumack CM, Wilson SR, Charboneau JW: *Diagnostic ultrasound,* St Louis, 1998, Mosby.

Sanders RC, James AE: *Ultrasonography in obstetrics and gynecology,* Norwalk, Conn., 1992, Appleton-Century-Crofts.

Tabar L, Dean PB: *Teaching atlas of mammography,* ed 2, New York, 1985, Thieme.

CHAPTER 11

Miscellaneous Diseases

■ **Prerequisite Knowledge**

The student should have a basic understanding of the physiology of the various body systems. In addition, proper learning and understanding of the material will be facilitated if the student has some clinical experience in general radiography.

■ **Goals**

To acquaint the student with the pathophysiology and radiographic manifestations of both common and unusual disorders caused by vitamin deficiencies, hereditary abnormalities, and some disease processes that do not fit neatly into a single body system, and to understand the use, positioning, and complications of various tubes, catheters, and wires in the chest

■ **Objectives**

1. To be able to describe nutritional disorders and their possible relationship to disorders of other organs
2. To be able to define terminology relating to nutritional disorders
3. To be able to describe the pathologic conditions caused by various vitamin deficiencies
4. To be able to describe the pathologic conditions associated with sarcoidosis
5. To be able to describe the pathologic conditions associated with muscular dystrophy
6. To be able to describe the pathologic conditions associated with melanoma
7. To be able to describe the pathologic conditions associated with systemic lupus erythematosus
8. To be able to describe hereditary abnormalities including chromosomal aberrations and genetic amino acid disorders

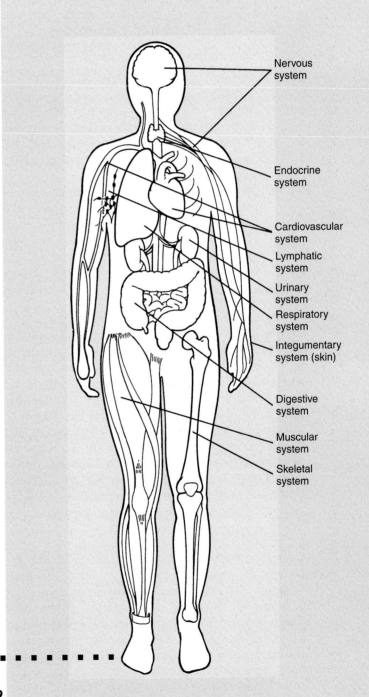

Nervous system

Endocrine system

Cardiovascular system

Lymphatic system

Urinary system

Respiratory system

Integumentary system (skin)

Digestive system

Muscular system

Skeletal system

■ Radiographer Notes

Radiography of patients with various nutritional diseases can be challenging because of the many effects these diseases have on all body systems. Some produce deformities; others can cause mental disorders. Obese patients can present unique problems in positioning and in selecting radiographic settings. The radiographer must be especially empathetic when dealing with these patients, who often are embarrassed because of their size and thus difficult to deal with. The manifestations of systemic lupus erythematosus cause considerable discomfort for patients. Patients with melanoma that has already metastasized or those who are facing extensive surgical intervention are usually very depressed and sometimes require special handling. Patients with muscular dystrophy can be easily agitated and are usually frustrated at their inability to control themselves. Hereditary diseases causing abnormalities require special understanding on the part of the technologist to attain optimal patient cooperation that will result in good diagnostic radiographs. In general, patients suffering from the various diseases in the miscellaneous category can be very demanding and require considerable patience on the part of the radiographer.

9. To be able to describe the correct location for an endotracheal tube, central venous catheter, Swan-Ganz catheter, and transvenous cardiac pacemaker
10. To be able to state the most common complications involved with improper placement of the aforementioned catheters and how chest radiography plays an important role in the diagnosis of these complications

■ Nutritional Diseases

Disorders of nutrition range from malnutrition and vitamin deficiency to obesity and hypervitaminosis. In addition to inadequate intake, nutritional deficiency may be related to disorders of the liver, pancreas, and gastrointestinal tract that result in an inability of the body to digest and properly use proteins, carbohydrates, and lipids. In diabetes mellitus the absence of insulin prevents entry of glucose into the cells and thus deprives the body of its major source of energy. Abnormalities of the pancreas, liver, and gastrointestinal tract causing nutritional diseases are discussed elsewhere; this section deals with diseases caused by vitamin deficiency, malnutrition, and obesity.

Vitamin deficiencies

Vitamins are an essential part of the enzymatic systems that are vital to the body's cellular metabolism. Vitamins are formed (synthesized) only by plants, not by animals. Therefore man's supply of vitamins comes directly from eating fruits and vegetables or from animals (including fish) that have eaten plants and have stored the vitamins. Vitamins are generally divided into two categories: fat soluble and water soluble. The fat-soluble vitamins (A, D, E, and K) can be

Figure 11-1   Beriberi. Diffuse pulmonary edema caused by severe high-output heart failure.

stored within body tissues. Water-soluble vitamins (B and C) cannot be stored and must be a regular part of the diet to prevent a deficiency. The major B vitamins include thiamine, riboflavin, niacin, pantothenic acid, cobalamin (vitamin B_{12}), and folic acid. Vitamin deficiency diseases are rare in the United States but are all too prevalent in underdeveloped countries.

BERIBERI (THIAMINE)

Beriberi results from a deficiency in thiamine (vitamin B_1), a coenzyme essential for carbohydrate metabolism that promotes growth and maintains muscle tone and heart function. Beriberi occurs primarily in rice-eating countries, such as China, where the main staple is polished rice that has had the vitamin-containing skin and germ removed. Noninflammatory degeneration of the myelin sheath caused by thiamine deficiency produces

Figure 11-2   Scurvy. Frontal projections of both knees demonstrate widening and increased density of the zone of provisional calcification, producing the characteristic white line of scurvy. Notice also the submetaphyseal zone of lucency and characteristic marginal spur formation (Pelken's spur). Epiphyseal ossification centers are surrounded by a dense, sharply demarcated ring of calcification (Wimberger's sign). (From Eisenberg R: *Atlas of signs in radiology,* Philadelphia, 1984, Lippincott.)

a peripheral neuropathy characterized by weakness of the limbs and a "pins and needles" sensation in the extremities.

Radiographic appearance

Initially, peripheral vasodilatation in beriberi causes increased cardiac output, which then produces a generalized enlargement of the cardiac silhouette and increased pulmonary vascular markings. With progression of disease, the myocardium becomes edematous and flabby and cannot function properly, leading to congestive heart failure and generalized edema (Figure 11-1).

PELLAGRA (NIACIN)

Pellagra, caused by a deficiency of niacin (vitamin B_3), is characterized by reddening and scaling of the skin on exposed parts of the body, vomiting and severe diarrhea, and nervous and mental disorders (ranging from chronic depression to violent, irrational behavior). The body requires niacin to complete the cellular process called respiration, in which nutrients and oxygen reach the cells through a series of chemical reactions.

SCURVY (VITAMIN C)

The deficiency of ascorbic acid (vitamin C) in patients with scurvy leads to an inability of the sup-

porting tissues to produce and maintain vascular endothelium and the cementing substances that hold epithelial cells together (collagen, osteoid, dentin). Scurvy was classically a disease of sailors and explorers deprived of fresh fruit and vegetables containing vitamin C.

Weakening of capillary walls in scurvy often results in bleeding into the skin, joints, and internal organs. The gums are especially affected and bleed easily. The open lesions provide an entry for bacteria, leading to necrosis of gum tissue and tooth loosening and loss. Impaired synthesis of collagen leads to poor and delayed wound healing.

Radiographic appearance

In children, disordered chondroblastic and osteoblastic activity cause radiographic bone changes that are most prevalent where growth is normally most rapid (especially about the knee and wrist). The bones are generally osteoporotic with blurring or disappearance of trabecular markings and severe cortical thinning. Widening and increased density of the zone of provisional calcification produce the characteristic "white line" of scurvy (Figure 11-2). A relatively lucent osteoporotic zone forms on the diaphyseal side of the white line. This osteoporotic zone is easily fractured, permitting the dense bone to become impacted on the shaft and to jut laterally beyond it, thus giving rise to characteristic marginal spur formation (Pelken's spur). The epiphyseal ossification centers are demineralized and surrounded by dense, sharply demarcated rings of calcification (Wimberger's sign of scurvy). If epiphyseal dislocations have not occurred, the appearance of the skeletal structures usually returns to normal after appropriate therapy.

Subperiosteal hemorrhage often occurs along the shafts of the long bones. Calcification of the elevated periosteum and underlying hematoma is a radiographic sign of healing.

RICKETS (VITAMIN D)

Rickets is a bone disease of young children in which a lack of vitamin D leads to decreased absorption of calcium from the gastrointestinal tract, resulting in weak, deformed bones. In adults, lack of vitamin D causes generalized softening of bones (osteomalacia). The radiographic findings of rickets and osteomalacia are found in Chapter 3.

VITAMIN A DEFICIENCY

Vitamin A, or retinol, is essential for vision because it is a vital component of the pigment that absorbs light in the rods of the retina. A lack of vitamin A results in night blindness, an inability to see in dim light. Vitamin A also is important for maintaining the integrity of the mucous membranes lining the respiratory, gastrointestinal, and urogenital tracts. A lack of vitamin A makes these membranes dry and susceptible to cracking, permitting infectious organisms to enter the underlying tissues.

Vitamin A is derived from β-carotene, a yellow plant pigment that is converted into vitamin A by the liver. Good sources of vitamin A include dairy products, egg yolks, fish, and vegetables such as carrots, spinach, and sweet potatoes.

VITAMIN K DEFICIENCY

Vitamin K, a fat-soluble vitamin, is necessary for the formation of prothrombin, an essential ingredient in the blood-clotting mechanism. It is primarily found in green leafy vegetables. A deficiency of vitamin K results in excessive bleeding.

Treatment of vitamin deficiencies

Three different approaches can be used to treat vitamin deficiencies: (1) the patient's diet is modified to include foods that contain the recommended daily requirements, (2) the patient is given synthetic oral supplements, or (3) vitamins are injected. Some deficiencies may be associated with absorption abnormalities resulting from a lack of the specific vitamins needed to absorb and process vitamins.

Dietary modifications for vitamin B deficiencies include increasing the intake of protein (meat), green leafy vegetables, and milk. For vitamin C deficiencies, an increase in consumption of fresh fruits and green leafy vegetables may help. Vitamin D deficiencies require adding cod liver oil, egg yolks, butter, and oily fish to the diet. To increase vitamin A, a diet including more liver, meat, eggs, milk, and dark green and yellow vegetables is of value. Eating more spinach, lettuce, broccoli, brussels sprouts, and cabbage increases dietary vitamin K.

Hypervitaminosis

Chronic excessive intake of vitamin A produces a syndrome characterized by bone and joint pain, hair loss, itching, anorexia, dryness and fissuring of the lips, hepatosplenomegaly, and yellow tinting of the skin. This condition usually affects young children, who become irritable and fail to gain weight.

Radiographic appearance

Excess vitamin D causes too much calcium to be absorbed from the gastrointestinal tract. The resulting hypercalcemia leads to the deposition of calcium in the kidney, heart, lungs, and wall of the stomach (Figure 11-3).

Treatment

Because there is an excess of vitamins, treatment requires a decrease in vitamin intake and monitoring of the patient to ensure that the levels are stable.

Protein-calorie malnutrition (kwashiorkor)

Severe protein-calorie malnutrition (kwashiorkor) affects millions of young children in developing coun-

Figure 11-3 Hypervitaminosis D. Huge masses of calcification near the shoulder joints bilaterally.

tries and produces abnormalities involving the gastrointestinal tract and nervous system. Fatty replacement of liver tissue and the resulting decreased levels of albumin lead to diffuse edema and ascites and the characteristic clinical appearance of a considerably protuberant abdomen. Damage to the pancreas and intestinal mucosa prevents proper digestion and absorption of nutrients.

Radiographic appearance

Retarded bone growth with thinned cortices usually occurs. Atrophy of the thymus gland and lymphoid tissues diminishes the child's resistance to infection from organisms that enter the body through skin lesions and the damaged mucous membranes of the gastrointestinal tract. Mental development is also impaired, and brain atrophy can be demonstrated radiographically.

Treatment

The initial approach is to correct the child's fluid and electrolyte balance. Milk and supplementary vitamins are added to the diet. The mortality rate of 15% to 40% results from the dangerous fluid imbalance.

Obesity

Obesity refers to an excess of adipose (fatty) tissue that develops when the caloric intake (from food) consistently exceeds the amount of calories required by the body to perform its daily activities. It may be related simply to personal habits of excessive eating combined with a lack of activity, or it may be a result of such conditions as hypothyroidism, Cushing's disease, insulinoma, and hypothalamic disorders.

Radiographic appearance

Excess adipose tissue can cause displacement of normal abdominal structures, producing such radiographic patterns as widening of the retrogastric (Figure 11-4) and retrorectal spaces. An extreme increase in the intraabdominal volume causes diffuse elevation of the diaphragm with a relatively transverse position of the heart (simulating cardiomegaly), prominence of pulmonary markings, and atelectatic changes at the lung bases. In the most severe form of obesity (pickwickian syndrome), the excursion of the diaphragm is limited and the lungs can barely expand with breathing. This results in profound hypoventilation, hypoxia, retention of carbon dioxide, secondary polycythemia, and pulmonary hypertension with right heart failure. An excessive deposition of fatty tissue can also appear radiographically as widening of the mediastinum and prominence of the pericardial fat pads.

Treatment

The simplest treatments include weight management by dieting, using nutritional counseling and behavioral therapy, and dietary drugs. Patients with morbid obesity may undergo surgical procedures in an attempt to lose large amounts of weight. Gastric restrictive operations attempt to limit gastric capacity and restrict gastric outflow, thus making the patient feel full after a small meal. This causes the patient to limit his or her oral intake and results in weight control. The major procedure is a gastroplasty, in which a small upper gastric remnant is connected to a larger lower gastric pouch by a narrow channel. Complications of gastric restrictive procedures can occur in the early and late postoperative periods and include leakage, perforation, widening of the channel, and obstruction.

Figure 11-4 Obesity. Enlargement of the retrogastric space caused by a massive deposition of fatty tissue.

Summary of Findings for Nutritional Diseases

DISORDER	CAUSE	RADIOGRAPHIC APPEARANCE	TREATMENT
Beriberi	Deficiency in vitamin B_1 Decrease in carbohydrate metabolism	Enlarged cardiac silhouette with increased pulmonary markings	Increase intake by diet modification Increase intake with synthetic supplements Receive injections of the specific vitamin Increase absorption of vitamin by association with other dietary products
Pellagra	Deficiency in vitamin B_3	Not specific	
Scurvy	Deficiency in vitamin C	Osteoporosis with blurring of trabecular markings and severe cortical thinning Widening and increased density of the zone of provisional calcification, producing a white line	
Rickets	Deficiency of vitamin D Leads to decrease in absorption of calcium	See Osteomalacia in Chapter 3	
Vitamin A	Deficiency of vitamin A Visual deficiencies and decreased integrity of mucous membranes	Not specific	
Vitamin K	Deficiency of vitamin K Decreased prothrombin production	Not specific	
Hypervita-minosis	Usually excessive vitamin A or D	Vitamin A—not specific Vitamin D—hypercalcemia leads to deposition of calcium in the kidney, heart, lungs, and wall of the stomach	Decrease vitamin intake
Protein-calorie malnutrition	Severe protein-calorie deficiency	Retarded bone growth Thinned cortices Brain atrophy	Balance fluids and electrolytes Provide milk and supplemental vitamins
Obesity	Excessive adipose tissue—due to caloric intake consistently exceeding calories required	Displacement of anatomic structures Elevated diaphragm Widened mediastinum	Weight management by dieting Nutritional counseling and behavioral therapy Dietary drugs Surgical resection to limit gastric capacity

Figure 11-5   Lead lines. Dense transverse bands of sclerosis *(arrowheads)* extend across the metaphyses of the distal femurs and the proximal tibias and fibulas. (From Eisenberg RL: *Diagnostic imaging in internal medicine,* New York, 1985, McGraw-Hill.)

■ Lead Poisoning

Lead poisoning results from the ingestion of lead-containing materials (especially paint) or from the occupational inhalation of lead fumes. The chronic form of lead poisoning may cause mental retardation, seizures, behavioral disorders, or delayed development.

Radiographic appearance

In children, because lead and calcium are used interchangeably by bone, high concentrations of lead are deposited in the most rapidly growing portions of the skeleton, especially the metaphyses at the distal ends of the femur. This results in classic lead lines, dense transverse bands extending across the metaphyses of the long bones and along the margins of flat bones such as the iliac crest (Figure 11-5). In young children who eat lead-containing paint (pica), plain abdominal radiographs may show extensive mottled opacities, which are suggestive of intestinal barium, even though no contrast material has been administered (Figure 11-6).

Treatment

First the source must be eliminated. Then, chelation therapy to aid in the urinary excretion of lead is prescribed for those who do not have kidney or liver disease.

Figure 11-6   Pica. Large amounts of lead-containing material ingested by a young child who had received no contrast material. (From Eisenberg RL: *Gastrointestinal radiology: a pattern approach,* Philadelphia, 1990, Lippincott.)

■ Sarcoidosis

Sarcoidosis is a multisystem granulomatous disease of unknown cause that is most often detected in young adults. Women are affected slightly more often than men, and the disease is far more prevalent

Figure 11-7   Sarcoidosis. Frontal **(A)** and lateral **(B)** projections of the chest demonstrate enlargement of the right hilar, left hilar, and right paratracheal lymph nodes, producing the classic 1-2-3 pattern of adenopathy. (From Eisenberg R: *Atlas of signs in radiology,* Philadelphia, 1984, Lippincott.)

among African Americans than among whites. Histopathologic findings include multiple epithelioid granulomas.

Radiographic appearance

Ninety percent of patients with sarcoidosis have radiographic evidence of thoracic involvement. Indeed, in most cases the presence of the disease is first identified on a screening chest radiograph of an asymptomatic individual.

Bilateral, symmetric, hilar lymph node enlargement, with or without diffuse parenchymal disease, is the classic radiographic abnormality in sarcoidosis. Usually, enlargement of the right paratracheal nodes occurs, producing the typical 1-2-3 pattern (Figure 11-7). Conventional tomography frequently reveals additional enlargement of the left paratracheal nodes, which usually cannot be seen on routine frontal radiographs because they are obscured by the superimposed aorta and brachiocephalic vessels. Unilateral hilar enlargement, which is a common manifestation of primary tuberculosis or lymphoma, is rare in sarcoidosis.

Diffuse pulmonary disease develops in most patients with sarcoidosis. Although hilar and mediastinal adenopathy is often involved, there tends to be an inverse relationship between the degree of adenopathy and the extent of parenchymal disease, with the latter increasing while the adenopathy regresses. The most common appearance is a diffuse interstitial pattern that is widely distributed throughout both lungs

Figure 11-8   Sarcoidosis. Diffuse coarse interstitial pattern.

(Figure 11-8). The alveolar pattern appears as ill-defined densities that may be discrete or may coalesce into large areas of consolidation. This pattern resembles an acute inflammatory process and may contain an air bronchogram. Infrequently, large, dense, round lesions may simulate metastatic malignancy.

The skeletal lesions in sarcoidosis involve primarily the small bones of the hands and feet. Granulomatous infiltration can cause destruction of the fine trabeculae, producing a mottled to lacelike, coarsely trabeculated pattern. Lytic destruction can produce sharply cir-

Figure 11-9 Sarcoidosis. Multiple osteolytic lesions throughout the phalanges produce the typical punched-out appearance. The apparent air density in the soft tissues is a photographic artifact.

Figure 11-10 Sarcoidosis. In end-stage disease, there is severe fibrous scarring, bleb formation, and emphysema.

cumscribed, punched-out areas of lucency (Figure 11-9). About 10% of patients with sarcoidosis have elevated levels of serum calcium, which may lead to nephrocalcinosis. Sarcoid involvement of the stomach can produce discrete masses or generalized luminal narrowing that predominantly involves the antrum.

Treatment

Although the pulmonary lesions usually regress spontaneously or after steroid therapy, irreversible pulmonary changes develop in up to 20% of the cases. Coarse scarring is seen as irregular linear strands extending outward from the hilum toward the periphery, often associated with bulla formation (Figure 11-10). Severe fibrosis and emphysema can cause pulmonary hypertension and right-sided heart failure.

■ Systemic Lupus Erythematosus

Systemic lupus erythematosus is a connective tissue disorder that involves primarily young or middle-aged women and most likely represents an immune-complex disease. The presentation and course of the disease are highly variable. Characteristic findings include a butterfly-shaped rash over the nose and cheeks and extreme sensitivity of the skin to sunlight.

Radiographic appearance

Pain in multiple muscles and joints is the most frequent clinical complaint in patients with systemic lupus erythematosus. A characteristic finding is subluxations and malalignment of joints in the absence of erosions (Figure 11-11). Cardiopulmonary abnormalities also frequently develop. Pleural effusions, usually bilateral and small but occasionally massive, occur in about half of the patients (Figure 11-12). Enlargement of the cardiac silhouette is generally the result of pericarditis and pericardial effusion.

Although kidney involvement, often leading to renal failure, is one of the most serious manifestations of systemic lupus erythematosus, no specific urographic findings are seen. Enlargement of the liver, spleen, and lymph nodes occurs in about one fourth of patients. In the gastrointestinal system, a necrotizing inflammation of blood vessels can result in massive bleeding, multiple infarctions, and bowel perforation.

Many of the radiographic manifestations of systemic lupus erythematosus tend to disappear during spontaneous remissions or after steroid therapy.

Treatment

Antiinflammatory drugs are used to treat pain in the muscles and joints. Systemic corticosteroids help

Figure 11-11   Systemic lupus erythematosus. Frontal and oblique projections of the hand show subluxation of the phalanges at the metacarpal articulations and hyperextension deformities of the proximal interphalangeal joints. Note the absence of erosive changes. (From Brown JC, Forrester DM: In Eisenberg RL, Amberg JR, editors: *Critical diagnostic pathways in radiology: an algorithmic approach,* Philadelphia, 1981, Lippincott.)

Figure 11-12   Systemic lupus erythematosus. Bilateral pleural effusions, more pronounced on the right, with some streaks of basilar atelectasis. Massive cardiomegaly is attributable to a combination of pericarditis and pericardial effusion.

prevent renal and central nervous system pathology. If skin lesions occur, antimalarial drugs are prescribed.

■ Melanoma

Melanoma is an extremely malignant skin cancer that metastasizes widely throughout the body. The tumor develops from a benign mole (nevus), which changes size and color and becomes itchy and sore.

Radiographic appearance

Metastases from malignant melanoma frequently involve the gastrointestinal tract, usually sparing the large bowel. They are typically well-circumscribed, round or oval nodules that may develop central necrosis and ulceration; in a barium study, this results in a dense, barium-filled central crater surrounded by a sharply marginated nodular mass (bull's-eye, or target, lesion) (Figure 11-13). Gastrointestinal metastases can be the first clinical manifestation of metastatic melanoma; at times it can be impossible to identify the primary tumor site.

Figure 11-13 Metastatic melanoma. Large central ulcerations in two sharply defined filling defects in the small bowel *(arrows)*.

Metastatic melanoma can also produce multiple nodules in the lung and destructive bone lesions with neither new bone formation nor reactive sclerosis.

Treatment

Carefully watching for changes in moles or the skin and having a biopsy to assess the lesion is the best prevention and is highly recommended. Also, continuous protection from the sun may reduce the development of these lesions. Surgical excision of the tumor and surrounding tissue may be all that is required. A lymph node biopsy determines whether chemotherapy is required for metastases. The prognosis depends on the size of the lesion and the results of the lymph node biopsy

■ Muscular Dystrophy

Muscular dystrophy refers to a group of chronic inherited conditions in which fat replaces muscle; this leads to generalized weakness and eventually death caused by respiratory muscle failure or pneumonia.

Radiographic appearance

On radiographs of the extremities, the extensive accumulation of fat within the remaining muscle bundles produces a fine striated, or striped, appearance (Figure 11-14). Because most of the muscle tissue is replaced by fat, the fascial sheath bounding the muscles may stand out as a thin shadow or as increased density as it is visualized on edge.

Figure 11-14 Muscular dystrophy. Thin, demineralized bones of the lower leg. Increased lucency, representing fatty infiltration in muscle bundles, makes fascial sheaths appear as thin shadows of increased density *(arrows)* surrounded by fat.

■ ■

Summary of Findings for Miscellaneous Disorders

DISORDER	CAUSE	RADIOGRAPHIC APPEARANCE	TREATMENT
Lead poisoning	Ingestion of lead-containing materials	Classic lead lines (dense transverse bands extending across the metaphyses of long bones)	Eliminate source Chelation therapy to aid in elimination
Sarcoidosis	Nonspecific or unknown cause of multisystem granulomatous disease	Chest film—bilateral hilar lymph node enlargement with or without diffuse parenchymal disease	No treatment if spontaneous recovery Steroid therapy
Systemic lupus erythematosus	Immune-complex disease (a connective tissue disorder)	Subluxations and malalignment of joints Pleural effusions, small and bilateral	Antiinflammatory drugs for muscle and joint pain Systemic corticosteroids help prevent renal and central nervous system pathology Antimalarial drugs for skin lesion
Melanoma	Widely metastasizing malignant skin cancer	Metastatic involvement of the GI tract; round or oval nodules with necrosis and ulceration	Prevention—watch for changes in skin and reduce sun exposure Surgical excision of lesion and surrounding tissue, biopsy needed to determine if chemotherapy is necessary
Muscular dystrophy	Replacement of muscle by fat	Fine striated (striped) appearance of remaining muscle bundles	Nonstrenuous exercise to maintain mobility and function

■ ■

Decreased muscular tone can lead to osteoporosis, bone atrophy with cortical thinning, scoliosis, and joint contractures.

An abnormal swallowing mechanism in muscular dystrophy can result in the failure to clear barium adequately from the pharynx; this may lead to tracheal aspiration and nasal regurgitation of contrast material (or other ingested substances).

Treatment

No curative therapy is known. A regimen of nonstrenuous exercise is recommended to maintain mobility and function for as long as possible.

■ Hereditary Diseases

Chromosomal aberrations

The chromosomes may mutate in many different ways and cause a multitude of disease processes. The following discussion of chromosomal aberrations include three trisomy disorders (Down syndrome, Turner's syndrome, and Klinefelter's syndrome) and an autosomal dominant disorder (Marfan's syndrome). A **syndrome** indicates the presence of a combination of symptoms that commonly occur together and are related to a single cause.

DOWN SYNDROME (MONGOLISM)

Down syndrome, the most common of the trisomy disorders (trisomy 21), is caused by an extraautosomal chromosome that results in an individual having three strands of chromosome number 21 instead of the normal two. Down syndrome is usually diagnosed at birth because of the characteristic clinical appearance—mental deficiency, short stature, poor muscle tone, short neck, and a straight skin crease that extends across the palm of the hand. The typical facial appearance includes widely set eyes, a short and flat nose, and a coarse tongue that often protrudes through a partially open mouth.

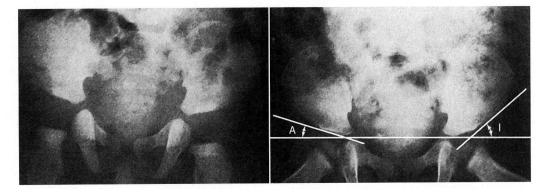

Figure 11-15   Down syndrome. Two examples of a typical pelvis in Down syndrome show flared iliac wings and diminished acetabular *(A)* and iliac *(I)* angles. (From James AE Jr et al: Radiological features of the most common autosomal disorders: trisomy 21-22 (mongolism or Down's syndrome), trisomy 18, trisomy 13-15, and the cri du chat syndrome, *Clin Radiol* 22:417-433, 1971.)

Congenital heart disease, especially septal defects, occurs in about 40% of patients with Down syndrome. There is also a greater-than-normal incidence of duodenal obstruction (duodenal atresia or annular pancreas) and Hirschsprung's disease, as well as a substantially increased likelihood of developing leukemia.

Radiographic appearance

The major skeletal abnormality in infancy is in the pelvis, where there is a decrease in the acetabular and iliac angles with hypoplasia and noticeable lateral flaring of the iliac wings (Figure 11-15). Other common skeletal abnormalities include shortening of the middle phalanx of the fifth finger, squaring of the vertebral bodies (superoinferior length becoming equal to or greater than the anteroposterior measurement), hypoplasia of the nasal sinuses, and delayed closure of the cranial sutures.

Treatment

The many different anomalies require various treatments, which generally provide a better quality of life for the afflicted person. Experimental dietary supplements (dimethyl sulfoxide [DMSO]–amino acid formula) are believed by some to slow the retardation process, but the Food and Drug Administration has not approved these drugs.

TURNER'S SYNDROME

Turner's syndrome (gonadal dysgenesis), a sex chromosome trisomy disorder, is characterized by primary amenorrhea (no ovulation or menstruation), sexual infantilism, short stature, and bilateral tiny gonads. Although the patient appears to be female, she has only one X chromosome as a result of faulty cellular division.

Various urinary tract anomalies, especially horseshoe kidney and other types of malrotation, are often seen in patients with gonadal dysgenesis. Coarctation of the aorta is the most common cardiovascular anom-

Figure 11-16   Turner's syndrome. Frontal projection of hand shows the short fourth metacarpal.

aly. Because coarctation of the aorta most often affects men, its appearance in a woman should indicate the possibility of underlying gonadal dysgenesis.

Radiographic appearance

A characteristic, but nonspecific, skeletal abnormality is shortening of the fourth metacarpal and sometimes also the fifth metacarpal (Figure 11-16). This produces a positive metacarpal sign, in which a line drawn tangentially to the distal ends of the heads of the fifth and fourth metacarpals passes through the head of the third metacarpal (indicating the disproportionate shortening of the fourth and fifth metacarpals), rather than extending distally to the head of the third metacarpal as in an unaffected person. Skeletal surveys performed serially at specified intervals during adolescence demonstrate changes in bone growth.

Treatment

Patients with Turner's syndrome can receive treatment for their short stature and for gonadal dysfunction. Human growth hormones have been available since 1994. Hormone replacement therapy of progesterone and/or estrogen may be prescribed to treat gonadal dysfunction (lack of ovulation) and to control female physical attributes (hair distribution and breast growth).

KLINEFELTER'S SYNDROME

Klinefelter's syndrome (testicular dysgenesis) is a disorder characterized by small testes that fail to mature or produce sperm and testosterone. The fundamental defect is the presence in a male of two or more X chromosomes, indicating that this disorder is another sex chromosome trisomy. The pituitary sends a signal for the body to produce testosterone, but the testes do not respond. At puberty, the breasts enlarge, and a female distribution of hair develops. The affected individual is tall, mentally deficient (often with language impairment), and sterile.

Radiographic appearance

Radiographically, the skeletal changes are both less common and less pronounced than in patients with Turner's syndrome, its female counterpart. A positive metacarpal sign presents in fewer than 25% of the patients. Hypogonadism may lead to delayed epiphyseal fusion and retarded bone maturation.

Treatment

Hormonal therapy provides treatment of the symptoms of Klinefelter's syndrome. When young men enter puberty, testosterone therapy assists the body in developing normal male attributes (male distribution of hair growth and muscular body type).

MARFAN'S SYNDROME

Marfan's syndrome is an inherited generalized disorder of connective tissue with ocular, skeletal, and cardiovascular manifestations. Most patients with this autosomal dominant disorder are tall and slender, appearing emaciated because of the decrease in subcutaneous fat. A typical feature of Marfan's syndrome is bilateral dislocation of the lens of the eye caused by weakness of its supporting tissues. A laxity of ligaments about the

Figure 11-17   Marfan's syndrome. Arteriogram shows the enormous dilatation of the aneurysmal ascending aorta. (From Ovenfors CO, Godwin JD: In Eisenberg RL, Amberg JR, editors: *Critical diagnostic pathways in radiology: an algorithmic approach*, Philadelphia, 1981, Lippincott.)

joints leads to loose-jointedness (or double-jointedness), recurrent dislocations, and flat feet.

Almost all patients with Marfan's syndrome have abnormalities of the cardiovascular system. Necrosis of the medial portion of the aortic wall causes a progressive dilatation of the ascending aorta that produces a bulging of the upper right portion of the cardiac silhouette (Figure 11-17) and an unusual prominence of the pulmonary outflow tract as it is displaced by the dilated aorta. Dissecting aneurysm, a serious complication, may kill the patient in early life.

Radiographic appearance

The major radiographic abnormality is elongation and thinning of the tubular bones (Figure 11-18), most pronounced in the hands and feet and seen clinically as **arachnodactyly** (spiderlike digits). Patients may exhibit pectus excavatum (concave sternum) on a lateral chest radiograph (Figure 11-19).

Treatment

Currently, no cure exists for Marfan's syndrome. The laxity of the joints makes these patients susceptible to scoliosis; monitoring the spine and treating any curvature early helps prevent spinal deformities. These patients are vulnerable to endocarditis resulting from dental procedures and commonly receive prophylactic antibiotics.

Figure 11-18   Arachnodactyly in Marfan's syndrome. Meta-carpals and phalanges are unusually long and slender.

Figure 11-19   Pectus excavatum. Lateral chest radiograph demonstrates a concave sternum.

Summary of Findings for Hereditary Diseases

DISORDER	CAUSES	RADIOGRAPHIC APPEARANCE	TREATMENT
Down syndrome	Extra autosomal chromosome—trisomy 21	Pelvis—decreased acetabular and iliac angles with hypoplasia and lateral flaring of iliac wings	Various treatments to provide a better quality of life
Turner's syndrome	Sex chromosome trisomy disorder—female with one X chromosome	Shortening of the 4th and 5th metacarpals	Growth hormones for stature Hormonal therapy for gonadal dysfunction
Klinefelter's syndrome	Sex chromosome trisomy disorder—male with two or more X chromosomes	Possible delayed epiphyseal fusion and retarded bone maturation	Hormonal therapy
Marfan's syndrome	Autosomal dominant disorder of connective tissue	Elongation and thinning of tubular bones (hands and feet), arachnodactyly	No cure

Genetic amino acid disorders

The genetic amino acid disorders result from the absence of an enzyme required to produce a biochemical reaction that the body requires for normal growth and physiologic function. This genetic defect causes a decrease or an interruption in amino acid metabolism.

HOMOCYSTINURIA

Homocystinuria, an inborn error of the metabolism of the amino acid methionine, causes a defect in the structure of collagen or elastin. The absence of the enzyme cysthionine synthase causes an elevation the level of methionine by not allowing the metabolic cycle to complete its process. Homocystinuria occurs only if both parents carry the gene (i.e., it is an autosomal recessive trait). Patients with homocystinuria have a tendency to develop arterial and venous thrombosis, and premature occlusive vascular disease is the major cause of death. Other common signs are similar to those of Marfan's syndrome (long limbs, arachnodactyly, and scoliosis). Additional symptoms include myopia (nearsightedness), dislocation of the lens of the eye, and mental retardation.

Radiographic appearance

The most frequent and striking radiographic feature of homocystinuria is osteoporosis of the spine, which is often associated with biconcave deformities of the vertebral bodies (Figure 11-20).

Treatment

As no cure has been found, treatment available today consists of a low methionine diet and increased doses of vitamin B$_6$ and folic acid. Not all patients have found this treatment effective.

PHENYLKETONURIA

Phenylketonuria (PKU) is an inborn error of metabolism in which an enzyme deficiency results in the impaired conversion of phenylalanine to tyrosine. Fortunately, routine screening enables diagnosis of this disease at birth. If the condition is not diagnosed and treated early, the excessive phenylalanine in the blood usually causes the patient to suffer profound retardation (microcephaly), hyperactivity, and seizures, all related to brain atrophy. Because of an inadequate amount of tyrosine, there is impaired production of the pigment melanin, and the patient is very light in color.

Radiographic appearance

The brain atrophy appears as dilatation of the ventricles and sulci on computed tomography (CT) scans or magnetic resonance (MR) images.

Figure 11-20   Homocystinuria. Striking osteoporosis of the spine is associated with biconcave deformities of the vertebral bodies. (From Thomas PS, Carson NA: Homocystinuria. The evolution of skeletal changes in relation to treatment, *Ann Radiol* 21:95-104, 1978.)

Treatment

Treatment includes a diet low in phenylalanine and protein. Dietary measures can control the disease process from progressing if the treatment begins before age 1. Treatment instituted later in life will not improve any destructive damage that has already occurred.

ALKAPTONURIA AND OCHRONOSIS

Alkaptonuria is a rare inborn error of metabolism in which an enzyme deficiency leads to an abnormal accumulation of homogentisic acid in the blood and urine. The urine is either very dark on voiding or becomes black after standing or being alkalinized. The disorder often goes unrecognized until middle age, when deposition of the black pigment of oxidized homogentisic acid in cartilage and other connective tissue produces a distinctive form of degenerative arthritis (ochronosis).

Radiographic appearance

The pathognomonic radiographic finding is dense, laminated calcification in multiple intervertebral disks (Figure 11-21); the calcification begins in the lumbar spine and may extend to involve the dorsal and cervical regions.

Figure 11-21 Ochronosis. Frontal projection of the lumbar spine shows the dense laminated calcification of multiple intervertebral disks *(arrows).*

Figure 11-22 Glycogen storage disease. Generalized globular cardiac enlargement with left ventricular prominence.

Treatment

Medical therapy can inhibit the rate of pigment deposit. A low protein diet and added vitamin C may retard the accumulation of homogentisic acid in older children and adults.

CYSTINURIA

Cystinuria is an inborn error of amino acid transport characterized by impaired tubular absorption and excessive urinary excretion of several amino acids. Large amounts of cystine in the urine predispose to the formation of renal, ureteral, and bladder stones.

Radiographic appearance

Pure cystine stones are not radiopaque and can be demonstrated only on excretory urography, where they appear as filling defects in the urinary tract. Stones containing the calcium salts of cystine appear radiopaque and can be detected on plain abdominal radiographs. Abdominal CT may define the filling defect better than intravenous urography.

Treatment

As no cure is currently available for cystinuria, therapy is designed to provide relief from symptoms and to prevent new stones from developing. One approach is to increase water intake to six to eight glasses a day, to dilute the increased excretion of cystine in the urine.

GLYCOGEN STORAGE DISEASES

The glycogen storage diseases are a group of genetic disorders that involve the pathways for the storage of carbohydrates as glycogen (in the liver) and for its use in maintaining blood glucose and providing energy. Normal or abnormal glycogen in an excess amount infiltrates and enlarges multiple organs, especially the heart and liver (Figure 11-22).

GAUCHER'S DISEASE

Gaucher's disease is an inborn error of metabolism characterized by the accumulation of abnormal quantities of complex lipids in the reticuloendothelial cells of the spleen, liver, and bone marrow. The adult (chronic) form of Gaucher's disease is most common; some cases arise in children or infants.

Aseptic necrosis (especially involving the femoral heads) is a common complication. The spleen is usually greatly enlarged, and hepatomegaly is common.

Radiographic appearance

The most striking changes occur in the skeletal system. Infiltration of the bone marrow with abnormal lipid-containing cells causes a loss of bone density with expansion and cortical thickening of the long bones, especially the femur. Marrow infiltration of the distal femur causes abnormal modeling, flaring, and the characteristic (but nonspecific) Erlenmeyer flask deformity (Figure 11-23).

Figure 11-23   Gaucher's disease. The distal ends of the femurs show typical underconstriction and cortical thinning. (From Levin B: *AJR Am J Roentgenol* 85:685-696, 1961.)

Summary of Findings for Genetic Amino Acid Disorders

DISORDER	CAUSE	RADIOGRAPHIC APPEARANCE	TREATMENT
Homocystinuria	Absence of cystathionine synthase	Osteoporosis of the spine—biconcave deformities of vertebral bodies	Low methionine diet; increase vitamin B_6 and folic acid
Phenylketonuria	Enzyme deficiency leading to excessive phenylalanine	CT or MRI—brain atrophy with dilatation of ventricles and sulci	Low phenylalanine and protein diet to control progression
Alkaptonuria/ochronosis	Enzyme deficiency leading to excessive homogentisic acid	Dense laminated calcification of multiple intervertebral disks	Therapy to inhibit rate of deposit
Cystinuria	Error of amino acid transport	CT—defines cystine stones in the urinary tract	No cure—increase water intake to help prevent stone formation
Gaucher's disease	Abnormal accumulation of complex lipids	Loss of bone density, with expansion and cortical thickening of long bones	Treatment to inhibit the accumulation of complex lipids

Treatment

In the past, the traditional treatment for Gaucher's was splenectomy. Today new experimental treatments are used in an attempt to inhibit the accumulation of complex lipids.

■ Internal Devices

Endotracheal tube

A chest radiograph should always be obtained immediately after endotracheal intubation to ensure proper positioning because clinical evaluation (bilateral breath sounds, symmetric thoracic expansion, palpation of the tube in the sternal notch) does not allow detection of the majority of malpositioned tubes. Daily radiographs are usually taken to make certain that the tube has not been inadvertently displaced by the weight of the respirator apparatus, by the patient's coughing, or by other unforeseen events. In addition, this permits prompt detection of complications of intubation and barotrauma (positive-pressure breathing) such as pneumothorax and pneumomediastinum.

The relationship between the tip of the tube and the carina (tracheal bifurcation) must be carefully assessed. When the head and neck are in a neutral position, the endotracheal tube tip ideally should be about 5 to 7 cm above the carina (Figure 11-24). With flexion and extension of the neck, the tip of the tube will move about 2 cm caudally and cranially, respectively.

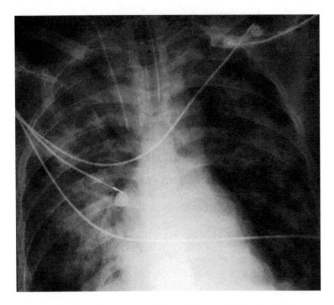

Figure 11-24   Proper position of the endotracheal tube.

Figure 11-25   Central venous pressure catheter in the right internal jugular vein. (From Dunbar RD: Radiologic appearance of compromised thoracic catheters, tubes, and wires, *Radiol Clin North Am* 22:699-722, 1984.)

About 10% to 20% of endotracheal tubes require repositioning after insertion. A tube positioned too low usually extends into the right main-stem bronchus, where it eventually leads to atelectasis of the left lung (see Figure 2-64). A tube positioned excessively high or in the esophagus causes the inspired air to enter the stomach, causing severe gastric dilatation and a high likelihood of regurgitation of gastric contents and aspiration pneumonia.

Central venous catheters

Central venous catheters inserted into the subclavian vein or a more peripheral vein in the upper extremity are extremely useful for measurement of the central venous pressure (CVP) and for providing a conduit for the rapid infusion of fluid or chronic hyperalimentation. So that the CVP may be correctly measured, the catheter must be located within the true central venous system, beyond all the valves, which interfere with direct transmission of right atrial pressure to the catheter. The optimal location is where the brachiocephalic veins join to form the superior vena cava (medial to the anterior border of the first rib on chest radiographs) or within the superior vena cava itself.

Because up to one third of CVP catheters are initially inserted incorrectly, the position of the catheter should be confirmed by a chest radiograph. The most common aberrant location of a CVP catheter is the internal jugular vein (Figure 11-25). CVP catheters that

extend to the right atrium are associated with an increased risk of cardiac arrhythmias and even perforation. Extension of the catheter into the hepatic veins may result in the infusion of potentially toxic substances (some antibiotics and hypertonic alimentation solutions) directly into the liver. Also, after successful placement, CVP catheters may change position as a result of patient motion or medical manipulation; therefore periodic radiographic confirmation of the catheter position is often recommended.

The anatomy of the subclavian region may lead to complications when a central catheter is introduced via the subclavian vein. Because the pleura covering the apex of the lung lies just deep to the subclavian vein, a pneumothorax may develop. As this may be difficult to detect clinically, a chest radiograph (if possible, with the patient in an upright position and in expiration) should be obtained whenever insertion of a subclavian catheter has been attempted. Another complication is perivascular CVP placement, which may result in ectopic infusion of fluid into the mediastinum or pleural space. This diagnosis should be suggested if there is rapid development of mediastinal widening or pleural effusion after CVP catheter insertion (Figure 11-26). Other complications include inadvertent puncture of the subclavian artery, air embolism, and injury to the phrenic nerve.

Catheter breakage and embolization can result from laceration of the catheter by the needle used to insert it, fracture at a point of stress, or detachment

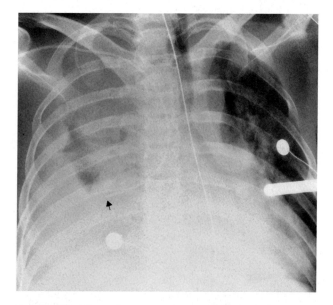

Figure 11-26   Central venous pressure catheter with its tip in the pleural space. A right subclavian catheter, which was introduced for total parenteral nutrition, perforated the superior vena cava and eroded into the right pleural space. Note the tip of the catheter projecting beyond the right border of the mediastinum *(arrow)*. The direct infusion of parenteral fluid into the pleural space has led to a large right hydrothorax. (From Eisenberg RL: *Diagnostic imaging in internal medicine,* New York, 1985, McGraw-Hill.)

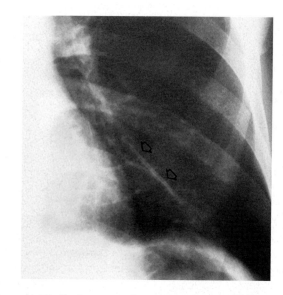

Figure 11-27   Broken central venous pressure catheter. The sheared-off portion of the catheter *(arrow)* is located in the left lower lobe. (From Eisenberg RL: *Diagnostic imaging in internal medicine,* New York, 1985, McGraw-Hill.)

of the catheter from its hub. The catheter fragment may lodge in the vena cava, in the right side of the heart, or in branches of the pulmonary artery (Figure 11-27), and the result may be thrombosis, infection, or perforation.

Swan-Ganz catheters

The flow-directed Swan-Ganz catheter consists of a central channel for measuring pulmonary capillary wedge (PCW) pressure and a second, smaller channel connected to an inflatable balloon at the catheter tip. Cardiac output and central venous pressure can also be measured by use of this catheter. It can be inserted at the bedside and floated to the pulmonary artery without the need for fluoroscopic monitoring.

Ideally, the catheter is positioned so that it lies within the right or left main pulmonary artery. Inflating the balloon causes the catheter to float downstream into a wedge position; deflating the balloon permits the catheter to recoil into the central pulmonary artery. Unlike standard intravenous catheters, the Swan-Ganz catheter has a radiopaque strip down its center.

The most common complication associated with the use of a Swan-Ganz catheter is pulmonary infarction distal to the catheter tip. Infarction may result from occlusion of a pulmonary artery by the catheter itself

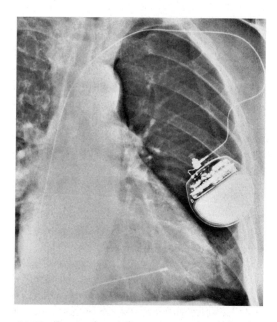

Figure 11-28   Pacemaker tip in coronary sinus. On the frontal projection, the tip of the electrode is angled slightly superiorly, traversing the heart in a higher plane than when it is located in the right ventricle. (From Dunbar RD: Radiologic appearance of compromised thoracic catheters, tubes, and wires, *Radiol Clin North Am* 22:699-722, 1984.)

(if it is wedged in a too-peripheral vessel) or from clot formation in or about the catheter. The pulmonary infarction appears as a patchy air-space consolidation involving the area of the lung supplied by the pulmonary artery in which the catheter lies. The appropriate treat-

Summary of Internal Devices

INTERNAL DEVICE	CORRECT PLACEMENT*	COMPLICATIONS
Endotracheal tube	Tip of tube 5-7 cm above the carina	Low placement—atelectasis High placement—air entering the stomach
Central venous catheters	Tip of catheter just beyond the joining of the brachiocephalic veins to form the superior vena cava	Internal jugular vein placement Right atrium—possible arrhythmias or perforation Pneumothorax with placement Infusion of fluid into mediastinum or pleural space
Swan-Ganz catheters	Right or left main pulmonary artery	Pulmonary infarction
Transvenous cardiac pacemakers	Overexpose to demonstrate the tip of the electrode at the apex of the right ventricle	Coronary sinus placement—needs a lateral chest film to distinguish Perforation at initial insertion

*Placement determined by chest radiograph.

ment is simply removal of the Swan-Ganz catheter; systemic heparinization is not required once this source of emboli or obstruction has been removed.

Transvenous cardiac pacemakers

Transvenous endocardiac pacing is the method of choice for maintaining cardiac rhythm in patients with heart block or bradyarrhythmias. Radiographic evaluation plays an important role in the initial placement of a pacemaker as well as in the detection of any subsequent complications. An overexposed film can demonstrate both the generator (for permanent pacemakers) and the course of the electrodes.

Ideally, the tip of the pacemaker should be positioned at the apex of the right ventricle. One common aberrant location is the coronary sinus. On a frontal radiograph, the tip often appears to be well positioned. A lateral projection is required to show that the tip is directly posterior in the coronary sinus, rather than in its proper position anterior in the right ventricle.

Although electrode fractures have become less common because of the development of new alloys, they are still a significant cause of pacing failure (Figure 11-28). The usual sites of fracture are near the pulse generator, at sharp bends in the wires, and at the point where the electrodes are inserted into the epicardium. Although most electrode fractures are easily detected on routine chest radiographs, some subtle fractures may be demonstrated only on oblique views or at fluoroscopy.

Figure 11-29 Fracture of a cardiac pacemaker wire *(arrow)*. (From Eisenberg RL: *Diagnostic imaging in internal medicine*, New York, 1985, McGraw-Hill.)

Perforation of the myocardium by an intravenous electrode usually occurs at the time of insertion or during the first few days thereafter. Perforation should be suspected when the pacemaker fails to sense or elicit a ventricular response. Plain radiographs show the electrode tip lying outside the right ventricular cavity (Figure 11-29).

QUESTIONS

1. A vitamin C deficiency that years ago was common among sailors because of their lack of fresh fruit and vegetables is termed _____.

2. _____ is a vitamin deficiency disease that occurs primarily in countries in which polished rice is the main staple.

3. A deficiency of niacin, characterized by reddening and scaling of exposed skin, vomiting, diarrhea, and nervous and mental disorders is termed _____.

4. A bone disease of young children who have been deprived of adequate vitamin D is termed _____.

5. Vitamin _____ is necessary in the blood clotting mechanism.

6. A lack of vitamin _____ can result in night blindness.

7. When caloric intake consistently exceeds the amount needed for the body to function, _____ occurs.

8. A granulomatous disease of unknown origin that usually affects women more than men and African Americans more than whites, and whose presence is most often identified on screening chest radiographs, is _____.

9. A disease of young to middle-aged women that is most likely an immune-complex disease, that can affect several systems of the body, and that is characterized by a butterfly-shaped rash across the nose and cheeks is _____.

10. A very malignant form of skin cancer, capable of metastasizing throughout the body, is _____.

11. An inherited muscular disease characterized by severe weakness and eventual death from respiratory muscle failure or pneumonia is _____.

12. The radiographer should be very alert to the possibility of _____ in patients with muscular dystrophy who lack normal swallowing ability.

13. Name three trisomy disorders: _____, _____, and _____.

14. The _____ syndrome occurs when a female has only one X chromosome.

15. Arachnodactyly, spiderlike digits, occurs in which two hereditary disorders?

16. Two common complications of intubation and barotrauma are _____ and _____.

17. A common catheter used to measure cardiac output and central venous pressure is the _____.

18. The optimal location for a central venous catheter is where the brachiocephalic veins join to form the _____.

19. An overexposed radiograph is often requested for visualizing transvenous endocardiac pacers to demonstrate both the _____ and the _____.

20. The most common complication associated with the Swan-Ganz catheter is _____ distal to the catheter tip.

21. Briefly describe why a lateral chest radiograph is very important for determining the correct position of the tip of the electrode of a transvenous cardiac pacer.

BIBLIOGRAPHY

Beers MH, Berkow R, editors: *The Merck manual of diagnosis and therapy,* ed 17, Rahway, N.J., 1999, Merck.

Goodman LR, Putman C: *Critical care imaging,* Philadelphia, 1991, Saunders.

Juhl JH, Crummy AB: *Essentials of radiologic imaging,* Philadelphia, 1987, Lippincott.

Kirks DR, McCormick VD, Greenspan RH: Pulmonary sarcoidosis, *AJR Am J Roentgenol* 117:777-786, 1973.

Lubowitz R, Schumacher HR: Articular manifestations of systemic lupus erythematosus, *Ann Intern Med* 74:911-921, 1974.

Glossary

aberration Deviation from normal

abscess Encapsulated collection of pus

achalasia Failure of the lower esophageal sphincter to relax because of absence or destruction of cells in the myenteric nerve plexus, which results in difficulty swallowing

adenoma Benign epithelial neoplasm that grows in a glandlike structure

adenopathy Enlargement of the lymphatic glands

adnexal Pertaining to the uterine appendages (ovaries, fallopian tubes, and ligaments)

afferent To carry toward the center

agenesis Absence of an organ

amorphous Without shape or definite form

anechoic Not producing internal echoes (on ultrasound)

angioma Tumor composed of blood vessels

ankylosis Immobility and consolidation of a joint caused by disease, injury, or surgical procedure

anticoagulant Substance that suppresses or delays coagulation of the blood

aplasia Lack of normal development resulting in a small size

arteriovenous malformation Abnormal communication between an artery and a vein

ascites Accumulation of fluid in the abdominal cavity

atresia Congenital absence or closure of a normal body orifice or tubular organ

atrophy Diminished size due to wasting away

Bence Jones protein Abnormal protein typically found in the blood of patients with multiple myeloma

bougienage Passage of an instrument through a tubular structure to increase its caliber (as in the treatment of a stricture of the esophagus)

bulla Large air-containing space

callus New bone tissue that reunites the parts of a fracture

caseation Form of necrosis in which the tissue is changed into a dry, amorphous mass resembling cheese

catamenial Pertaining to menstruation

cavitation Formation of cavities, as in pulmonary tuberculosis or neoplasm

centesis Puncture and aspiration

chondroblastic Forming cartilaginous tissue

chordae tendineae Thin cords that connect each cusp of the two atrioventricular valves to papillary muscles in the heart ventricles

coalesce To merge into a single mass

colic Intermittent abdominal pain whose fluctuation corresponds to smooth muscle peristalsis

collaterals Blood vessels that develop or enlarge to provide an alternative route around an obstruction

congenital Existing at birth

conjunctivitis Inflammation of the delicate membrane that lines the eyelids and covers the exposed surface of the sclera (white part) of the eye

contracture Shortening or shrinkage of a muscle or tendon resulting in persistent flexion or distortion at a joint

cortex Outer portion of a bone or internal organ (kidney, adrenal gland, brain)

curvilinear Having a curved configuration

cyst Saclike structure usually filled with fluid

cytology Microscopic examination to determine cell structure

demarcate To set or mark the limits of

de novo From the beginning; anew

diaphysis Shaft of a long bone

dilation and curettage Dilation of the cervix to allow the scraping of the uterine wall

diploic space Loose osseous tissue between the two tables of the skull

dissection Separation of layers

dysphagia Difficulty swallowing

dysplasia Disordered growth or faulty development of various tissues or body parts

dyspnea Shortness of breath

echogenic Producing a relatively strong reflection in ultrasound

ectopic Abnormally positioned

effaced Wiped out or obliterated

efferent To carry away from the center or part

effusion Accumulation of fluid

embolus Any foreign matter, such as a blood clot or an air bubble, carried in the bloodstream

emphysema Pathologic accumulation of air in tissues or organs (especially as applied to a disease of the lungs)

empyema Accumulation of pus in a cavity

endemic Present in a particular country, nation, or region

endogenous Originating from within the body

engorgement Congestion of a blood vessel or tissue with blood or other fluid

epiphysis End of a long bone that at first is separated from the main part by cartilage but later fuses with it by ossification

erythropoietin Protein serving as the humoral regulator of red blood cell formation

etiology The study of disease causes (*not* a synonym for *cause*)

eventration Diaphragmatic—elevation of the diaphragm; abdominal—protrusion of the bowel or removal of abdominal viscera

exacerbation   Increase in the severity of a disease or any of its symptoms

exenteration   Removal of all organs to debulk a tumor

exogenous   Arising from outside the body

exophthalmos   Abnormal protrusion of the eyeball

extramedullary hematopoiesis   Formation of red blood cells outside the bone marrow

exudate   Material (fluid, cells, or cellular debris) that has escaped from blood vessels and has been deposited in tissues or on tissue surfaces, usually as a result of inflammation

fecalith   Intestinal stone formed around a center of fecal material

fibrin   Essential portion of a blood clot

fibrinolysis   Breaking up of a blood clot

fistula   Abnormal connection, usually between two internal organs or from an internal organ to the surface of the body

focal   Localized

fusiform   Spindle shaped

grading   Assessment of malignant tumor to determine the degree of aggressiveness or malignancy

Gram's method   Technique for staining microorganisms

granuloma   Tumorlike mass of tissue caused by a chronic inflammatory process

Heberden's nodes   Small, hard nodules at the distal interphalangeal joints of the fingers produced by calcific spurs of the articular cartilage and associated with osteoarthritis

hematogenous   Spread by means of the bloodstream

hemodynamic   Pertaining to the movements involved in the circulation of the blood

hemoptysis   Coughing up blood or bloodstained sputum

hereditary   Transmitted to offspring through genes

heterogeneous   Composed of materials that have different structures or qualities

histology   Microscopic examination to determine tissue structure

homogeneous   Composed of material of similar or identical structure or quality

hydrocephalus   Enlargement of the head resulting from an abnormal increase in fluid within the ventricular system

hyperlucency   Overly black appearance on a radiograph

hyperplasia   Abnormal increase in the number of cells composing a tissue or organ

hypertension   High blood pressure

hypocalciuria   Abnormally low calcium in the urine

hypotension   Low blood pressure

hypoxia   Deficiency (lack) of oxygen

iatrogenic   Resulting from the activity of diagnosis or treatment by medical personnel

idiopathic   Having an unknown cause for underlying disease

indolent   Causing little or no pain; slow to heal

infarction   Death of tissue because of interruption of the normal blood supply

infundibulum   Funnel-shaped organ or passage

inguinal   Pertaining to the groin

insidious   Developing in a slow or unapparent manner; more dangerous than seems evident (e.g., an insidious disease)

in situ   Confined to the site of origin

intima   Innermost layer of an organ or blood vessel

intraluminal   Within the empty space (lumen) of a hollow viscus

intramural   Within the wall of an organ

intrinsic   Belonging to the real nature of a thing

ipsilateral   Relating to the same side (antonym: contralateral)

ischemia   Lack of blood supply in an organ or tissue

juxtaarticular   Adjacent to a joint

kyphosis   Anterior convexity in the curvature of the thoracic spine, sacrum, and coccyx, as viewed from the side

leukocytosis   Abnormal amount of white blood cells in the blood

lipoma   Tumor composed of fat

lordosis   Anterior concavity in the curvature of the lumbar and cervical spine, as viewed from the side

lymphangitic   Spread by means of the lymphatic system

lymphoma   Neoplastic disorder of lymphoid tissue

lytic   Destructive

malaise   Vague feeling of physical discomfort or uneasiness, as early in an illness

matrix   Basic material from which a substance (such as tissue) develops

medulla   Inner substance of a bone (bone marrow) or an internal organ (kidney, adrenal gland)

megahertz (MHz)   One million waves per second

mesentery   Peritoneal folds that attach the small and large bowel to the back wall of the peritoneal cavity

mesothelioma   Tumor that develops from the surface of the pleura, pericardium, or peritoneum

metaphysis   Wider part at the end of the shaft of a long bone, adjacent to the epiphyseal plate; located between the epiphysis and the diaphysis

metastasis   Spread of disease to another organ or tissue in the body

monoclonal immunoglobulin   Antibodies that are formed against a specific cell type

Morgagni hernia   Protrusion of abdominal contents into the anterior and lateral aspects of the thoracic cavity

morphologic   Pertaining to the form and structure of an organ

multilocular Having many cells or compartments

mycoplasma Colloquial usage for any of a genus of tiny microorganisms, smaller than bacteria but larger than viruses, that appear to be the causative agents of many diseases

mycosis Fungal infection

myxedema Puffy thickening of the skin with slowing down of physical and mental activity caused by failure of the thyroid gland

necrosis Death of tissue

necrotic Dead or decayed

neoplasm Any new and abnormal growth, especially when the growth is uncontrolled and progressive

nephrocalcinosis Calcium deposits within the substance of the kidney

neurogenic Originating in the nervous system

nidus Focal point, especially of a stone or an inflammatory process

octreotide Radioactive peptide tracer; a long-acting analog of the hormone somatostatin

oligemia Decreased blood volume

osteoblastic Forming bony tissue

osteoclastic Bone resorption

osteolytic Destroying bone

palpitations Rapid or fluttering beating of the heart, of which one is aware

paradoxical Seeming to contradict the known facts

parenchyma Essential tissue of an organ

pathognomonic Especially distinctive or characteristic of a disease or pathologic condition

pedunculated Having a stalk (pedicle)

peripheral Outside or away from the central portion of a structure

peristalsis Wormlike movement by which the alimentary canal or other tubular organ propels its contents

permeative Diffusely spreading through or penetrating a substance, tissue, or organ, as by a disease process such as cancer

pinna Cartilaginous portion of the external ear

Pneumococcus Genus of gram-positive bacteria

pneumoperitoneum Presence of free gas in the peritoneal cavity

postpartum After childbirth

proliferate To multiply rapidly, increase profusely

punctate Marked with dots or tiny spots

purpura Spontaneous hemorrhages in the skin or mucous membrane

resection Partial surgical removal of a organ or bone

rudimentary Imperfectly developed

saccular Resembling a pouchlike sac

sclerosis Conversion of a portion of bone into an ivory-like, densely opaque mass; an abnormal hardening of body tissues or parts, especially of the walls of arteries

sequestrum Piece of dead bone that has become separated from the surrounding healthy bone

serosa Outer layer of a viscus (especially in the alimentary tract)

shock Acute peripheral circulatory failure

silhouette (cardiac) Outer border of the heart, seen against the radiolucent lungs

spirochete Spiral type of bacterium of the genus *Spirochaeta*

staging Determination of the amount of spread of a neoplasm, necessary to select appropriate therapy and to predict the future course of a disease

stasis Stagnation of some fluid in the body (as of blood in veins); reduced peristalsis of the intestines resulting in the retention of feces

subchondral Just beneath the articular margin

subluxation Incomplete or partial dislocation

surfactant Agent that lowers the surface tension

telangiectasia Vascular lesion formed by dilatation of a group of small blood vessels

teratoma Neoplasm composed of various kinds of embryonic tissue

tertiary Third in rank or order

thymoma Tumor originating from the thymus gland

tortuous Full of twists, turns, or curves

trabeculae Supporting or anchoring strands of connective tissue within body structures

triradiate Radiating in three directions

trisomy Presence of an additional (third) chromosome

trophoblastic Relating to the layer by which the fertilized ovum is attached to the uterine wall and from which the developing embryo receives its nourishment

ulceration Destruction of tissue creating an opening within a structure

urate Salt of uric acid

valvulae conniventes Circular folds of the small bowel

vasculitis Inflammation of a vessel

virus One of a group of minute infectious agents characterized by a lack of independent metabolism and by the ability to reproduce only within living host cells

viscous Thick, sticky

viscus Any large internal organ, especially in the abdomen

APPENDIX A

Prefixes/Suffixes/Roots

PREFIX/SUFFIX/ROOT	MEANING	EXAMPLE
a-, ab-	away from	abduction
a-, an-	without; not	asymmetric, anencephalic
ad-	toward	adduction
-algia	pain	arthralgia
ana-	up, back again	anaplastic
ante-	before, in front of	antecubital
anti-, ant-	against	antibody, antitoxin
auto-	self	autoimmune
bi-	two	bilateral, bidirectional
-blast	budding	osteoblast
cardi-	heart	cardiology, cardiac; pericardium
caudal	tail	caudal
cephal-	head	cephalic; hydrocephaly
chondro-	cartilage	chondroma, chondrosarcoma
-clast	destroyer, breaker	osteoclast
contra-	opposite	contralateral
crani-	skull	cranium, cranial
cyano-	dark blue	cyanotic
cyto-	cell	cytoplasm; erythrocyte, leukocyte
-dactyl-	finger, toe	polydactyly, arachnodactyly
deci-	tenth	decimal
derm-	skin	dermatology; epidermis
dys-	bad; difficult	dysplasia, dysuria
ecto-	outside of	ectoderm, ectopic
endo-, ento-	within	endoderm, endometrium
erythr-	red	erythrocyte
gastr-	stomach	gastric
-genic	causing	carcinogenic, pathogenic
gyn-, gyneco-	woman	gynecology
hem-, haem-	blood	hemorrhage, hemolytic
hemi-	half	hemisphere, hemidiaphragm
hetero-	different	heterogeneous
homo-	same	homogeneous
hyper-	over; excessive	hyperthyroidism, hypertension, hyperintense
hypo-	under; too little	hypothyroidism, hypotension, hypointense
iatro-	healer, healing	iatrogenic; psychiatry
infra-	below	infratemporal
intra-	within	intramural, intradermal
ipsi-	same	ipsilateral
iso-	equal	isointense
-itis	inflammation	appendicitis, diverticulitis
juxta-	near, next to	juxtaarticular
kilo-	thousand	kilogram
leuko-, leuco-	white	leukocyte, leukemia
lipo-	fat	lipoma, liposarcoma
-lysis, -lytic	dissolve	lytic, osteolytic
macro-	large	macroadenoma
magn-	great, large	magnify, magnum (foramen)

PREFIX/SUFFIX/ROOT	MEANING	EXAMPLE
mal-	bad, ill	malunion, malalignment
mega-, megalo-	large	megadose
melan-	black	melanoma, melanin
micro-	small	microscope, microadenoma, microcirculation
milli-	thousandth	milligram, milliliter
mono-	one	monostotic, monoclonal
multi-	many	multilocular, multifaceted
myelo-	marrow	myelogram; osteomyelitis
myo-	muscle	myoma, myositis
necro-	dead	necrosis
neo-	new	neovascularity, neoplasm
non-	not	nonunion, nonviable
ocul-	eye	ocular, oculomotor (nerve)
oligo-	few	oligemia
-ology	study of	radiology, pathology
onco-	tumor	oncology
ophthalm-	eye	ophthalmology
-osis	condition of	diverticulosis
osteo-	bone	osteomyelitis, osteosarcoma
pan-	all	pansinusitis, pancytopenia
par-, para-	beside	paraaortic, paravertebral
patho-	disease	pathology; adenopathy
peri-	around	periarticular, periventricular, pericardium
plasm-, plast-	shape, form	neoplasm; anaplastic
pleur-	rib; side	pleural, pleurisy
pneumo-	air, breath	pneumothorax, pneumonia
poly-	many	polycystic, polyostotic
post-	after, later; behind	posttraumatic, postsurgical, postoperative
pre-	before; in front of	premenstrual, prepontine
pseudo-	false	pseudotumor, pseudopolyp
psych-	mind, spirit	psychiatry, psychology
re-	again, anew	reoperate, recalcify
retro-	backward; behind	retroperitoneum
-rrhea	flow, gush	diarrhea
schizo-	split	schizophrenia
sclero-	hard	sclerotic; atherosclerosis
semi-	half	semicircular
sub-	under, below	suborbital, subphrenic, subhepatic
super-, supra-	above; more than	suprarenal, supraorbital
syn-, sym-	with, together	synthesis, symmetric
tachy-	fast	tachycardia
techn-	art, skill	technology, technique
terti-	third	tertiary
tetra-	four	tetralogy (of Fallot)
thermo-	heat	thermometer
tomo-, -tome	cut	tomography; microtome
trans-	across	transverse (colon), transvenous (pacer)
tri-	three	trimalleolar, trisomy
ultra-	beyond	ultrasound
uni-	one	unilateral

APPENDIX B

Laboratory Values	Significance of Laboratory Values
↑ Acid phosphatase	Prostate cancer, metastatic to bone
↑ Alkaline phosphatase	Liver disease; Paget's disease; bone tumor
↑ Amylase	Pancreatitis
↑ Bilirubin	Liver disease
↑ Calcium	Hyperparathyroidism, bone destruction
↑ Cholesterol	Tendency toward atherosclerosis
↑ Creatinine phosphokinase (CPK)	Myocardial infarction; pulmonary infarction
↑ Creatinine	Kidney disease
↑ Glucose	Diabetes mellitus; Cushing's syndrome; glucagon-secreting pancreatic tumor
↑ Lactic dehydrogenase (LDH)	Myocardial infarction; pulmonary infarction; liver disease
↑ Total protein	Dehydration; immunoglobinopathy
↑ Serum glutamic-oxaloacetic transaminase (SGOT)	Liver disease
↑ Serum glutamic-pyruvic transaminase (SGPT)	Myocardial infarction; liver disease
↑ Blood urea nitrogen (BUN)	Kidney disease
↑ Uric acid	Gout; antidiuretic therapy
↓ Calcium	Hypoparathyroidism; malabsorption; osteomalacia/rickets
↓ Total protein	Chronic liver disease; malnutrition; nephrotic syndrome
↓ Cholesterol	Malnutrition; liver disease
↓ Glucose	Insulin-secreting pancreatic tumor; liver disease; hypopituitarism

APPENDIX C

Chapter 1 Key

1. edema		11. F		21. D	
2. phagocytosis		12. I		22. J	
3. keloid		13. Q		23. E	
4. suppurative		14. B		24. N	
5. ischemia		15. H		25. L	
6. infarct		16. O		26. K	
7. hematoma		17. T		27. S	
8. atrophy		18. P		28. A	
9. neoplasia		19. C		29. R	
10. adenoma		20. G		30. M	

Chapter 2 Key

1. patient inhales, then exhales, then inhales again to full inspiration
2. alveoli
3. pleura (visceral)
4. hyaline membrane disease
5. cystic fibrosis
6. lung abscess
7. bronchography
8. emphysema
9. silicosis, asbestosis, antracosis
10. pulmonary arteriovenous fistula
11. tension pneumothorax
12. empyema
13. diaphragm
14. to demonstrate air fluid levels
15. B
16. + +
    + −
    + +
    + +
    − +
17. low-pressure, low-resistance system through which oxygen enters and carbon dioxide is removed
18. high-pressure systemic circulation by which oxygenated blood is supplied to nourish lung tissue
19. parietal pleura
20. pneumonia
21. histoplasmosis, coccidioidomycosis
22. coughing, droplets
23. pneumothorax
24. emphysema
25. pneumoconiosis
26. mesothelioma
27. septic embolism
28. atelectasis
29. larger and more vertical main-stem bronchi
30. subcutaneous emphysema
31. expiration, lateral decubitus
32. less air in lungs, more lung tissue to pass through increase by 25% to 30% mAs or +1 density if using AEC
33. C
34. lateral decubitus
35. mediastinal emphysema (pneumomediastinum)
36. C

Chapter 3 Key

1. B
2. A
3. D
4. D
5. B
6. A
7. B
8. A
9. B
10. C
11. A
12. D
13. B
14. D
15. C
16. B
17. C
18. B
19. D
20. B
21. C
22. A
23. C
24. D
25. B
26. B
27. I   I
    I (initially), D (later)   D
    D   D
    D   I

Chapter 4 Key

1. B
2. C
3. A
4. B
5. C
6. A
7. B
8. D
9. C
10. C
11. C
12. B
13. B
14. D
15. D
16. A
17. B
18. A
19. D
20. tracheoesophageal fistula
21. B
22. B
23. D
24. B
25. C
26. A

Chapter 5 Key

1. C
2. D
3. B
4. A

5. C
6. D
7. C

8. D
9. C
10. A

Chapter 6 Key

1. D
2. A
3. B
4. D
5. D
6. C
7. B
8. D

9. A
10. A
11. C
12. C
13. A
14. B
15. A
16. C

17. B
18. C
19. B
20. B
21. B
22. B
23. D
24. D

Chapter 7 Key

1. C
2. C
3. B
4. D
5. D
6. B
7. A
8. C
9. B
10. C
11. CT
12. CT, MRI
13. transient ischemic attack
14. MRI
15. epilepsy

16. Alzheimer's disease
17. Parkinson's disease
18. horizontal, erect
19. hydrocephalus
20. cross-table lateral, horizontal
21. D
22. J
23. N
24. G
25. T
26. P
27. I
28. M
29. C
30. R

31. O
32. A
33. H
34. V
35. F
36. S
37. W
38. U
39. X
40. L
41. Q
42. B
43. Y
44. K
45. E

Chapter 8 Key

1. C
2. A
3. C
4. B

5. B
6. C
7. C
8. C

9. A
10. C
11. B
12. B

Chapter 9 Key

1. C
2. C
3. A
4. B
5. B
6. C
7. B
8. B
9. C
10. B
11. D
12. B
13. C
14. B
15. B
16. B
17. B
18. A
19. C
20. B
21. D

Chapter 10 Key

1. nonionizing
2. hysterosalpingography, mammography
3. spermatogenesis
4. testosterone
5. vasectomy
6. cancer of the prostate
7. ultrasound
8. T
9. ivory vertebra
10. ultrasound
11. testicular torsion
12. testicular, lymphatic
13. ovulation
14. ectopic
15. hysterosalpingography
16. syphilis
17. dermoid/teratoma
18. fibroids
19. breast
20. carcinoma of the cervix

Chapter 11 Key

1. scurvy
2. beriberi
3. pellagra
4. rickets
5. K
6. A
7. obesity
8. sarcoidosis
9. systemic lupus erythematosus
10. melanoma
11. muscular dystrophy
12. aspiration
13. Down syndrome, Turner's syndrome, Klinefelter's syndrome
14. Turner's syndrome
15. Marfan's syndrome, homocystinuria
16. pneumothorax, pneumomediastinum
17. Swan-Ganz
18. superior vena cava
19. generator, electrodes
20. infarction
21. In AP and PA radiographs, the tip may *appear* to be in the proper position, but a lateral view is needed to ensure that the tip is in the anterior portion of the right ventricle—the correct position.

Index

Note: Page numbers followed by f indicate figures; those followed by t indicate tables.